POISON ON TAP

HOW GOVERNMENT FAILED FLINT, AND THE HEROES WHO FOUGHT BACK

By the staff of Bridge Magazine

Poison on Tap Editor: Bob Campbell

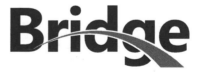

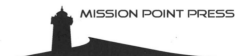

MISSION POINT PRESS

Poison on Tap
How Government Failed Flint,
and the Heroes Who Fought Back

By the staff of Bridge Magazine
Timeline and Truth Squad Analysis by
John Bebow

Poison on Tap editor: Bob Campbell
Designer: Heather Lee Shaw
Copy editors: Doug Weaver and
Anne Stanton

Cover photo: Jake May/MLive.com

ISBN: 9781943995080

Library of Congress Control Number:
2016908961

Published by Mission Point Press,
Traverse City, Michigan.

Printed in the United States of Amercia.

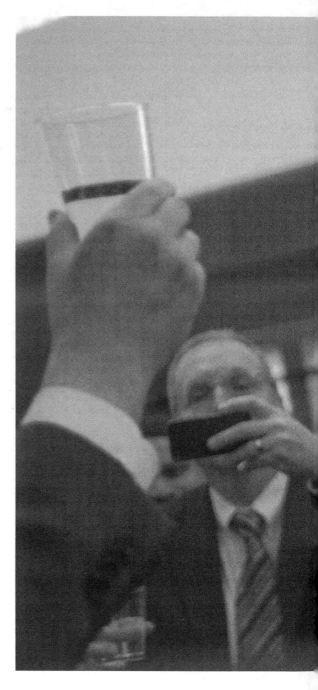

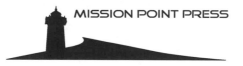
MISSION POINT PRESS

About the cover photograph:
A Flint protester holds a plastic bottle
of tainted water at a session in Lansing,
where about 150 protesters demanded
Gov. Rick Snyder's resignation. The
picture was taken by Flint Journal chief
photographer Jake May on Jan. 14, 2016.

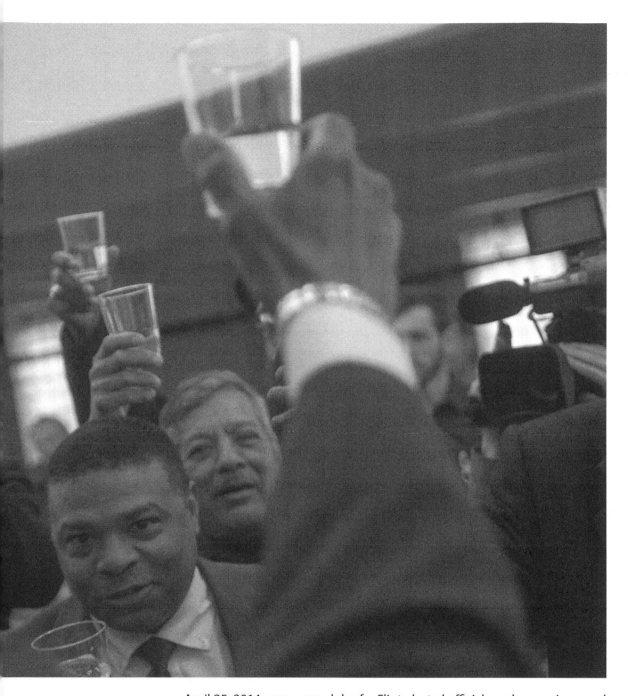

April 25, 2014, was a proud day for Flint elected officials and supervisors and employees of the city's water plant. They toasted the switch of the city's drinking water from Lake Huron water purchased from Detroit to Flint River water treated and pumped from their own plant. Closest to the camera is Howard Croft, director of Flint's Department of Public Works, which oversees the water plant operations.

Photo by Samuel Wilson/MLive.com

The heroes

Logan Wallace, a Virginia Tech photographer, was assigned to document the work professor Marc Edwards was doing with Flint's water crisis and his group of researchers, students and volunteers called flintwaterstudy.org. She was in the right place at the right time in early March 2016 when four critical heroes, credited with turning the tide of bureaucratic indifference to the travails of Flint, met face-to-face for the first time.

It was a joyous moment for (from left) Lee-Anne Walters, the mom whose son was lead poisoned, Miguel Del Toral, the EPA Region 5 regulations manager who was the first to challenge the state's failure to treat Flint River water with corrosion controls, Dr. Mona Hanna-Attisha, the pediatrician whose study of blood-lead levels provided an undeniable link to lead poisoning in Flint's children, and Edwards, who brought a team of researchers and students to Flint to sample for lead in tap water and showed serious problems.

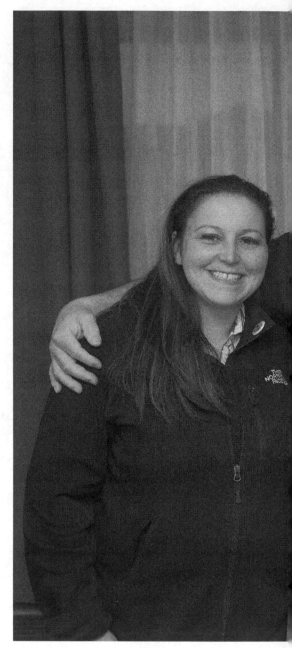

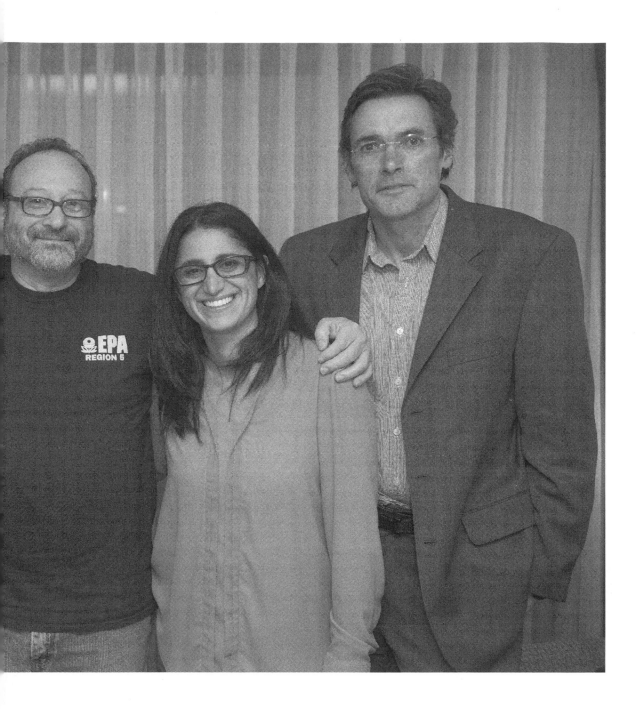

ABOUT BRIDGE MAGAZINE AND THE CENTER FOR MICHIGAN

Bridge Magazine is published online, four times weekly, at bridgemi.com. Launched in 2011, Bridge is Michigan's leading nonprofit news source, having earned more than 50 state and national journalism awards before its fifth birthday. The publication is staffed by professional journalists with nearly 200 years of experience covering the people, public policy and politics of Michigan.

Bridge is the only Michigan-based member of the Institute for Nonprofit News, a trade organization for a nationwide trend of news organizations stepping in to fill the gaps in coverage as traditional newspapers face increasing financial and staff cutbacks. The number of professional journalists in Michigan has declined by nearly 40 percent in the past generation.

More than 700,000 people read Bridge in 2015. As a nonprofit, Bridge is entirely supported by philanthropy from foundations, corporations and individual readers who voluntarily pay for the publication's journalism. Bridge's journalism strategy focuses mainly on six coverage components: talent and education; public sector watchdogging, Michigan quality of life, vulnerable children and families, economy and competitive position, and success in its many forms.

Bridge Magazine's parent is The Center for Michigan, a nonprofit "think and do tank" founded in 2006 by retired newspaper publisher Philip Power and his wife, Kathy. The Center for Michigan's mission is to improve quality of life in the state through broad public engagement, in-depth journalism, and nonpartisan public policy research and framing. The Center holds more than 100 statewide community meetings each year to understand and amplify citizen priorities for the future of the state.

The Center's combined public engagement, journalism, and policy framing has contributed to a wide range of policy improvements in Michigan, including the nation's largest expansion of public pre-schools; intensified teacher certification testing, teacher evaluation and other education reforms; and $250 million in taxpayer savings through prison reforms.

For more information, please visit thecenterformichigan.net and bridgemi.com.

TABLE OF CONTENTS

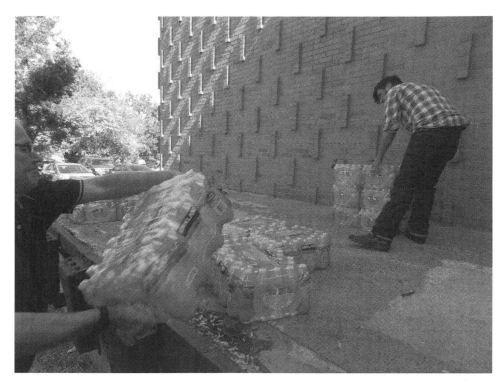

Donated water bottles arrive at a Flint church.

Photo courtesy of Michigan Radio

HOW TO HELP IN FLINT

The Flint water crisis has inspired thousands of individuals, groups, churches, organizations and businesses to help. In early May 2016, 10 foundations based in Michigan or with Michigan roots pledged $125 million to address immediate and long-term needs of residents. Earlier in the crisis, celebrities from Madonna to Aretha Franklin to Jimmy Fallon to rapper The Game, plus professional and college athletes, joined the crusade to help Flint. The biggest donor has been the Flint-based Charles Stewart Mott Foundation, which pledged $100 million as part of the May 2016 announcement. Detroit Pistons' owner Tom Gores, a Flint native, formed FlintNow, a foundation focused on raising money from the private sector. It has committed at least $10 million.

Here's how you can help:

Flint Child Health & Development Fund of the Community Foundation of Greater Flint
www.flintkids.org

The founding donors, including Dr. Mona Hanna-Attisha, created the fund to help with the current and long-term health needs of those most vulnerable to lead exposure – children 6 years old and younger. "The creation of this Fund will further ensure that our children are afforded the resources and interventions to overcome this population-wide exposure to lead," said Hanna-Attisha. To host an event or fundraiser, call Sandra Murphy at 810-767-3653. The fund is administered by the Community Foundation of Greater Flint.

Mission Point Press, the publisher of this book, and Bridge Magazine are donating $1 for every book sold to this fund.

United Way of Genesee County
www.unitedwaygenesee.org

The United Way of Genesee County has set up this fund for the purchase of filters, bottled water, emergency support services and prevention efforts. One-hundred percent of the fund is used for these projects and no administrative fee is assessed. You can donate through the website.

The Salvation Army
http://centralusa.salvationarmy.org/emi/flint_water_crisis

The Salvation Army of Genesee County is working with other Flint-based service organizations to help purchase water, filters and pay delinquent water bills for residents facing shutoff. Donations can be made online by calling 1-877-SAL-MICH or sending checks to The Salvation Army Flint Water Crisis, 211 W. Kearsley, Flint, Mich. 48502.

To volunteer your time
www.flintvolunteer.com or flint.voly.org

Because of the numbers of people interested in helping, volunteers are coordinated through these websites. Follow the instructions on the site. If a group wants to volunteer, identify a leader. Leaders can search the site for a project that meets the group's schedule. Groups may search for projects by zip code. Individuals also can choose opportunities that match their availability.

For more information: go to http://www.helpforflint.com.

FOREWORD

By Phil Power
Bridge Magazine

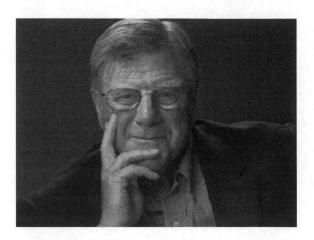

F lint.

It's rare when one word crystallizes a complex tragedy of human anxiety and suffering, governmental failure and incompetence at all levels, bureaucratic bungling, political exploitation, municipal catastrophe and a systemic breakdown of simple good governance in the provision of public goods to American citizens. But "Flint" does it.

It's rare, but not unknown. Kent State. Ferguson. Watergate.

These words resonate down the corridors of our history. Over time, they become milestones in our collective memory, events whose consequences run far beyond their immediate fallout. They become symbols packed with meaning, receptacles of time and place, markers of failure and lessons in our system of governance.

Some of us were fortunate – what an odd term! – to see them at close range. That was the job for us at the Center for Michigan and its publication, Bridge Magazine, as week by week we traced the myriad twists and turns of the catastrophe in Flint as it played out from early 2015 to the present day.

How could entire Flint neighborhoods suffer for months the brown, smelly drinking water that turned out to be poison, especially to little kids? How could it be that entire layers of government – local, state, regional and national – either failed to understand what was going on or, understanding it all too well, systematically tried to cover up their mistakes? How could it be that politicians of all stripes converted a human and municipal crisis into a convenient punching bag for political gain?

It boggles the mind. The only way we could un-boggle our collective minds at Bridge Magazine was to make Flint one of the largest stories of our careers. We squinted our way through thousands and thousands of emails, trying to make sense of the story as it mutated ... and as nearly every participant tried to spin it to their advantage. We read with growing astonishment the self-serving messages of indifference from "public servants" at the Michigan Department of Environmental Quality and the federal Environmental Protection Agency.

We devoted countless hours and 30,000 words to teasing out a comprehensive timeline that tracked the story as it grew. We learned how a whole series of state-appointed emergency financial managers followed the financial-only component of their job description and how this blinkered perception affected common sense. And we realized how state policy in Michigan had tolerated – even accelerated – the gradual descent into poverty and helplessness of what 40 years ago had been a thriving community.

We profiled the heroes who collectively struggled to make Flint into a story of courage, honesty, dedication and guts: Dr. Mona Hanna-Attisha, the local pediatrician who helped uncover the threat of lead poisoning; professor Marc Edwards, the national expert on drinking water contamination from Virginia Tech who – with researchers, students and volunteers – proved high levels of lead in tap water; Lee-Anne Walters, the mom from Flint's south side who noticed hair loss and rashes on her kids and raised hell; EPA regulator Miguel Del Toral, who risked his career in memos that told the truth that his superiors tried to suppress. Dozens of journalists who jumped through hoops to pierce the veil of secrecy and deception and the many citizens who protested loudly about the foul taste, odor and color of their tap water.

And we sent our reporters to the front lines of a scared city. They came back with the simple and tragic story that virtually every Flint resident was now no longer prepared to trust ANY person in ANY position of governmental authority.

We came to the conclusion that the poisoning of Flint was a cautionary tale for our times that has featured the pulling together of public skepticism of the utility of good government, of a tax and spend ideology that understood all too well the cost of everything and the value of nothing, and of a political system that insulated bureaucrats and office-holders from accountability.

And we realized that this story wasn't just about Flint; it was about far too much of America. And that it deserved to be told over and over again, and in detail.

One of the central political and policy debates of our times has been over the proper size and scope of government. Those of us who live and work close to Flint know better. We don't need more government. Or less government.

We need – desperately – capable and effective government. We hope readers of this book will realize just why … and act accordingly.

Phil Power is the founder and chairman of Center for Michigan,
publisher of Bridge Magazine.

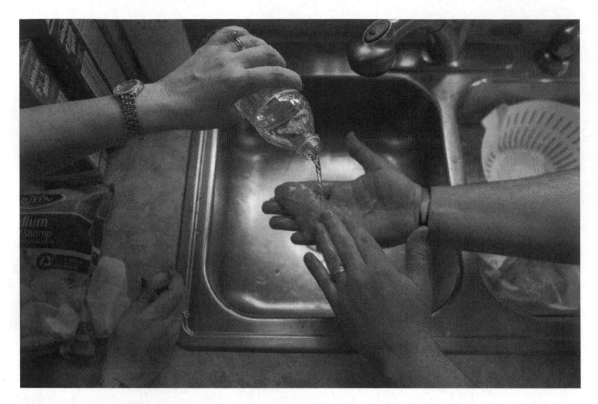

Melissa Mays helps her husband, Adam, wash chicken over the sink with bottled water as they prepare jambalaya for dinner at their home on May 12, 2015 in Flint. The meal for Mays and her family took over 10 bottles of water to prepare as they feared using tap water to wash their food.

Photo courtesy of Brittany Greeson

WHAT FLOWS FROM FLINT: AN INTRODUCTION TO THIS BOOK

THEMES THAT PROVIDE LASTING LESSONS

By John Bebow
Bridge Magazine

The water stunk. What flowed from some faucets in Flint, Mich., looked like it came straight from the river. Yet all the authorities entrusted to safeguard the public assured citizens the water was safe to drink. Even after issuing boil-water alerts. After heavy treatment led to temporarily dangerous chemical levels in the water. After the water corroded General Motors' engine parts. After state government quietly used taxpayer money to provide purified water coolers in a Flint office building. The authorities repeated their steadfast reassurances: Drink the water. It's safe.

If you lived in Flint in early 2015, none of it made sense. How could some Flint neighborhoods get perfectly fine water while others suffered a fetid flow? How, when neighbors told of skin sores and hair loss after showering and sickness after drinking the stuff, could the water possibly be safe? The people of Flint knew better. They stormed city hall and held milk jugs of dirty water in the air. They felt, smelled and tasted the coming disaster long before many in power acknowledged it.

IF YOU LIVED IN FLINT IN EARLY 2015, NONE OF IT MADE SENSE.

"The very first time we get validation from the medical community that there was an illness—or God forbid a death—that can be attributed to this water, I cannot tell you how bad it's going to be," Flint minister Byron Moore told Bridge Magazine in January 2015.

Moore sensed the foreboding but couldn't possibly foresee the tragedy coming: How government at every level failed a fundamental duty to deliver clean and safe drinking water. How gross errors poisoned the city's youngest and most vulnerable children with lead. How Legionnaire's bacteria festered at a highly unusual rate after people began drinking from the Flint River. How government leaders far and wide failed to act on and even degraded Flint residents' pleas for help, wrongly prolonging the danger for months. How sticking a pipe into the river, a money-saving move, ultimately cost far more than it ever could have saved. How a band of heroes emerged to begin righting the wrongs.

1

How the crisis will stubbornly linger well into the futures of growing children and in the neighborhoods and business corridors of an already challenged city. How tough lessons took shape but then led to other questions: Will we really learn? Will we change enough to prevent it from happening again?

This book documents the essentials of what happened in the first year-plus of the Flint water crisis, analyzes the root causes and begins to interpret the lessons. This is a collection of journalism first published in Bridge Magazine at www.bridgemi.com. Named "Newspaper of the Year" in 2016 by the Michigan Press Association, Bridge is part of a national movement of nonprofit news organizations growing in response to years of cutbacks at struggling newspapers. Bridge is staffed by a team of professional journalists with nearly 200 years of combined experience covering the people, public policy, and politics of Michigan.

FLINT IS A STORY OF COMPLETE GOVERNMENT FAILURE AND DISRESPECT FOR THE PEOPLE.

Beginning in early 2015 and continuing today, Bridge reporters have documented key themes that we hope become lasting lessons to prevent Flint's drinking water crisis from repeating:

If you threw a lead-soaked dart at a map of the United States, you couldn't hit a more direct bullseye than Flint. An after-action task force of experts declared the Flint disaster a case of "environmental injustice." The roots of that injustice trace back decades. Dr. Mona Hanna-Attisha, a pediatrician who helped uncover the threat in Flint, explained in the American Journal of Public Health in February 2016:

"Increased lead-poisoning rates have profound implications for the life course potential of an entire cohort of Flint children already rattled with toxic stress contributors (poverty, violence, unemployment, food insecurity).... As our aging water infrastructures continue to decay, and as communities across the nation struggle with finances and water supply sources, the situation in Flint may be a harbinger for future safe drinking-water challenges. Ironically, even when one is surrounded by the Great Lakes, safe drinking water is not a guarantee."

When lead gets in the bloodstream, it eats at developmental and biological processes, especially in the youngest children. Lead can literally rob infants and toddlers of intelligence. The effects are largely irreversible and life-altering. Lead poisoning is most common in aging cities, where it circulates in the air from decaying industrial sites, and from old lead paint chips off the walls and windowsills and frames of decrepit homes. So lead was already in Flint. But when lead flowed through the city's drinking water in 2014 and 2015, it struck a population of children already facing some of America's toughest odds.

Roughly 7,900 children under the age of 6 live in Flint. Many of them were born with scant economic or educational opportunity. Flint consistently ranks among the most violent cities in America. In the past six years, 316 people were murdered in the city. By sad comparison, 314 students graduated from Flint's two traditional public high schools in 2015. More than one quarter of Flint's housing units are vacant. More than 40 percent of the city's residents are in poverty. As the water crisis festered, Flint's unemployment rate of nearly 10 percent nearly doubled the state's rate. Property values and personal incomes in the city have plummeted for years.

Then poison flowed through the drinking water.

As in many declining manufacturing hubs across the country, it wasn't always this way. Flint was a thriving and prosperous city of 200,000 people in 1960. Incomes were high. Neighborhoods thrived. People had futures. Over time, industry and many prosperous residents pulled out and crisis steadily filled the void. In the late 1970s, more than 80,000 people worked for General Motors in the Flint area. By 2006, 90 percent of those GM jobs were gone. Left behind was a city in shambles—few new jobs, troubled schools, a quickly shrinking tax base, rising pension obligations for city workers hired in more prosperous times, rising crime, and the hangover of a crumbling water and sewer infrastructure built for a much larger city.

FLINT IS A STORY OF A WORST FAILURE, IN A WORST PLACE, AT A WORST TIME. IT IS A CONFOUNDING INJUSTICE – AN AMERICAN PARABLE.

Flint suffered its seventh straight budget deficit in 2014. Years of state oversight, municipal service and job cuts had not fixed the city's bottom line. Flint businesses and residents paid more for less. They faced the highest property tax rates, by far, in their region. In the turmoil, the city leaned on an unusual source of cash. As Michigan State University municipal finance expert Eric Scorsone told Bridge Magazine, "Flint used water and sewer funds as a bank. In one sense it made sense: That's where the cash is."

Money, as well as regional rivalry, motivated the 2014 switch from Detroit's drinking water system to what would turn out to be the very problematic Flint River. Through it all, Flint businesses and residents faced unbelievably high prices for what would prove to be unbelievably bad water. The average residential water bill in Flint in 2015 was $864. The highest in the nation, and about $300 higher than any other city in Michigan. It was a system based on user fees, with a shrinking population of users. The users who remained had a shrinking ability to pay.

Largely neglected in all of this was the condition of the water system itself. By 2014, Flint's water pipes lost between 20 and 40 percent of their load due to leaks. After years of budget cuts, talent and resources in city government were slim—and not up to the task of a complex and rare change in a drinking-water source. The miles and miles of old water pipes needed millions and millions of dollars of repairs and replacement.

In retrospect, it is easy to see how some kind of Flint water disaster was just a matter of time.

Anywhere on the political spectrum you reside, the Flint water crisis can accommodate your distrust, disgust and disaffection with government and politics. Only, these weren't talk show bragging rights at stake. This was public safety at stake. This was the most basic of 21st Century First World assumptions—clean

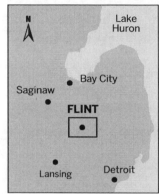

drinking water—at stake. Forty-five years after America put a man on the moon, the residents of an American city drank Third World water.

The essentials of what went wrong:

For decades, Flint bought clean, safe drinking water from Detroit, whose massive system pumps Lake Huron water to dozens of communities in southeastern Michigan. Leaders in the Flint region grew tired of Detroit price increases and wanted control of their own water destiny. They made plans to build their own Lake Huron pipeline.

Flint was under the control of a state-appointed emergency manager, so Gov. Rick Snyder's team was heavily involved in the discussions. Negotiations with Detroit frayed. State bean counters concluded the Flint region might save money with its own pipeline. The emergency manager announced Flint would eventually leave the Detroit water system. Detroit responded in kind, essentially giving Flint a water eviction notice with one year's notice. The new pipeline to Lake Huron wouldn't be finished by then. So the emergency manager turned to the city's old back-up water plant to tap the Flint River.

Oversight of safe drinking water was in the hands of the Michigan Department of Environmental Quality. After years of cutbacks, the MDEQ drinking-water division was under-staffed, under-experienced, and sometimes lax in its oversight of lead and other safety issues. Studies raised concerns about the Flint River. The plant intake was "very susceptible" to contamination. The river wasn't nearly as clean as Lake Huron. "Aesthetic" problems were likely. And MDEQ safety regulators feared that continuous use of the river posed increased public-health risks ranging from microbes that might make people sick to increased exposure to carcinogens in water disinfectants. Still, the MDEQ approved the Flint River switch.

Flint demographics

City of Flint

City land area:
33.42 (sq. miles)

Median household income:
2014 $24,679; (MI-$49,087)

Poverty rate:
41.6%; (MI-16.2%)

Unemployment rate:
JAN. 2016: 5.5%; (MI-5.1%)
(PEAKED AT 26.5% JULY 2009)

Owner occupied homes:
55.5% (MI-71.5%)

Median home value:
$36,700 2010-14
(MI-$88,300)

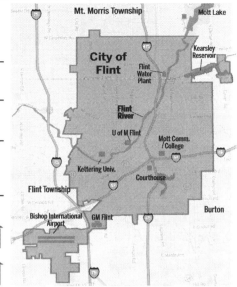

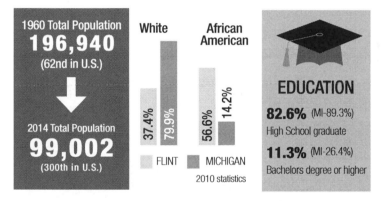

1960 Total Population
196,940
(62nd in U.S.)

↓

2014 Total Population
99,002
(300th in U.S.)

White — FLINT 37.4%, MICHIGAN 79.9%
African American — FLINT 56.6%, MICHIGAN 14.2%
FLINT   MICHIGAN
2010 statistics

EDUCATION
82.6% (MI-89.3%)
High School graduate

11.3% (MI-26.4%)
Bachelors degree or higher

Noteworthy about Flint:

Education: Home to the University of Michigan-Flint (one of three U-M campuses); Kettering University (formerly GMI); Mott Community College and Michigan School for the Deaf.

Books: Flint is the setting for "Rivethead: Tales from the Assembly Line" by Ben Hamper and "Teardown: Memoir of a Vanishing City" by Gordon Young.

Philanthropy: The Charles Stewart Mott Foundation was ranked 95th in the nation for its philanthropy in grant-giving in 2014. The Foundation contributed $4 million to help Flint switch back to Detroit water in October 2015.

Natives

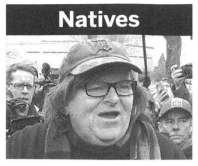

Filmmaker **MICHAEL MOORE**

Born in Flint and raised in nearby Davison. Flint was the focus of many of his films and other ventures, most notably "Roger and Me," a documentary about GM's closure of Flint auto plants.

BOB BELL (Bozo the clown)

BOB EUBANKS
(The Newlywed Game host)

CASEY KASEM
(radio DJ/host of American Top 40)

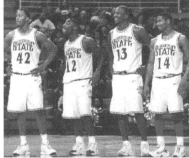

Photo courtesy of MSU

THE FLINTSTONES

We're not talking about Fred and Wilma. Flint's Flintstones are (as pictured above from left to right) Morris Peterson, Mateen Cleaves, Antonio Smith and Charlie Bell. In 1999, the four Michigan State University basketball players from Flint helped take MSU to the NCAA's Final Four. Smith graduated that year but in 2000, the three remaining Flintstones led the Spartans to the NCAA championship.

Flint history

1819: Founded as a village by fur trader Jacob Smith

1855: Incorporated as a city.

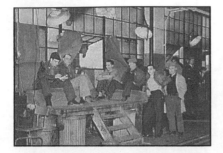

1936-37: Flint sit-down strike led to formation of the United Auto Workers union.

Post WWII: Buick and Chevrolet divisions of GM founded in Flint.

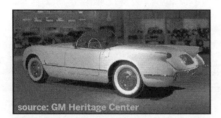

source: GM Heritage Center

1951: Harley Earl, GM's top designer, decides Chevrolet division must respond after seeing a Jaguar XK120. Two years later Chevy unveils the Corvette.

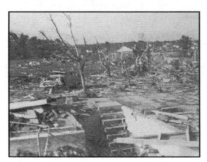

1953: The eighth deadliest U.S. tornado killed 115 people and injured 844 in and around Flint.

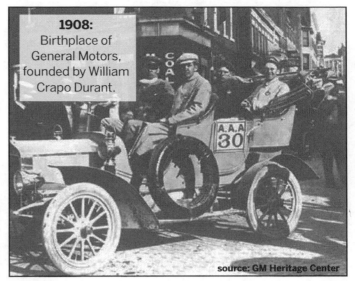

1908: Birthplace of General Motors, founded by William Crapo Durant.

source: GM Heritage Center

1978-2010: GM employment in and near Flint falls from 80,000 to 8,000. In 1996 greater Flint had 46,000 manufacturing jobs, and in 2015 only about 12,000 remained.

1984: Autoworld, a Six Flags outdoor theme park, opened with great expectations to usher in a city turnaround.

1994: Autoworld closed.

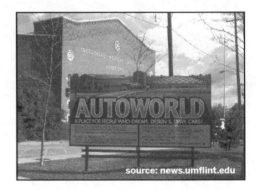

source: news.umflint.edu

2002: As the city faced a $30 million debt, voters recalled Mayor Woodrow Stanley.

2007-2013: Flint makes headlines as one of the nation's most violent cities based on FBI statistics.

2011: With Flint deep in debt again, Gov. Rick Snyder appoints the first of several financial managers.

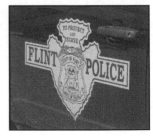

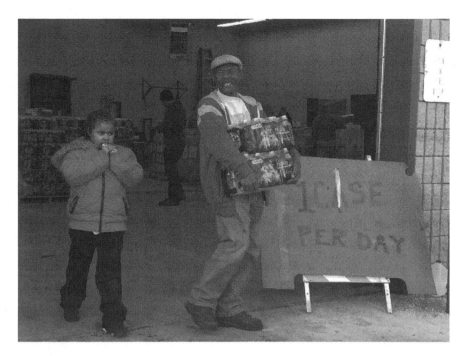

Flint residents Curtis West, 57, and his daughter, Brooklyn Pratcher, 7, get cases of free bottled water at a fire station near their home.

Photo by Chastity Pratt Dawsey/Bridge Magazine

Few cities just up and switch their drinking-water sources. This was new territory, and the MDEQ made the crucial mistake. Flint River water was highly corrosive. Water systems almost everywhere use treatment techniques to prevent water from corroding water mains, because, when old water mains corrode, they can release dangerous levels of lead into drinking water. The Detroit water system, like so many others, used corrosion control for years. But MDEQ didn't require corrosion control as Flint switched to the river.

Just days before the switch, a Flint water-treatment plant supervisor complained MDEQ wasn't giving him clear direction and warned, "If water is distributed from this plant in the next couple of weeks, it will be against my direction." Days later, in April 2014, the valves turned and city officials literally toasted the Flint River switch.

Citizen complaints about dirty, smelly, foul-tasting water rolled in almost immediately. Then came boil-water alerts over sickening bacteria in the water, followed by notices that the water contained elevated levels of potentially carcinogenic disinfectants meant to treat the bacteria. In October 2014, a GM engine plant pulled off the Flint system. GM's move alarmed two of the governor's top aides, who surmised if the water wasn't good enough for GM's parts, how could it be good enough for people? "I see this as an urgent matter to fix," the governor's top environmental adviser declared in email to several colleagues but not to the governor, who was in the last weeks of a re-election campaign. The governor's chief legal counsel, a Flint native, added: "(T)he notion that I would be getting my drinking water from the Flint River is downright scary....

They should try to get back on the Detroit system as a stopgap ASAP before this thing gets too far out of control."

Instead, the situation grew way out of control.

Local, state and federal officials privately wrung their hands via email about an uptick in Legionnaires' disease in the Flint area. MDEQ regulators scoffed: there was no way the drinking water caused the Legionnaires' spike. At least one federal Environmental Protection Agency expert disagreed, and said the drinking water was a possible culprit. Nobody, the governor would claim, told him about the Legionnaires' until the end of 2015. To this day, the full source of the Legionnaires' spike, which killed a dozen people, is not fully known.

Citizen outrage intensified. But at every turn, the MDEQ publicly insisted the water met drinking-water standards. And Flint officials repeated those assurances.

In late February 2015, the EPA started questioning MDEQ regulators about corrosion control, because of fears that rusting water lines were causing a lead problem. At first, MDEQ regulators said corrosion control was in place. Then they admitted it wasn't. Then they engaged in a months-long and byzantine defense—by their interpretation, regulations didn't require corrosion control in Flint. EPA disagreed but didn't act.

Flint just wouldn't calm down. Snyder's chief of staff reacted in fits and starts. He explored a switch back to Detroit water but was told it was too expensive. He helped Flint ministers deliver bottled water and filters. The email correspondence was voluminous. But rarely did the correspondence include the governor himself.

In March 2015, the Flint City Council voted to return to Detroit drinking water. But the vote didn't mean anything. Such decisions were under the control of the latest in a revolving door of state-appointed emergency managers. The emergency manager called the council vote "incomprehensible" because the city couldn't afford the switch, especially when MDEQ continued to assure that the Flint River water met drinking water standards. So the unfolding crisis prolonged, against the will of the city's elected officials.

In mid-summer 2015, the MDEQ's don't-worry narrative began to crumble. Journalists reported high lead levels in tap water in some Flint homes; they wrote about leaked documents suggesting some in the EPA worried the drinking water was dangerous.

In September 2015, independent water-quality scientists and doctors proved the water wasn't safe to drink. MDEQ was dead wrong. Other state regulators charged with monitoring lead dangers also waved off concerns. They were dead wrong. The city's children did, indeed, have elevated blood lead levels.

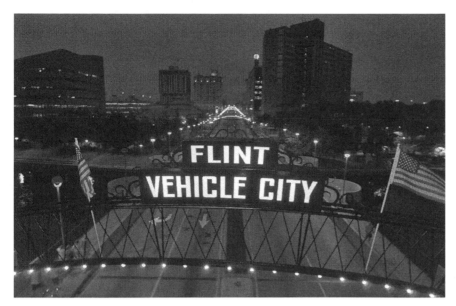

Entering downtown Flint on Saginaw Street, drivers are reminded of the city's heritage as a capital of the automotive industry, and before that, the buggy business. The current city archways and signs are modeled after those that spanned the street until 1919. The new arches and signs went up in 2004.

Photo courtesy Dan Crannie, owner Signs by Crannie

Only then did authorities finally tell Flint residents their water wasn't safe to drink. Only then did Snyder finally stop believing the bungling bureaucrats in state government and swing into action with a blizzard of recovery plans that couldn't possibly extinguish the public anger and damage.

Circle-the-wagons inaction, denials and disrespect for the public, throughout the saga, served as a bitter exclamation point.

"There are 'hiccups' with Flint drinking water, but it's not like an imminent threat to public health," the MDEQ declared in a briefing to the governor in February 2015.

That same month, when the EPA worried in emails to MDEQ that very high lead in the tap water in one Flint home might represent a city-wide problem, a MDEQ water-safety regulator remarked to colleagues that he didn't understand why EPA "sees this one sample as such a big deal." That regulator now faces criminal charges and has been suspended from his job.

Another MDEQ regulator took offense when a state agency trucked purified water into a state office building in Flint with the rationale that it had "high public traffic." The regulator, in turn, emailed colleagues and asked: "Why does 'public traffic' deserve a higher consideration than concern for state workers? How does that reasoning appear to state employees?"

In July 2015, MDEQ's chief spokesman assured on public radio, "Let me start here—anyone who is concerned about lead in the drinking water in Flint can relax." Weeks later, the same spokesman fired off this email missive to a Snyder aide: Flint residents are "confused, in no small part because various groups have worked hard at keeping them confused and upset.… (I)t's been rough sledding with a steady parade of community groups keeping everyone hopped up and misinformed." The spokesman resigned under pressure at the end of 2015.

In September 2015, as a Flint pediatrician announced conclusive evidence of elevated blood levels in Flint children, a manager in the Michigan Department of Health and Human Services scoffed, "This is definitely being driven by a little science and a lot of politics." MDHHS monitors lead poisoning, but only the Flint pediatrician adequately did the job in Flint.

Flint demonstrates how this country is not fully broken—as long as its people wrest control of the truth when those in power don't tell it. Citizen heroes emerged—from the neighborhoods and the ranks of medicine, academia and the media, and even from deep within otherwise dysfunctional government.

From city hall, to houses of worship, to the state capitol, to the White House, Flint residents demanded answers. The voice of one mother on Browning Avenue, on Flint's south side, rose above all. In early 2015, Lee-Anne Walters' family experienced hair loss and rashes. She suspected the tap water. Somehow, against all odds, this anonymous mother reached deep into an imposing bureaucracy, the EPA regional headquarters in Chicago, and found a single water-safety expert willing to provide real help.

While so many bureaucrats remained paralyzed in a regulatory haze throughout the Flint crisis, EPA regulator Miguel Del Toral traveled to Browning Avenue. He tested Walters' water. He discovered astronomically high lead levels. He gave Walters the test results. He fired off alarming memos throughout the EPA and the MDEQ. He boldly concluded the MDEQ seriously blundered by failing to require corrosion control. He accurately surmised Flint could be in a drinking water crisis. MDEQ regulators discounted Del Toral and painted him as a lone rogue acting beyond his authority. The EPA sat on Del Toral's conclusions for months. The EPA regional administrator even apologized for his work. But Del Toral was dead on the mark.

Soon, his memos and Walters' scary lead test results leaked to the media. Curt Guyette, a reporter for the American Civil Liberties Union, broke the story in July 2015. More investigations by Michigan Public Radio, the Detroit News, the Detroit Free Press and MLive.com followed.

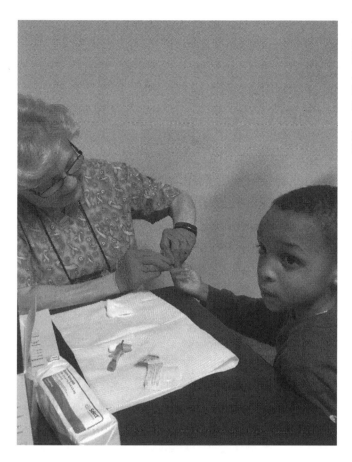

There's not a tear in sight after JaCarie, 5, of Flint had his finger pricked for a blood test in early 2016. His mother JaMise Wash-Lang took her son in for the test to find out if he had lead in his bloodstream.

Photo by Chastity Pratt Dawsey/Bridge Magazine

Along came Marc Edwards. A civil engineering professor at Virginia Tech University, Edwards is like a one-man National Guard who calls himself to duty on drinking-water crises. A dozen years earlier, he uncovered a lead poisoning crisis in Washington, D.C. In 2007, he received a MacArthur Genius grant for "playing a vital role in ensuring the safety of drinking water and in exposing deteriorating water-delivery infrastructure in America's largest cities." To the numerous and stubborn Flint-water-crisis deniers in state government, Edwards became their worst nightmare when he arrived in Flint in summer 2015. His Flint Water Study blog (http://flintwaterstudy.org/) rapidly published undeniable bombshell after bombshell: Flint River water was highly corrosive. The river water corroded city water lines. The deteriorating water mains leached dangerous amounts of lead into the drinking water. The water wasn't safe to drink. And government regulators were either incredibly incompetent or covered up the truth. Edwards quickly and loudly refuted nearly a year's worth of bureaucrats' water safety wave-offs. *(Continued on page 16)*

> ## FLINT ILLUSTRATES HOW ANY POLITICAL LEGACY IS JUST ONE UNSEEN CRISIS FROM DESTRUCTION.

(Continued on page 16)

THE PLAYERS: Governor's office

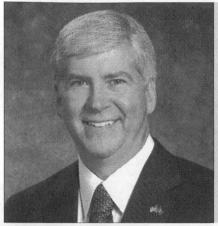

GOVERNOR
RICK SNYDER

Despite earlier successes as governor, the Flint water crisis may prove his greatest — and most damning — legacy. He has apologized many times to Flint residents and said he got bad information from state bureaucrats that the water was safe. He acknowledges his failure to ask tough questions, even as key staffers raised red flags as early as October 2014.

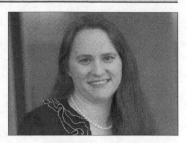

DEPUTY LEGAL COUNSEL
VALERIE BRADER

She urged Snyder staff in October 2014 to push Flint's emergency manager to return to Detroit water immediately.

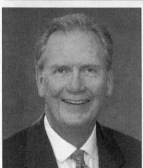

CHIEF OF STAFF
DENNIS MUCHMORE

He got emails from two of Snyder's top attorneys in October 2014 urging return to Detroit water before lead was in issue. He wrote an email in July 2015, saying that he felt the state was blowing off legitimate concerns from residents. He left his job at the end of 2015.

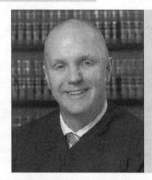

CHIEF LEGAL COUNSEL
MICHAEL GADOLA

He grew up in Flint and his mom still lives there. In response to Brader's email, he wrote: "Nice to know she's drinking water with elevated chlorine levels and fecal coliform." He also urged return to Detroit water.

THE PLAYERS: Emergency managers

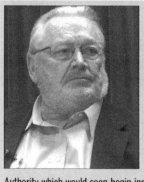

ED KURTZ
(AUG. '12-JULY '13)

He made the decision in June 2013 to use Flint River water while the new pipeline was being built. With support from elected officials, he asked State Treasurer Andy Dillon for permission in late 2012 to allow Flint to join the Karegnondi Water Authority which would soon begin installing a new water line from Lake Huron. Other communities and counties near Flint were joining Karegnondi to gain local control and cut costs charged by Detroit. In June 2013, Kurtz moved to prepare to use the Flint River as the interim source while Karegnondi is completed.

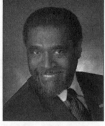

DARNELL EARLEY
(OCT. '13-JAN. '15)

He was in charge during the switch to the Flint River. He didn't challenge regulators' assertions that the water was safe. He wrote a guest column for the Detroit News in October 2015, saying: "This was a local decision that was made by local civic leaders. Anyone who says otherwise is being disingenuous."

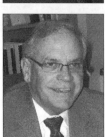

JERRY AMBROSE
(JAN. '15-APRIL 30, '15)

He rejected Detroit's offer in January 2015 to waive a $4 million fee to reconnect to its water. Two months later he rejected the Flint City Council's demand to reconnect to Detroit water. He said the treated water from the Flint River met all standards and that reconnecting would cost $1 million a month.

THE PLAYERS: Michigan Department of Environmental Quality

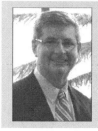

Director
DAN WYANT
(resigned 12/29/15)

He consistently supported the regulators on his staff that Flint water was safe, until issuing a statement on Oct. 19, 2015, saying: "It recently has become clear our drinking water staff made a mistake."

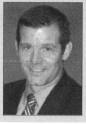

Communications director
BRAD WURFEL
(resigned 12/29/15)

He made many comments to reporters to discredit an EPA official who raised lead concerns and the Virginia Tech professor whose water tests showed high lead levels. He said a Flint pediatrician's comments about her study of blood-lead levels in children were "unfortunate."

STEPHEN BUSCH
(suspended 1/22/16; charged with six criminal counts 4/19/16)

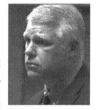

District supervisor. He repeatedly said Flint River water didn't need corrosion control, and on Feb. 27, 2015, wrongly told EPA that corrosion control was in use. Busch warned colleagues, unrelated to lead issues, that Flint River quality was problematic in 2013, before the city switched to using it for drinking water.

MICHAEL PRYSBY
(suspended 4/19/16, charged with six criminal counts)

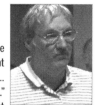

District drinking water engineer. On Sept. 18, 2014, he jokingly remarked in an email to a colleague about Flint residents' complaints: "....off to physical therapy... perhaps mental therapy with all these Flint calls...lol." Later, he said in an email that it "felt prudent" to put purified water coolers in a state office building in Flint because it was "high traffic."

THE PLAYERS: Michigan Department of Health and Human Services

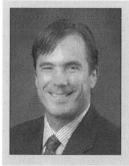

Director
NICK LYON

Before a press conference in September 2015, he sent staff an email: "I would like to make a strong statement with a demonstration of proof that the lead-blood levels seen are not out of the ordinary and are attributable to seasonal fluctuations." He couldn't – it wasn't true.

Director of division of environmental health
LINDA DYKEMA

Called upon in late July 2015 to look into the Flint lead issue, she talked to MDEQ's Busch and parroted his responses – Flint complies with regulations.

CRISTIN LARDER, epidemiologist. Found evidence that blood-lead levels in the three summer months after water switch were higher and concluded it "does warrant further investigation."

ROBERT SCOTT, data manager. He saw the same summer uptick as his colleague Larder, but said it also happened in 2010. He concluded: "I think the water was not a major factor here."

NANCY PEELER, director of program for child home visits. She sent an email based on the work of Larder and Scott that concluded the data didn't support the link from drinking water to blood-lead levels in children.

WES PRIEM, manager of Healthy Homes group. He sent an email Sept. 24, 2015 – the day Dr. Mona Hanna-Attisha's study was released – concluding: "This is definitely being driven by a little science and a lot of politics."

"FLINT WATER IS SAFE TO DRINK."

APRIL 25, 2014, news release from the City of Flint

THE PLAYERS: Flint officials

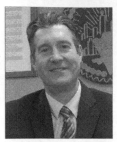

Mayor
DAYNE WALLING
(elected Aug. '09, re-elected '11; powers removed 12/1/11-4/30/15 when Emergency Managers were in control)

On July 9, 2015, he went on TV and drank Flint water, saying it was safe. This came after he raised questions with EPA's top regional official and was given no sense water was dangerous. He lost his re-election bid.

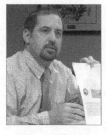

Flint Utilities Administrator
MICHAEL GLASGOW
(pleaded no contest to misdemeanor charge in deal to drop felony in exchange for cooperation with prosecutors) As a water plant supervisor he raised objections a week before the switch to Flint River water. Later, pressured to meet a deadline, he wrongly affirmed that water samples came from taps in homes known to have lead service lines, as testing protocol required.

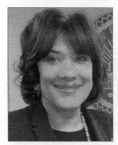

Mayor
KAREN WEAVER
(took office 11/9/15)

A strong critic of the Snyder administration's handling of the water crisis, she complained of poor communication. She joined Hillary Clinton at a rally before the Michigan presidential primary. Clinton called for Snyder to resign.

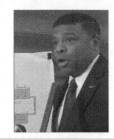

DPS Director
HOWARD CROFT
(resigned 11/15)

He seemed to show little concern about the water, as residents protested and his water plant supervisor said he needed more time to prepare for the switch to the Flint River as the city's drinking water source.

THE PLAYERS: U.S. Environmental Protection Agency

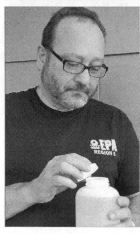

Region 5 regulations manager
MIGUEL DEL TORAL

He was the first to demand MDEQ order corrosion treatment and suggest that the state's failure to do so likely caused lead leaching into drinking water from old pipes. He wrote the blistering memo about lead in Flint water and MDEQ's unwillingness to act. His memo was leaked to an ACLU reporter. A day later, he told a colleague that he was weary of the EPA's unwillingness to step in when "bad actors" put children's health at risk.

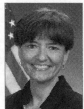

Region 5 Administrator
SUSAN HEDMAN (resigned 1/21/16)

She left to protect the agency, she said, which was being unfairly attacked. Told Mayor Walling on July 1, 2015 when he asked about Del Toral's memo that it was preliminary, required review and shouldn't have been released.

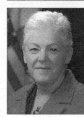

EPA National Administrator
GINA MCCARTHY

In testimony before a U.S. House committee, she wouldn't acknowledge that EPA had made mistakes, but said the agency could have done more in Flint. She supported Hedman until and after her resignation, saying she was "courageous."

"

THIS IS NO SURPRISE. LEAD LINES + NO TREATMENT = HIGH LEAD IN WATER = LEAD POISONED CHILDREN.

~ Sept. 22, 2015 email from Miguel Del Toral to his EPA boss Thomas Poy and others

"

EPA Michigan manager
JENNIFER CROOKS

After learning in late February 2015 of a test taken by the city and showing high lead levels in Lee-Anne Walters' home, she wrote in an email to MDEQ's Busch and Prysby. "Wow, did he find the LEAD! 104 ppb. She has 2 children under the age of 3... Big worries here."

EPA supervisor
THOMAS POY

Miguel Del Toral's supervisor who was the recipient of the 8-page memo. Beginning in July, Poy increasingly pressured MDEQ's Liane Shekter Smith to order and speed up the start of corrosion controls in Flint's drinking water. In an August 31, 2015 conference call with MDEQ he made clear that Marc Edwards' water study supported Del Toral's assertions about lead in the water.

THE PLAYERS: Governor Snyder's Flint water task force

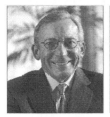

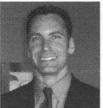

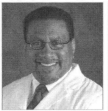

KEN SIKKEMA

senior policy fellow with Public Sector Consultants of Lansing; former Republican legislator

CHRIS KOLB

president of Michigan Environmental Council former Democratic legislator

DR. LAWRENCE REYNOLDS

Flint pediatrician and president of Mott Children's Health Center

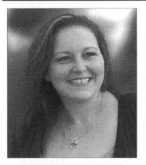

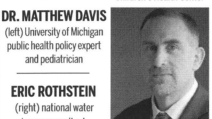

DR. MATTHEW DAVIS

(left) University of Michigan public health policy expert and pediatrician

ERIC ROTHSTEIN

(right) national water issues consultant

Task Force: MDEQ most at fault

The Flint Water Advisory Task Force didn't sugarcoat its findings. Its first report assigned primary blame to MDEQ. A day later the MDEQ director and spokesperson resigned. Over the next five weeks, Liane Shekter Smith was fired and Stephen Busch was suspended. In its conclusions, the task force cited MDEQ as most at fault. "...confronted with evidence of its failure, MDEQ responded publicly through formal communications with a degree of intransigence and belligerence that has no place in government." The task force also said Snyder, his staff, the Michigan Department of Health and Human Services, the EPA, emergency managers, Flint and Genesee County officials share blame that added to or prolonged the crisis. It said Flint residents were victims of "environmental unjustice" – the majority black citizens didn't get the same treatment as those in other communities would have. And it asked for review of the state's Emergency Manager law to allow more citizen input.

(see appendix A for full executive summary)

THE PLAYERS: They fought back and won

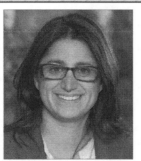

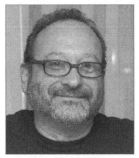

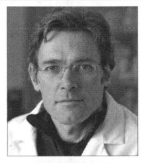

LEE-ANNE WALTERS

The Flint mother of four and Navy wife who after noticing physical and behavioral changes in her children, pushed for answers and got the city to take water tests from her home taps. The testing confirmed high lead levels. She contacted EPA's Del Toral and started events that brought credibility to MDEQ's critics.

DR. MONA HANNA-ATTISHA

The Flint pediatrician who - after the Michigan Department of Public Health and Human Resources dismissed concerns about lead in Flint's water - did her own ground-breaking study (released Sept. 24, 2015) which showed blood levels of lead in young children had more than doubled in some areas since the water source switch. Soon after, the state confirmed her findings and Gov. Snyder ordered a return to Detroit water.

MIGUEL DEL TORAL

Region 5 regulations manager in the drinking water branch, first to demand MDEQ order corrosion treatment and suggest that state's failure to do so likely caused lead leaching into drinking water from old pipes.

(see description under EPA)

MARC EDWARDS

Virginia Tech professor and national expert on public water supplies and lead. He directed research team which found much higher lead levels than city tests. He was befuddled by MDEQ decisions. In testimony before a congressional committee, he was one of the harshest critics of the EPA, especially Susan Hedman.

(Continued from page 11)

If so much lead was in the water, what was it doing to Flint's kids? No problem, the Michigan Department of Health and Human Services kept repeating. Their epidemiologists ran the numbers, and the talking heads insisted there was no uptick in Flint lead poisoning—until Flint pediatrician Mona Hanna-Attisha ran her own numbers and called a press conference to independently repeat what Marc Edwards was shouting. The water wasn't safe. Since the switch to the Flint River, the percentage of infants and children with elevated blood-lead levels had nearly doubled—and nearly tripled in high-risk neighborhoods.

Without Lee-Anne Walters, Miguel Del Toral, Marc Edwards, Dr. Mona Hanna-Attisha, some in the media, and citizens who raised hell, Flint might still be drinking poison water.

Fresh from his 2014 re-election, Gov. Snyder traveled from California to New York in spring 2015 to tout "Michigan's Comeback Story." Flint—which represents only 1 percent of the statewide population—was not a high point in Snyder's relentlessly positive narrative.

Five years earlier, Snyder, a multi-millionaire business executive and venture capitalist, burst into public consciousness with Super Bowl ads. Declaring himself "One Tough Nerd," Snyder prescribed "jobs" as job one. Unemployment in the Great Lakes State reached 15 percent during the height of the Great Recession. Michigan's fall was a national story—its July 2009 unemployment rate was the highest seen in any state in a quarter century.

Many pundits at first discounted Snyder's 2010 candidacy as an odd sideshow. His political chops were questionable at best. He ran as a Republican while living in the ultra-liberal college town of Ann Arbor. "As a past board member of Nature Conservancy's Michigan chapter, he wasn't exactly a conservative poster child. And his high-pitched voice implied inexperience and discomfort with press conferences and public speeches.

But Snyder was a winner. He grew up in Battle Creek, where his father owned a modest window-cleaning business. Early on, Rick pointed toward big things. In the time it took most college students to earn one degree, Rick Snyder earned two, a bachelor's in accounting and a MBA, both from the University of Michigan. By age 31, he was partner in a major accounting firm and in charge of its mergers and acquisitions office in Chicago. In the 1990s, he ran Gateway Computers. He came back to Ann Arbor and launched two successful venture capital firms.

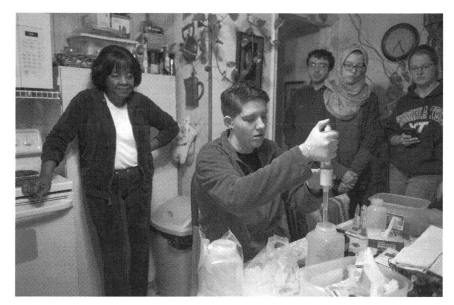

In early March, many Virginia Tech graduate and undergraduate students joined professor Marc Edwards in Flint to conduct follow-up water tests to determine if the switch back to corrosion-treated Detroit water was reducing lead levels in the city's water.

Photo courtesy of Logan Wallace/Virginia Tech

Then he won in 2010, running as a moderate among a crowd of conservatives in the Republican primary. He easily won the general election against Democrat Virg Bernero, the mayor of Lansing, whose mercurial campaign never overcame his moniker as "America's Angriest Mayor." Suddenly, the Nerd was a governor with a mandate. Snyder carried 79 of Michigan's 83 counties. Genesee County—home to Flint—was among the four exceptions. But even in Genesee, a Democratic bastion, Snyder won nearly half of the vote.

In the high-minded times of early 2011, the political newbie governor urged his appointees to work in "dog years," implying he wanted to spur change at roughly seven times normal human speed. They got off to a fast and sometimes controversial pace. They reformed the state's much-hated business tax. They led the nation in expansion of early childhood learning programs. They wrote special messages and launched task forces on dozens of issues. They signed right-to-work and various forms of controversial hot-button social-issue legislation not originally on Snyder's agenda. They passed state budgets on time and grew the state's rainy-day reserves. They helped engineer a unique infusion of public and philanthropic investment to pull Detroit out of the nation's largest-ever municipal bankruptcy. And they sent state-appointed emergency managers into Michigan's most financially troubled cities. Like Flint.

Four years in, the November 2014 election was a litmus test of Snyder's technocratic, numbers-heavy, business-styled leadership. The media steadily reported public rage over right-to-work, social issues, and state-emergency-manager control over troubled cities and school districts. But Snyder won re-election by four percentage points.

By spring 2015, Michigan's economy was well-thawed in many places (not Flint). The state unemployment rate was 5.6 percent, a third of what it was in the dark days of 2009. And the governor wanted the world to know.

"I will continue to tell Michigan's comeback story nationally because our reinvention should not be unique to just our state," Snyder declared. He appeared positioned for a possible cabinet position if a Republican won the White House in 2016.

How quickly the mighty can fall.

By the end of 2015, the Flint crisis eclipsed every glimmer of Snyder's economic-recovery narrative. There was no denying—Flint happened on Snyder's watch. In early 2016, Snyder gave his state-of-the-state address, humbly apologized to Flint and essentially pledged to use what was left of his second term to fix it.

The backlash was the fiercest any Michigan governor has faced in modern times. Protesters marched in front of his downtown Ann Arbor home, declaring "you're not welcome here." Some all but accused the governor of murder. Journalists at home and across the country vilified him, with even business-friendly voices like Detroit News columnist Daniel Howes accusing Snyder of "butt covering, not leadership." In the political theater of Congressional hearings, Democrats smashed the Snyder piñata.

"Plausible deniability only works when it's plausible," Pennsylvania Rep. Matt Cartwright lectured Snyder. "And I'm not buying that you didn't know about any of this until October 2015. You were not in a medically-induced coma for a year, and I've had about enough of your false contrition and phony apologies."

Snyder positioned his entry into politics as a post-partisan crusade of government reinvention. Now he faced a Flint scarlet letter on his sport coat. The intensity of the public rage puzzled some of his friends. On the eve of the Flint debacle, Snyder devoted his 2015 state-of-the-state address to the plight of those living in poverty. He envisioned reinventing welfare and human services programs to be far more effective and people-friendly. It sounded more like Bill Clinton than Ted Cruz. Snyder called it the "River of Opportunity." Then the Flint River drowned him.

Flint native Chris Rizik, a longtime friend of the governor, offered a passionate defense via Facebook:

"First of all, I mourn for my hometown and am appalled at the events that happened to a city and to people I love… Second, I am saddened by the unfair treatment that Governor Rick Snyder has gone through by those who wish to ignore the facts or who have no understanding of how an organization (such as The State of Michigan) with 50,000 employees runs…(T)hose who have threatened the Governor with violence, who have hung him in effigy, who have picketed in front of his house demanding that he be jailed, who have called him everything from an elitist to a racist, don't know or don't care to know him. That is simply not who he is or who he ever was. Were they cheering him two years ago when he successfully pushed a hesitant legislature to expand Medicaid to 500,000 more Michigan low-income citizens and to adopt the Affordable Care Act? Or when he helped allocate nearly $200 million to shore up Detroit City pensions as part of the "Grand Bargain"? Or when he created Community Ventures and funded it with tens of millions of dollars to help ex-offenders and the structurally unemployed to find work? The greatest irony is that a man whose mantra is 'relentless positive action,' and who has never said one bad word about a political opponent, is now the subject of one of the worst smear campaigns I have ever seen…."

FLINT IS A STORY OF AMERICAN HEROES.

Politicians are *not* the victims of Flint. But the tolls the crisis takes on elected leaders have implications.

"I'm kicking myself every day," Snyder acknowledged in February 2016. A month later, he topped a Fortune Magazine list of the "world's most disappointing leaders."

The Flint crisis also left its mayor feeling powerless and defeated. Dayne Walling graduated from now-closed Flint Central High School, became a Rhodes Scholar and won election in 2009, giving him the privilege to preside over worst-in-the-nation crime and economic misfortune. Then came the Flint River water switch, which he toasted, and the Flint water crisis, in which he repeatedly failed to gain significant state and federal help.

In fall 2015, a Flint priest ripped Walling in an email, declaring the lead problem "unconscionable." Walling forwarded the email to MDEQ Director Dan Wyant, and added: "I have searched myself over and over on this. I don't know what more I could have done given the guidance coming from EPA and DEQ and subsequently city staff but this major health issue did come up anyway and our community is paying a huge price." Walling urged an "explanation for how this happened" and "steps that ensure it will never happen again." Two months later, Flint residents voted Walling out of office.

It's a common refrain: Where are the leaders today? In the wake of Flint, perhaps it is understandable if thoughtful, rational, experienced leaders recoil from public office in greater numbers. Why sacrifice everything to run for office when, if you win, you win the obligation to work enormous hours, often for much lower pay than in the private sector, attempting to lead in a climate where so much could go wrong, and hangmen in every political corner are poised to noose you?

O bviously, this book is not the last word on the Flint water crisis. Surely we are many years from a last word on a crisis with tentacles as tangled as these. Congressional investigations… Hearings in the Michigan Legislature… State and federal criminal probes… Civil lawsuits too numerous to count... Attempts to fight the potential long-term damage of lead poisoning and fix the Flint water system… Political rivalries stoked by the tension of the crisis… Impacts on the Flint economy, its real estate market, and its business competitiveness… Impacts on the statewide Pure Michigan tourism economy.

And the thousands of stories of how Flint residents, especially young children, endure a tragedy they did not cause or deserve.

The news seems sure to flow as predictably as the Flint River has flowed through the city for generations.

We hope readers, leaders and the people of Flint will benefit from this volume, which is anchored only in the headwaters of the still-unfolding Flint disaster.

ABOUT THE TIMELINE AND TRUTH SQUAD

Bridge Magazine's detailed timeline of the Flint water crisis, which follows, is the heart of "Poison on Tap." Our objective is to present concerned citizens and policymakers the full weight, detail and context of the water crisis in Flint and its implications beyond. We hope readers find it useful in sorting fact from fiction, and credible analysis from spin.

In some places, our Truth Squad adds clarifying commentary and poses questions to help readers understand and interpret entries – and ask their own questions. Center for Michigan President and CEO John Bebow compiled the timeline and authored the Truth Squad analyses. He did so with the help of thousands of pages of public documents and published reports, including:

- *Michigan Department of Environmental Quality and Michigan Department of Health and Human Service email records first obtained under the Freedom of Information Act and published by Virginia Tech professor and water expert Marc Edwards.*

- *Email records released by Michigan Gov. Rick Snyder.*

- *Other local, state and federal documents from the City of Flint, Michigan Department of Treasury, Michigan Auditor General, and U.S. Environmental Protection Agency.*

- *A peer-reviewed study published in a February 2016 medical journal.*

- *Media reports, especially from MLive, Michigan Radio and the Detroit Free Press and Detroit News.*

We recognize that the story is far from over. State criminal charges were announced as we neared completion of this book and state and federal investigations were continuing. And lawsuits are outstanding.

We expect to periodically update the timeline at bridgemi. com. And we expect to publish updated editions of this book as events unfold.

— Bob Campbell, "Poison on Tap" editor

2013

SPRING 2013: Flint joins Karegnondi Water Authority that's building new pipeline to Lake Huron.

2014

APRIL 2014: Flint switches to Flint River from Lake Huron (Detroit) water until Karegnondi is online. MDEQ tells plant operators corrosion controls not needed.

REST OF 2014: Residents complain water smells, tastes, looks bad

OCT. 2014: Gov. Snyder's deputy legal advisor urges reconnect to Detroit water; Snyder not in her email loop.

OCT. 2014: GM plant stops using Flint water because it's corroding parts.

REST OF 2014: MDEQ regulators insist water meets standards.

2015

JAN. 2015: Protests grow; activist Erin Brockovich weighs in.

JAN. 2015: Flint Emergency Manager says no to Detroit offer to reconnect.

FEB. 2015: High lead found in water of Lee-Anne Walters' home.

FEB. 2015: EPA's Miguel Del Toral asks if MDEQ required corrosion control. MDEQ says Flint has optimized corrosion control.

MARCH 2015: Emergency Manager says no to City Council demand to reconnect to Detroit water.

APRIL 2015: MDEQ admits there is no corrosion control.

JUNE 2015: Del Toral writes memo to EPA bosses fearing widespread lead poisoning of Flint's children.

JULY 1, 2015: EPA Region 5 administrator gives Flint's mayor no sense of alarm about Del Toral's memo.

JULY 9, 2015: ACLU reporter publishes report based on Del Toral memo.

JULY 9, 2015: Mayor Dayne Walling drinks Flint water on live TV, says it's good.

JULY 13, 2015: MDEQ spokesman tells Michigan Radio: "Anyone who is concerned about lead in the drinking water in Flint can relax."

JULY 21, 2015: Snyder's chief of staff writes email to heads of MDEQ and MDHHS that Flint residents "are basically getting blown off by us."

AUG. 17, 2015: MDEQ tells Flint to use corrosion control, but gives the water plant operators two years to implement.

SEPT. 2, 2015: Virginia Tech Professor Marc Edwards says his team found much higher lead levels in water than city tests.

SEPT. 9, 2015: MDEQ's Brad Wurfel is dismissive of Edwards results in MLive.com interview.

SEPT. 24, 2015: Pediatrician Dr. Mona Hanna-Attisha releases study: Blood-lead levels in young kids sharply increased after switch to Flint River water.

OCT. 1, 2015: MDHHS confirms Hanna-Attisha's results, Snyder's staff works on switch back to Detroit water.

OCT. 2, 2015: Snyder announces massive plan to help Flint residents

OCT. 16, 2015: Flint reconnects to Detroit water.

OCT. 18, 2015: MDEQ director acknowledges "staff made a mistake" that led to Flint crisis.

DEC. 29, 2015: Snyder task force issues preliminary report citing MDEQ as "primarily responsible" and says department must be held accountable.

DEC. 29, 2015: MDEQ's Dan Wyant and Brad Wurfel resign.

2016

JAN. 12, 2016: Snyder activates National Guards troops to distribute bottled water.

JAN. 13, 2016: Snyder announces 87 cases of Legionnaires' disease, including nine deaths.

JAN. 19, 2016: Snyder apologizes to Flint citizens: "I'm sorry and I will fix it."

JAN. 21, 2016: EPA Region 5 administrator Susan Hedman announces resignation.

FEB. 2, 2016: U.S. Attorney's office announces FBI investigation.

FEB. 3, 2016: First of three congressional hearings on Flint.

FEB. 5, 2016: Snyder fires Liane Shekter Smith, head of MDEQ's drinking-water program, and suspends Stephen Busch, a district supervisor.

REST OF FEBRUARY: Snyder's office releases two huge dumps of Flint emails.

MARCH 23, 2016: Task force final report find lots of blame for state government, including governor, but especially MDEQ.

APRIL 20, 2016: Two MDEQ and one Flint water-plant supervisor charged with crimes for Flint water crisis.

MAY 4, 2016: President Obama visits, drinks Flint water and tells residents "I've got your back."

MAY 10, 2016: Mott Foundation and nine other foundations pledge $125 million to meet short- and long-term Flint recovery needs.

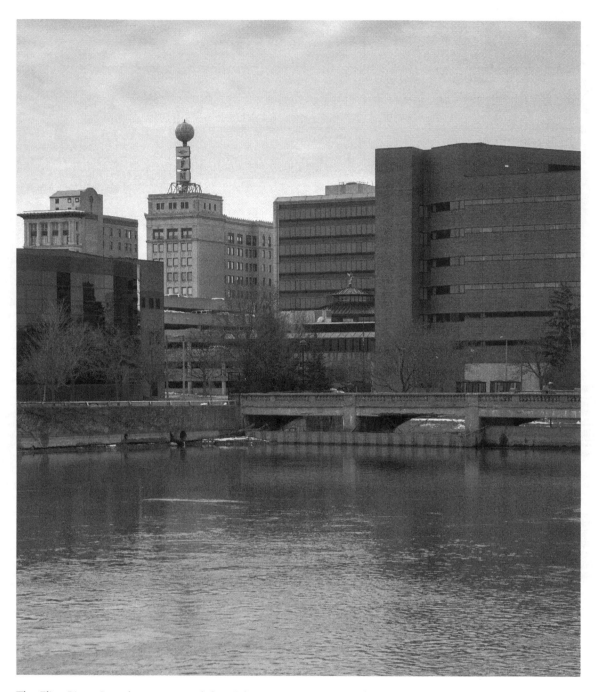

The Flint River. Regulators warned that "The source water area for the Flint emergency intake includes 96 potential contaminant sources."

Photo courtesy of Logan Wallace/Virginia Tech

2004-2013

A FLAWED IDEA

FLINT SEEKS NEW WATER SOURCE; STUDIES AND REGULATORS RAISE QUESTIONS

Editor's summary: The city of Flint enters the new decade saddled with a decimated tax base caused by a hollowed-out economy.

Among Flint's financial issues is the high cost of water it is purchasing from the Detroit Department of Water and Sewerage, which is pumped from Lake Huron. But as far back as 2004, the alternative of the Flint River as a drinking water source is problematic. A multi-agency report cites farm and urban runoff as big problems.

Seven years later, Flint's financial collapse prompts Gov. Rick Snyder to name an emergency manager to run the city. A few months later, Flint agrees to join the new Karegnondi Water Authority, which had formed to build a new pipeline to Lake Huron for communities in Genesee, Lapeer and Sanilac counties.

With strong support from Flint's elected officials, the emergency manager cites local control over water cost as a key reason for the change. In 2013, Michigan Department of Environmental Quality staff raises concerns about using Flint River as the main source for drinking water while the new water pipeline is being built.

"AS YOU MIGHT GUESS WE ARE IN A SITUATION WITH EMERGENCY FINANCIAL MANAGERS SO IT'S ENTIRELY POSSIBLE THAT THEY WILL BE MAKING DECISIONS RELATIVE TO COST."

TIMELINE: 2004 – 2013

By John Bebow
Bridge Magazine

2004

FEBRUARY: A technical assessment of the Flint River raises concerns about using the river for drinking water. The key points of the "Source Water Assessment Report for the City of Flint Water Supply – Flint River Emergency Intake" prepared by the U.S. Geological Survey, Michigan Department of Environmental Quality, and Flint Water Utilities Department:

"(T)he emergency intake for the Flint Water Treatment Plant has a very high degree of sensitivity to potential contaminants. When the effects of agricultural and urban runoff in the Flint River watershed are considered, the Flint intake is categorized as very highly sensitive."

"The source water area for the Flint emergency intake includes 96 potential contaminant sources."

"The potential contaminant sources, in combination with the very highly sensitive intake, indicate that the Flint emergency intake source water is very highly susceptible to potential contamination."

"However, it is noted that when operating, the City of Flint Water Treatment Plant has effectively treated this source water to meet drinking water standards."

> **TRUTH SQUAD ANALYSIS:** For many years, the City of Flint bought water from the Detroit drinking water system. But the Flint Water Treatment plant retained access to the Flint River for emergency backup. As this timeline fully outlines, Flint – with official approval from its state-appointed manager and State Treasurer Andy Dillon, but also with support of local officials – switched to the Flint River as its drinking water source in April 2014. This was to be a temporary move, until the new Karegnondi Water Authority regional water pipeline from Lake Huron opened in late 2016.)

2011

JULY: Report from Rowe Engineering titled "Analysis of the Flint River as a Permanent Water Supply for the City of Flint." Prepared for the City of Flint. Key points:

"Preliminary analysis indicates that water from the river can be treated to meet current regulations' however, additional treatment will be required than for Lake Huron water. This results in higher operating costs than the alternative of a new Lake Huron supply…. (A)esthetics of the finished water will be different than from Lake Huron. As an example, the temperature of water supplied to customers during the summer will be warmer than the present Lake Huron supply, because of the increased summer temperature in the relatively shallow river."

"A detailed investigation of potential sources of contamination has not been completed."

NOV. 29: Flint becomes Michigan's fourth city under the control of an emergency manager. A review team finds accumulated deficits of $25.7 million.

2012

MAY 9: Letter from Flint Department of Public Works Director Howard Croft to Michigan Department of Environmental Quality District Engineer Mike Prysby: "The Karegnondi Water Authority has the potential to be a major factor in our region's economic development efforts. The City of Flint is pleased to be a partner in the process and we pledge to offer our assets to support the development. We appreciate your technical support as we develop our components of the project."

JUNE: Flint emergency manager Mike Brown asks the Detroit Water and Sewerage Department (DWSD) for permission to blend Flint River water with DWSD water to save Flint between $2 million and $3 million annually.

NOVEMBER: New Flint emergency manager Ed Kurtz writes to state Treasurer Andy Dillon suggesting that the Karegnondi Water Authority (KWA) is the best long-term option for Flint water due to rising costs from the Detroit Water and Sewerage Department (DWSD). The KWA positions itself as an example of local government control for entities in Genesee, Lapeer, and Sanilac counties – all about an hour's drive north of Detroit. The KWA website states: "By joining the group it will give you more control over the costs and the water. Currently, you purchase finished water from the DWSD with no input as to the cost. As a member of the group, you will purchase raw water and treat it to your own standards. As a member, you will participate in establishing the cost and rates for the water." Karegnondi is the name the Huron-Petun native Americans (later known as Wyandot), gave to Lake Huron. It means Big Lake.

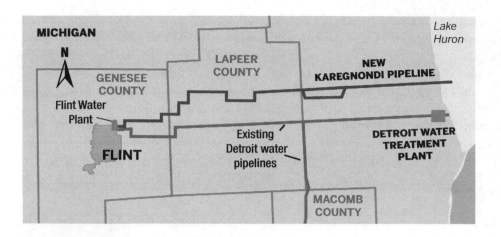

2013

JAN. 23: MDEQ's Mike Prysby to colleague Liane Shekter Smith and others about the feasibility of Flint switching to the Flint River: "I agree that the city should have concerns of fully utilizing the Flint River (100%) for the following: the need to soften, the potential for more advanced treatment after next round of crypto monitoring, available capacity in Flint River at 100-year low flow, residuals management (disposal of lime sludge)."

FEBRUARY: Engineering study ordered by state Department of Treasury concludes KWA is the cheaper option for Flint water.

MARCH: Flint City Council endorses joining the Karegnondi Water Authority. MLive.com coverage is headlined: "Flint City Council approves resolution to buy water from Karegnondi, state approval still needed." The story quotes local officials support for the switch:

Flint City Councilman Joshua Freeman: "We got there, that's the important thing."

Rebecca Fedewa, Flint River Watershed Coalition: "Going with Karegnondi is the best decision."

Flint Mayor Dayne Walling: "It's a historic night for the city of Flint."

The only dissenting vote was from Councilman Bryan Nolden: "I just feel like the Flint River is our best option."

TRUTH SQUAD ANALYSIS: The council's vote is symbolic; with the city under control of an emergency manager, the council vote is not binding. State Treasurer Andy Dillon made the final decision to switch from DWSD to KWA.

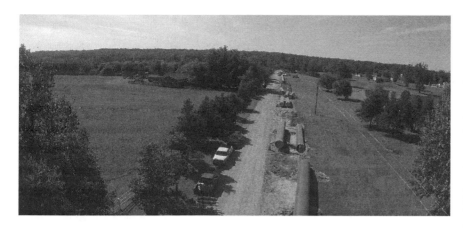

Construction of the new 36-inch Karegnondi Water Authority line that will serve residents in Sanilac, Lapeer and Genesee County, including Flint, began in late 2014.

Photo courtesy Karegnondi Water Authority

MARCH 26: Genesee County Drain Commissioner Jeff Wright, who is not party to the water contract, nevertheless writes a letter of support for the decision: "I have said from the beginning that this decision must be made by Flint's City Council and Mayor. I appreciate the council voting the way they did, but even more than that, I am glad the residents of Flint were able to have their voices heard via their elected officials…. There is a basic tenet of government is best when it has local control. We saw that with the council vote. Nobody, whether they live in Flint, Grand Blanc, Davison, Fenton, or anywhere in Genesee County, should have these types of decisions made by people who live outside their community."

MARCH 26: An email from MDEQ's Michael Alexander to colleagues Stephen Busch, Christine Alexander and William Creal points out issues about the "Flint River Intake Location":

"Based on the listing from Michigan's 2012 Integrated Report, the Flint River from just upstream of the City of Flint to the upstream end of the Holloway Reservoir is not meeting designated uses for:

"Fish consumption due to PCB in fish tissue and water column.

"Total and partial body contact due to E. coli in water column.

"Other indigenous aquatic life due to nutrients and phosphorus in the water column.

"These are just the major categories for the designated uses currently not being met within this subject stretch of the Flint River."

MARCH 26: An email from Stephen Busch, an MDEQ district supervisor, to MDEQ Director Dan Wyant with Liane Shekter Smith and other MDEQ staff copied. Citing water quality, it warns about using Flint River as an interim water source until the Karegnondi pipeline is connected. The memo is written "in preparation for a call" the same day with the office of State Treasurer Andy Dillon:

"All contract options with DWSD that are considered semi-competitive with the KWA contract do not fully supply the City of Flint, and would require the City of Flint to meet a significant, if not majority, of its water demands by treating water from the Flint River. Continuous use of the Flint River at such demand rates would: "Pose an increased microbial risk to public health (Flint River vs. Lake Huron source water)

"Pose an increased risk of disinfection by-product (carcinogen) exposure to public health (Flint River vs. Lake Huron source water)

"Trigger additional regulatory requirements under the Michigan Safe Drinking Water Act."

MARCH 27: MDEQ's Jim Sygo responds to colleague Stephen Busch about a possible interim switch to use Flint River as a drinking-water source:

"As you might guess we are in a situation with Emergency Financial Managers so it's entirely possible that they will be making decisions relative to cost. The concern in either situation is that a compliant supply of source water and drinking water can be supplied."

MARCH 28: State Treasurer Andy Dillon sends an email to Gov. Rick Snyder and copies many Treasury officials and MDEQ Director Dan Wyant:

"Governor, based upon today's presentations to the DEQ by the City of Flint, KWA and the engineering firm (Tucker Young) Treasury hired to vet the options as to whether Flint should stay with DWSD or join KWA, I am recommending we support the City of Flint's decision to join KWA. The City's Emergency Manager, Mayor, and City Council all support this decision. Dan Wyant likewise concurs and will confirm via email.

"We have a briefing call tomorrow morning with Dennis and John to provide more background as to why we reached this conclusion. Flint's Emergency Manager wants to sign the resolution ASAP as the project is moving forward with or without them and their participation affects the design and the construction season is upon them. I assume DWSD will make a last ditch effort to save the customer but I will not advise them of my recommendation until we brief Dennis and John."

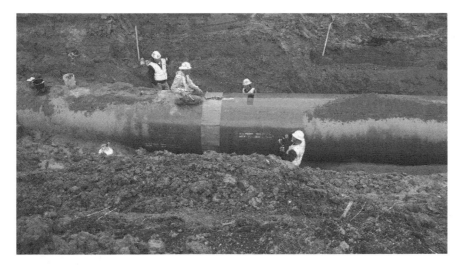

The Karegnondi Water Authority pipeline is expected to be completed in 2016, but Flint officials, the MDEQ and the U.S. EPA want to make sure everything is in order to deliver clean, safe water before switching away from Detroit water.

Photo courtesy Karegnondi Water Authority

APRIL 1: DWSD "responds to Flint's decision, issuing a statement that Flint's plans will not save money. The statement says Flint has 'launched the greatest water war in Michigan history' and that it will result in higher prices for the department's other customers." (As reported by the Detroit Free Press, January 2016.)

APRIL: State Treasurer Andy Dillon gives state emergency manager Ed Kurtz permission to notify the Detroit Water and Sewerage Department that it would be terminating service in the future and contracting with the KWA.

APRIL 15: "The Detroit Water and Sewerage Department provides a best and final offer to the City of Flint. Analyses by Flint Emergency Manager Ed Kurtz, the Department of Environmental Quality and Treasury's Office of Fiscal Responsibility independently conclude that the Karegnondi Water Authority option is cheaper for the City of Flint." (As reported in the Michigan Department of Treasury Flint Water Timeline, September 2015.)

APRIL 16: "Flint Emergency Manager Ed Kurtz informs the State Treasurer that the city will join KWA. This decision was officially announced May 1, 2013." (As reported in the Michigan Department of Treasury Flint Water Timeline, September 2015, and in a December 2015 Michigan Auditor General investigation report.)

APRIL 17: DWSD transmits letter to Flint emergency manager Kurtz terminating service to the City of Flint, effective exactly one year later, April 17, 2014.

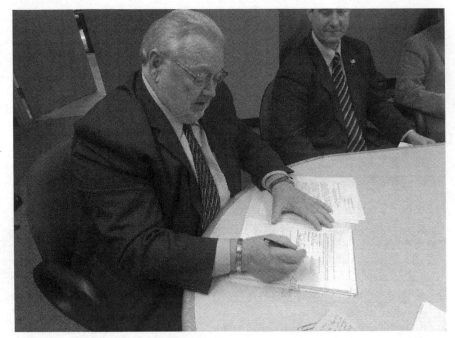

Ed Kurtz, Flint's emergency manager who ran the city when the decision was made to switch to Flint River water as the city's drinking water sources.

Photo courtesy of Michigan Radio

JUNE: KWA breaks ground with completion expected in late 2016.

JUNE 21: Emergency Manager Kurtz signs contract with an engineering company to prepare the Flint water treatment plant to begin using the Flint River as primary interim source of water.

JUNE 29: All-day meeting of Flint, Genesee County Drain Commissioner and MDEQ officials where they discuss feasibility of using Flint River until KWA is ready. (As reported by the Detroit Free Press, January 2016)

AUGUST: Rowe Professional Services completes an engineering proposal for improvements that would allow Flint to draw water continuously from the Flint River in lieu of DWSD service.

CHAPTER 3

2014

THE SHORT-LIVED TOAST

CITIZENS QUICKLY CRY FOUL
OVER FLINT RIVER DRINKING-WATER SWITCH

Editor's summary: Negotiations fail to reach a deal to continue Detroit water and in late April Flint switches to the Flint River as its drinking water source.

A week before that happens, a Flint water-lab supervisor says his staff is unprepared for the move. No one seems to pay attention. A city press release touts the water's high quality, but citizens complain within weeks about its smell and taste.

Over three weeks in late August and September, the city issues boil-water advisories to residents because of fecal bacteria. In October, General Motors officials stop using Flint water at an engine plant because it's corroding car parts. The same month, several key aides to Gov. Snyder urge a quick return to Detroit water.

"IF WATER IS DISTRIBUTED FROM THIS PLANT IN THE NEXT COUPLE OF WEEKS, IT WILL BE AGAINST MY DIRECTION. I NEED TIME TO ADEQUATELY TRAIN ADDITIONAL STAFF AND TO UPDATE OUR MONITORING PLANS BEFORE I WILL FEEL WE ARE READY. I WILL REITERATE THIS TO MANAGEMENT ABOVE ME, BUT THEY SEEM TO HAVE THEIR OWN AGENDA."

— MICHAEL GLASGOW

TIMELINE: 2014

By John Bebow
Bridge Magazine

2014

MARCH 7: The latest Flint Emergency Manager, Darnell Earley, sends a letter to DWSD saying Flint will switch to the Flint River as its primary source of water and disconnect from DWSD.

MARCH 26: Email from MDEQ water safety regulator Stephen Busch to Liane Shekter Smith and Richard Benzie, MDEQ chief of field operations for the Office of Drinking Water and Municipal Assistance: "One of the things we didn't get to today that I would like to make sure everyone is on the same page on is what Flint will be required to do in order to start using their plant full time. Because the plant is setup for emergency use, they could startup at any time, but starting up for continuous operation will carry significant changes in regulatory requirements so there is a very gray area as to what we consider for startup."

APRIL 16: Warning in an email sent from Michael Glasgow, a water treatment plant operator for the City of Flint, to Adam Rosenthal at MDEQ:

"I am expecting changes to our Water Quality Monitoring parameters, and possibly our DBP on lead & copper monitoring plan.… Any information would be appreciated, because it looks as if we will be starting the plant up tomorrow and are being pushed to start distributing water as soon as possible… I would like to make sure we are monitoring, reporting and meeting requirements before I give the OK to start distributing water."

APRIL 17: Second email warning from Glasgow to Adam Rosenthal, Mike Prysby and Stephen Busch at MDEQ:

"I have people above me making plans to distribute water ASAP. I was reluctant before, but after looking at the monitoring schedule and our current staffing, I do not anticipate giving the OK to begin sending water out anytime soon. If water is distributed from this plant in the next couple of weeks, it will be against my direction. I need time to adequately train additional staff and to update our monitoring plans before I will feel we are ready. I will reiterate this to management above me, but they seem to have their own agenda."

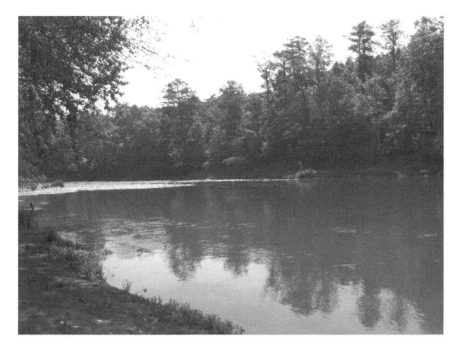

The Flint River had been the water source for the City of Flint until the mid-1960s, when Flint signed an agreement to get water from a new pipeline Detroit built to Lake Huron to service its northern suburbs and Flint. In April 2014, Flint again became the drinking-water source as officials sought to save money until the new Karegnondi Water Authority line was complete.

Photo by Bridge Magazine

APRIL 23: Email from Stephen Busch to MDEQ spokesman Brad Wurfel discussing talking points for a public meeting in Flint regarding drinking water. Busch raises this talking point: "While the Department is satisfied with the City's ability to treat water from the Flint River, the Department looks forward to the long term solution of continued operation of the City of Flint Water Treatment Plant using water from the KWA as a more consistent and higher quality source water."

APRIL 24: Email from Daugherty Johnson, City of Flint Utilities Administrator, to Flint colleague Howard Croft, and Mike Prysby and Busch at MDEQ:

"As you are aware, the City has undergone extensive upgrades to our Water Treatment Plant and its associated facilities. Our intentions and efforts have been to operate our facility as the primary drinking water source for the City of Flint. Through consultation with your office and our engineering firm we've developed a system of redundant electrical systems, treatment processes and adequate finished water storage to negate the need for a signed backup agreement with DWSD due to their termination of our contract. Upon inspection of these facilities would you convey your concurrence that there is no regulatory requirement for us to sign up a backup agreement with DWSD."

APRIL 25: Flint officially begins using Flint River as an interim primary water source. City press release touts that "officials from the City of Flint, the Genesee County Drain Commission, and the Michigan Department of Environmental Quality were all on hand to witness the historic event."

The press release notes that the city used the Flint River as a temporary source of drinking water at numerous points in the past and said, "Each temporary stint on local water proved three things to city employees and residents alike: That a transition to local river water could be done seamlessly, and that it was both sensible and safe for us to use our own water as a primary water source in Flint," Flint DPW Director Howard Croft states in the press release,

"The test results have shown that our water is not only safe, but of the high quality that Flint customers have come to expect. We are proud of that end result."

Flint Mayor Dayne Walling states: "It's regular, good, pure drinking water, and it's right in our backyard. This is the first step in the right direction for Flint, as we take this monumental step forward in controlling the future of our community's most precious resource."

MLive publishes photos showing Flint officials toasting the switch to the Flint River.

MAY 15: Email from Jennifer Crooks, U.S. EPA's Michigan drinking water liaison, to EPA colleagues Mindy Eisenberg, Thomas Poy and Tinka Hyde:

"A Mr. Lathan Jefferson has talked with Tinka, and also with me just now about his drinking water quality. Flint has just switched from Detroit water (from Lake Huron) to Flint River water within the past couple of weeks. Flint River quality is not great, but there is a surface water treatment plan producing water that is currently meeting SDWA standards, according to the MI DEQ district engineer, Mike Prysby. The water has more hardness, and pH and alkalinity may be different from Detroit water…. Mr. Jefferson said he and many people have rashes from the new water. He said his doctor says the rash is from the new drinking water, and I told him to have his doctor document this and he can bring to the attention of the MI DEQ, since lab analyses to date show that the drinking water is meeting all health-based standards. He has no interest in speaking with Mike Prysby; he doesn't trust anyone in MI government. He asked me for free drinking water lab analyses, which I was unable to provide. He only wants to speak with someone from EPA headquarters."

TRUTH SQUAD NOTE: Eisenberg was a high-ranking official at EPA in Washington, D.C.

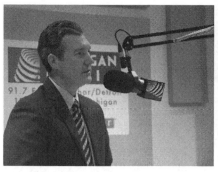 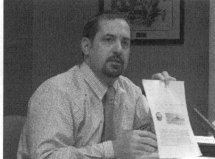

Left: Dayne Walling, Flint's mayor 2009-2016.

Photo courtesy of Michigan Radio

Right: Michael Glasgow, Flint water plant supervisor.

Photo Courtesy Steve Carmody/Michigan Radio

JUNE 2014: Complaints are now coming in regarding Flint drinking-water quality. Flint Mayor Dayne Walling and state-appointed emergency manager Darnell Earley keep telling residents the water is safe. "It's a quality, safe product," Walling is quoted in MLive.com. "I think people are wasting their precious money buying bottled water."

JULY 2014: Michigan Department of Environmental Quality begins the first six-month testing and monitoring of Flint water under the department's interpretation of the federal Lead and Copper rule.

> **TRUTH SQUAD ANALYSIS:** A wide range of documents, including a January 2016 order from the U.S. EPA, will eventually determine that the City of Flint and MDEQ did not anticipate or provide for corrosion control. As a result, the highly corrosive Flint River water in city water lines would cause hazardous lead to leach into city drinking water supplies and into the homes of Flint residents.

AUG. 15: Flint issues boil-water advisory after fecal coliform bacteria is found in the water. The city adds chlorine to treat.

SEPT. 5: Second boil-water advisory issued because of coliform bacteria.

OCT. 13: MLive.com reports: "General Motors said it will no longer use the river water at its engine plant because of fears it will cause corrosion" due to high chloride levels. GM instead buys Lake Huron water from Flint Township.

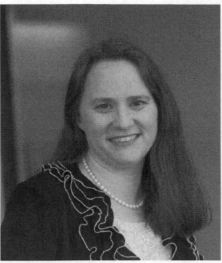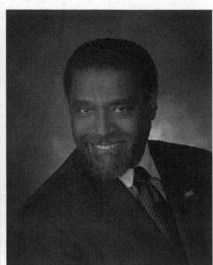

Left: Valerie Brader, deputy legal counsel to Gov. Rick Snyder.

Right: Darnell Earley, Flint Emergency Manager from October 2013 to January 2015.

Photos courtesy State of Michigan

OCT. 13: Email from DEQ's Prysby to colleagues Busch, Shekter Smith and others at MDEQ regarding an inquiry from Ron Fonger at the Flint Journal/MLive.com concerning GM getting off Flint water. Prysby notes that Flint water is elevated for chlorides but downplays the issue.

"Although not optimal" he said, it's "satisfactory…"

"I stressed the importance of not branding Flint's water as 'corrosive' from a public health standpoint simply because it does not meet a manufacturing facility's limit."

OCT. 14: In the final weeks of Gov. Rick Snyder's re-election campaign, two key Snyder aides raise alarms about Flint water. Snyder deputy legal counsel Valerie Brader emails Snyder's chief of staff, Dennis Muchmore, Communications Director Jarrod Agen, legal counsel Michael Gadola, and Deputy Chief of Staff Beth Clement. She urges them to ask the Flint emergency manager to consider moving Flint off the Flint River and back to the Detroit drinking water system "as an interim solution to both the quality, and now the financial, problems that the current solution is causing."

At the time, Flint residents had been complaining about the water for months, GM had stopped using it at an engine plant and Flint had issued boil water advisories. Meanwhile, there were growing concerns about the amount of chemicals Flint needed to use to treat the river water.

"I see this as an urgent matter to fix," Brader wrote.

The governor's chief legal counsel, Michael Gadola, responds 12 minutes later to everyone on Valerie Brader's original email string.

"… (T)o anyone who grew up in Flint as I did, the notion that I would be getting my drinking water from the Flint River is downright scary. Too bad the (emergency manager) didn't ask me what I thought, though I'm sure he heard it from plenty of others. My Mom is a City resident. Nice to know she's drinking water with elevated chlorine levels and fecal coliform. I agree with Valerie. They should try to get back on the Detroit system as a stopgap ASAP before this thing gets too far out of control."

"Can you guys step into this?" Muchmore asks state Treasury Department officials the same day.

OCT.: Snyder requests and receives a briefing paper from MDEQ. It blames September 2014 boil-water advisories due to e coli bacteria in Flint drinking water on several factors, notably the worn, 75-year-old cast iron water pipes subject to corrosion and bacteria. Lead concerns are not raised at this time.

OCT. 21: Susan Bohm of the Michigan Department of Health and Human Services alerted officials in Genesee County in an e-mail that there were concerns that Flint's water would be linked to an outbreak of Legionnaires' disease, a pneumonia that can be caused by inhaling water. Liane Shekter Smith, the head of the Office of Drinking Water and Municipal Assistance for the state Department of Environmental Quality, had contacted state health officials "a couple of times" to discuss the outbreak, the emails show. "She was concerned that an announcement was going to be made soon about the water as the source of the infection; I told her the Flint water was at this point just a hypothesis," Bohm wrote. (As reported by the Detroit Free Press in early 2016).

NOVEMBER: Dick Posthumus, senior adviser to the governor, asks Snyder in an email if he wants to support a bill to allow Flint to boost its income tax from 1 percent to 1.5 percent (a rate some other cities have). There is no clear response from Snyder in publicly released emails, but other emails show the idea has momentum in the administration. A December 2014 email from Snyder's deputy director of legislative affairs, Sally Durfee, to Executive Director to the Governor Allison Scott and Posthumus says such a bill would raise $6.5 million per year, has the support of the Flint emergency manager and the state Treasury Department. But, according to the email, State Rep. Jeff Farrington, R-Utica, said, "he would take up this bill over his dead body."

Erin Brockovich, the Los Angeles-based environmental activist, was one of the first to raise concerns about Flint's water to a national audience. Her Facebook post on Jan. 20, 2015, began "Dangerous Undrinkable Drinking Water."

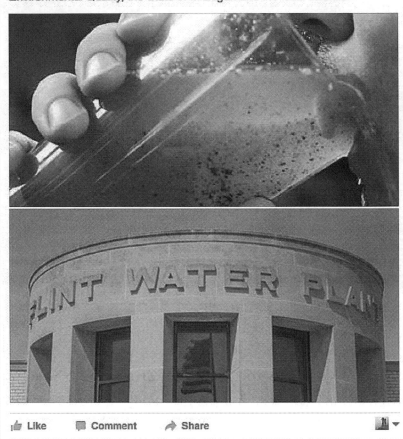

 Erin Brockovich ✓ added 2 new photos.
January 20, 2015 · 🌐

👍 **Like Page** ⌄

Dangerous Undrinkable Drinking Water

Flint, Michigan adds its name to the list of hundreds of cities, towns and community water systems that are failing. Bottomline, they have made many bad choices... and yet there are real solutions.

EXCUSES... EXCUSES... EXCUSES

Until the Safe Drinking Water Act is really enforced... Drinking Water if the United States will be equal to a third world country.

Today Mayor Dayne Walling says access to clean, safe, affordable water is a basic human right, and Governor Rick Snyder has the responsibility for helping to deliver it. Now is not the time for the blame game...Detroit has failed and Flint jumped ship. So much for local control... everyone is responsible from the top down: USEPA, Michigan Department of Environmental Quality, the State of Michigan and the local officials.

👍 Like   💬 Comment   ↪ Share

👍 3.5K

5,326 shares   693 comments

CHAPTER 4

JANUARY 2015

'A PR CRISIS WAITING TO EXPLODE'

PUBLIC OUTCRY GROWS.
OFFICIAL HAND-WRINGING INTENSIFIES - BEYOND PUBLIC VIEW.

Editor's summary: As Flint residents carry jugs of brown and smelly tap water into public meetings, environmental activist Erin Brockovich weighs in on Facebook in one of the first examples of nationwide concern over Flint's drinking water.

State water regulators see an uptick in lead in the city's drinking water, but the increase isn't high enough to spur action.

State and local officials begin a months-long and private dialogue about a Legionnaires' disease outbreak but don't take serious steps to confront the possibility that the drinking water may be a factor.

Flint's city manager declines a new opportunity to return to Detroit drinking water.

And a Snyder administration special projects manager, Ari Adler, issues a prescient email warning: "This is a public relations crisis… waiting to explode nationally."

> "IT WOULD BE UNUSUAL FOR WATER LEAVING THE PLANT TO HAVE COLOR LIKE PEOPLE ARE SEEING AT THEIR TAPS. GENERALLY THIS IS A DISTRIBUTION SYSTEM PROBLEM OR A PREMISE PLUMBING ISSUES. SINCE IT APPEARS WIDE-SPREAD, IT'S MOST LIKELY A DISTRIBUTION SYSTEM PROBLEM."
>
> — LIANE SHEKTER SMITH

TIMELINE: JANUARY 2015

By John Bebow
Bridge Magazine

2015

JAN. 1: MDEQ begins second six-month lead/copper monitoring period. The first testing period shows a 90th percentile reading of six parts per billion of lead in Flint's tap water.

> **TRUTH SQUAD ANALYSIS:** Lead is a potent human toxin and can cause lifelong harm to intelligence, and developmental problems, especially in children 5 and younger. With the federal "action level" for lead in drinking water at 15 parts per billion, MDEQ takes no action beyond beginning the second six-month monitoring period.

JAN. 2: "The city mails a notice to its customers saying it is in violation of the Safe Water Drinking Act due to elevated presence of trihalomethanes" – a byproduct of disinfecting the water, according to an MLive.com timeline published later in the year.

JAN. 7: An email from Richard Benzie to MDEQ colleagues Mike Prysby, Liane Shekter Smith and Stephen Busch discusses Benzie's impressions after talking about Flint issues with State Rep. Sheldon Neely, D-Flint, and other legislators:

"(T)hey indicated that based on the number of calls they are receiving and the tenor of the callers, there appears to be a significant (I think they used the word complete) loss of public confidence in the drinking water quality in Flint. Mike indicated that we would be working with the city to try to restore that confidence... Maybe there are some lessons to be learned from how the Lansing Board of Water and Light is trying to recover from the loss of public confidence as a result of their response to the ice storm a year ago."

JAN. 9: The University of Michigan – Flint finds lead in water in some campus drinking fountains. The Detroit Free Press reports this in January 2016.

JANUARY: Snyder administration emails show a growing awareness and concern about Flint water. Dick Posthumus writes on Jan. 22 that "we have two meetings coming up on this next week," including Snyder Director of Strategy John Walsh, top urban affairs aide Harvey Hollins and many others in the administration. "Later that day we are meeting with several people from Flint, including the EM, Mayor, and Senator Ananich."

JAN. 12: DWSD offers Flint's emergency manager a waiver of a $4 million reconnection fee to switch back to Detroit water.

JAN. 12: An email from Mike Prysby to numerous MDEQ colleagues discusses the provision of "alternative" drinking water supplies to a Flint office building housing state government workers:

".. given that this state building has high public traffic (Flint citizens); it was felt prudent to offer an alternative supply of drinking water to citizens entering the building."

Richard Benzie at MDEQ responds the same day:

"Why does 'public traffic' deserve a higher consideration than concern for state workers? How does that reasoning appear to state employees? A visitor may take one drink of water from this site in their lifetime. State workers (like any employees) may get half of the water they consume each day at their place of employment.

"Which group faces the greater health risk from drinking water in state-occupied premises?....How does this action by DTMB impact the answer when ODWMA district staff are asked by others in the media or from the general public about whether Flint residents should continue to consume Flint's drinking water with elevated disinfection by-products? No doubt it will make it more difficult from a perception standpoint for ODWMA staff."

The exchange followed a Jan. 7 advisory from the Michigan Department of Treasury, Management and Budget indicating the state is "in the process of providing a water cooler on each occupied floor, positioned near the water fountain, so you can choose which water to drink."

MDEQ's Shekter Smith sends Benzie's email to numerous DEQ colleagues on Jan. 12 and says: "The decision to provide bottled water when the public notice was not a 'do not drink' causes us some concern."

JAN. 20: Environmental activist Erin Brockovich weighs in on Facebook, an indication that Flint's water troubles are beginning to break into the national consciousness. MLive.com quotes her: "Now is not the time for the blame game....Detroit has failed and Flint jumped ship. So much for local control.... everyone is responsible from the top down: USEPA, Michigan Department of Environmental Quality, the state of Michigan, and the local officials."

JAN. 21: "Frustrated residents attend a meeting with scientists at City Hall, bringing with them jugs of discolored water – water they say tastes funny and smells terrible." (As reported by the Detroit Free Press.)

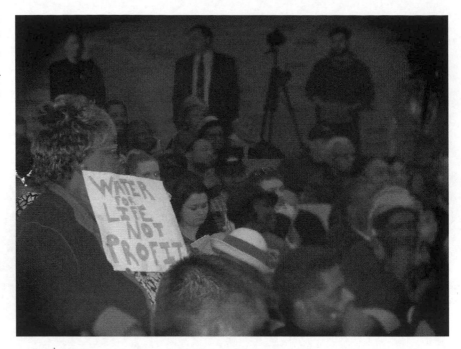

Residents jam a meeting inside Flint's city hall.

Photo courtesy of Michigan Radio

JAN. 21: An email from Liane Shekter Smith to MDEQ colleagues Stephen Busch, Mike Prysby, Richard Benzie, Maggie Datema, Sara Howes, Brad Wurfel, and Jim Sygo (the agency's deputy director):

"Our position has always been that we do not dictate which acceptable option(s) a water supply may choose. Our responsibility is to see that operations are managed properly, regulations are met, and safe water is delivered. For example, when Flint decided to leave Detroit and operate using the River, our role wasn't to tell them our opinion; only what steps would be necessary to make the switch."

TRUTH SQUAD ANALYSIS: What a manifesto for safeguarding public health! In the end, MDEQ would fail in all aspects of its duties that Shekter Smith mentioned. Despite concerns about Flint River quality raised as early as 2004 and as late as 2013, MDEQ allowed the Flint River switch to go forward, even as a Flint water treatment plan supervisor warned the plant wasn't ready. It's clear, too, that MDEQ failed to grasp the challenges in an old urban city with many lead service pipes of switching from mild Lake Huron-sourced water to highly corrosive Flint River water. The result: Flint children were poisoned, and two MDEQ employees and one Flint water plant employee would eventually face criminal charges for their official acts.

JAN. 23: Flint Mayor Dayne Walling spreads blame for the growing water crisis in a report published by MLive.com:

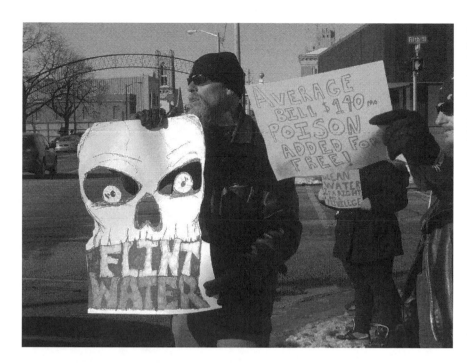

Protesters stand outside Flint's city hall, upset about the quality and cost of the city's water.

Photo courtesy of Michigan Radio

"Walling said the decision to use river water last year was made by emergency manager Darnell Earley, but the mayor said he was involved in the decision for the city to join the Karegnondi Water Authority in 2013. 'The governor and the (state) treasurer to their credit recognized it was important for the city's elected representatives to be included in the decision about the long-term source (of water) because we would be living with it,' he said. 'But once the decision was made in April 2013, it became an operational issue … and I wasn't directly involved.… I wasn't directly involved in the city's (decision) to use the Flint River as a source.… It's now clear that the challenge was underestimated.'

"Walling blamed the Detroit Water and Sewerage Department for terminating Flint's contract to purchase Lake Huron water while the KWA pipeline was under construction," said the Mlive.com account.

"'I do think it bears repeating that it was DWSD that terminated the contract with the city of Flint,' Walling said. 'DWSD put the city of Flint in a difficult position when they terminated that contract we had for decades and decades.… My goal had always been to have a cooperative relationship with DWSD but every opportunity that was looked at ended with a barrier.'"

JAN. 23: Snyder administration Special Projects Manager Ari Adler raises concerns about Flint with Communications Director Jarrod Agen: "This is a public relations crisis – because of a real or perceived problem is irrelevant – waiting to explode nationally. If Flint had been hit with a natural disaster that affected its water system, the state would be stepping in to provide bottled water or other assistance. What can we do given the current circumstances?"

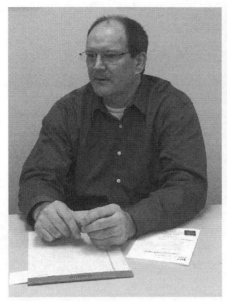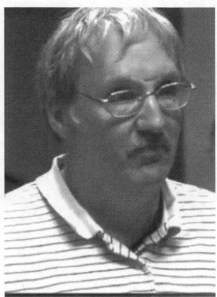

JAN. 27: Shannon Johnson, a Michigan Department of Health and Human Services epidemiologist, emails the Genesee County Health Department about the county's Legionnaires' outbreak.

"At this point, the priorities in the public health investigation are to determine the scope of the outbreak and to define as clearly as possible the characteristics of the cases of Legionnaire's disease …," she wrote, according to emails obtained by the Detroit Free Press. "A current map of the municipal water system needs to be obtained and cases' residences mapped in relation to the water system."

JAN. 29: Flint Emergency Manager Jerry Ambrose declines DWSD water-source reconnection.

JAN. 29: In response to a Bridge Magazine story about residents' complaints about Flint water, MDEQ Deputy Director Jim Sygo forwards the story to drinking water chief regulator Shekter Smith.

Sygo writes that he's never seen trihalomethane issues (one of the early water-safety violations in Flint) "cause such discoloration" in drinking water.

Shekter Smith responds: "I'm theorizing here, but most likely what they are seeing is a result of differing water chemistry. A change in water chemistry can sometimes cause more corrosive water to slough material off of pipes as opposed to depositing material or coating pipes in the distribution system. This may continue for a while until things stabilize.

"It would be unusual for water leaving the plant to have color like people are seeing at their taps. Generally this is a distribution system problem or a premise plumbing issues. Since it appears wide-spread, it's most likely a distribution system problem."

TRUTH SQUAD ANALYSIS: Shekter Smith's theories prove quite accurate. As an independent drinking water quality expert, Virginia Tech's Marc Edwards, later proves, corrosive Flint River water is breaking down Flint distribution lines. Shekter Smith is also correct that materials are sloughing off the Flint pipes. In fact, those materials include very harmful lead. In essence, Shekter Smith's private theories to an MDEQ colleague are consistent with the alarms about pipe corrosion and lead that EPA water expert Miguel Del Toral brings to MDEQ a month later. But for months more, MDEQ discounts Del Toral's warnings.

JAN. 30: The same week Bridge Magazine and other publications are reporting about public uprisings over Flint's discolored, smelly water, MDEQ Communications Director Brad Wurfel emails Snyder Deputy Press Secretary Dave Murray:

"I don't want my director (MDEQ's Dan Wyant) to say publicly that the water in Flint is safe until we get the results of some county health department epidemiological trace back work on 42 cases of Legionnaires disease in Genesee County since last May."

29 JANUARY 2015

CRINGE OVER TROUBLED WATER:

Flint's smelly dilemma

By Chastity Pratt Dawsey
Bridge Magazine

Editor's summary: Here, staff writer Dawsey takes readers into the home of Ineatha Waters, who has stopped drinking her tap water and explains why so many residents are fed up with what they perceive as the state's indifference to the obvious taste, smell and color issues with the their water. Residents started complaining about the water within a month of the city's switch to Flint River water. At the time this report was published, the lead issue hadn't come up, and media beyond the Flint Journal/MLive.com were only starting to take notice.

Ineatha Waters pays for water she does not drink.

She goes through about two cases of water a week because a notice sent to Flint residents this month left her frightened to drink what comes from her tap – even though the city has said it was safe to drink.

When she bathes, she adds a few drops of bleach, says a prayer and hopes that it and her immune system can fight off any harm – real or perceived – from contact with the city's water. The Flint River has been the source of the city's tap water since Flint ended its contract to buy water from the Detroit Water and Sewerage Department last April.

Officials say they are working to improve water quality as Flint transitions to a new water system in 2016.

"I feel like I'm living in a third-world country," said Waters, 45. "I want to have safe, clean water to drink like every other American should in the United States of America. The mayor has written a letter, but he's not in control of the city. We don't know where to go next for help. Who do we go to?"

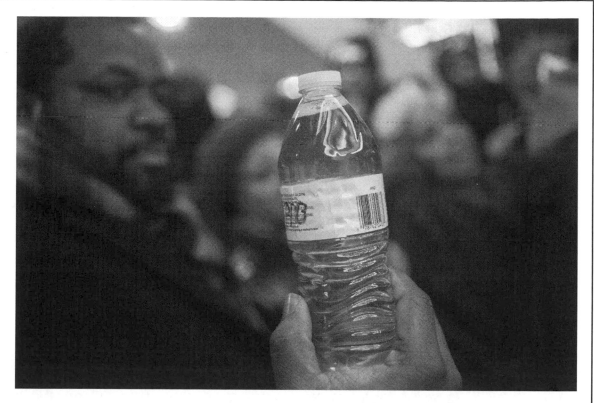

A Flint protester holds a plastic bottle of tainted water at a session in Lansing.

Photo courtesy of Jake May/Mlive.com

In response to residents' angst, Flint Mayor Dayne Walling recently wrote Gov. Rick Snyder asking for help. Walling wants the state to dip into resources earmarked for water improvements and distressed cities across Michigan to help Flint through its water debacle.

Frustrated residents say the state owes Flint as much, considering that a state-appointed emergency manager for the cash-short city made the decision to switch Flint's water source. The water Detroit pumped to Flint came from Lake Huron – cold and relatively free from impurities. By contrast, the Flint River is much more difficult to treat.

Walling's requests and the demands of frustrated Flint residents, if heeded, could have effects across the state.

"More than any other issue, water affects almost everything," said Eric Lupher, president of the Citizens Research Council of Michigan, a nonprofit, nonpartisan research group.

Walling and residents are looking to the right person for answers, Lupher said. In the line of accountability, Flint residents hold Gov. Rick Snyder responsible for the emergency manager's decisions because the people of Michigan voted for governor; they did not vote for emergency manager.

"On the issue of responsibility, there probably isn't any legal responsibility for the state," Lupher said, "but there certainly is a moral responsibility."

Low-quality, but safe?

Flint residents have thronged to public meetings and protests since the state Department of Environmental Quality reported last month that the city's drinking water exceeded federally permitted levels of trihalomethane, or TTHM, a byproduct of chlorine-treated water. Excess trihalomethane over many years can cause liver, kidney or central nervous system problems, and an increased risk of cancer, according to the U.S. Environmental Protection Agency.

The MDEQ's notice of excess TTHM indicated that problems existed almost from the start of Flint's switch to treating its river water last spring. In late August and early September, the city issued boil-water advisories because of bacterial contamination in city water.

City and state officials say that, despite high TTHM levels, the water, which residents say tastes, smells and looks bad, is safe to drink, though they've also noted that the most vulnerable residents (infants, the elderly and those with compromised immune systems) should seek medical advice before drinking the water.

In his Jan. 18 letter to the governor, Walling said "there is nothing more important in Flint right now" than fixing problems with the drinking water.

In an interview, Walling said he drinks the city-treated water, but understands why residents such as Waters does not. "The city is taking steps to improve the quality of the water, while steps are taken to ensure the safety," he said.

Government officials acknowledge that water quality is a problem, but say the excessive TTHM levels are neither an emergency nor public safety threat in the short term.

"The quality of the water does need improvement, but that is not to be confused with safety of the water," the city's online explainer about the water issue says.

Jill Thiare, spokesperson for the nonprofit Water Research Foundation based in Denver, echoed that finding, and noted, after reviewing the MDEQ notice to Flint residents, that "all (water) samples taken during the last sample date of the year, were at the lowest levels across all test sites, which may be an indicator of progress. The increased levels may have been caused by a temporary fluctuation in the water source."

LINGERING MISTRUST

Still, such comments don't satisfy residents who toted jugs and bottles of their discolored tap water to a public meeting last week and said they are planning more action. In the meantime, local stores are stocking up and reducing prices for bottled water, while local charities and businesses are giving it away to the poor.

If Walling has his way, the state will help underwrite Flint's water recovery while also taking steps to help the state's most vulnerable residents in the future. In his letter, Walling requested:

That the state approve Flint's request for $2 million in Distressed Cities grants: $1 million to pay for leak detection in the Flint water system and $1 million to shift to a more economical way of disposing of waste water byproducts.

Federal and state support for forgiving Flint's debt payments to the Drinking Water Revolving Fund.

Creating a drinking water emergency fund to help low income and vulnerable elderly citizens and families, much like agencies such as The Heat and Warmth Fund help needy people with utility bills. Flint has one of the nation's highest poverty rates.

That water testing dates be reported to all Michigan communities at least quarterly. Such reporting would be more frequent than the annual reporting required under federal law.

"We need the governor to respond," Walling said, referring to his letter. "But we're not waiting for others to realize that this is serious before we do what we can."

U.S. Rep. Dan Kildee, D-Flint, also said that the city's loan payments might need to be revisited. Michigan's Drinking Water Revolving Fund helps water suppliers meet the requirements of the Safe Drinking Water Act by offering low-interest loans.

A COSTLY PRECEDENT

Walling's suggestion that the state forgive a municipality's debt is a long shot because of the precedent it would set.

If the state took on Flint's loan payments, said Lupher of the Citizens Research Council, "a hundred units of government would be putting their hands up saying, 'Me next!'"

So far, Snyder's office has made no promises. In a statement, the state says it's working closely with Flint on water. "Flint residents deserve clean, safe water," the statement said.

State Sen. Jim Ananich, D-Flint, said he understands some of his poor constituents in Flint may fear the water but drink it because they can't afford bottled water. He won't drink it himself, though. The state, he said, must allay fears and expedite a solution, because the city is run by a state-appointed emergency manager.

"The state clearly broke the system – if you break it, you should have to buy it," Ananich said. "If that means debt forgiveness, technical or financial assistance, the state (appointed emergency manager) should not leave without fixing this."

PAYING THE PRICE

Flint's water woes started as a plan to cut the financially-troubled city's high cost for Detroit water.

Using the Flint River was seen as a temporary, cost-cutting alternative to continuing with Detroit water, while the city waits for the new Karegnondi Water Authority it joined in 2013 to be completed. Like Detroit, Karegnondi, made up primarily of Genesee County communities, is building a pipeline to Lake Huron.

Flint River water is more of a treatment challenge because of fluctuations in water temperature and other factors, such as agricultural and road salt pollution.

The city may have troubled waters, but the change is helping clear up the budget. Before and after the city left the Detroit water system, Flint raised water and sewerage rates. Last year, Flint customers paid $35 more per month in water and sewer fees than nearby municipalities.

As a result, a Flint city audit released Monday shows income jumped by $4.7 million raised mostly by a 25 percent increase in sewerage rates in 2013. Rates rose by an average 6 percent in 2014 and will increase by another 6 percent this year.

Rev. Byron Moore, a member of Concerned Pastors for Social Action, said higher water rates have made tempers boil.

"We're paying more for something that can be detrimental to you," Moore said. "People are scared….There's fear of long-lasting impact on health and the ecology. And anger over the lack of a democratic process. The emergency manager made this decision."

The city must file an evaluation report with updated water sample results by March 1, according to the notice from the MDEQ.

Flint's Emergency Manager Jerry Ambrose hopes by Feb. 9 to hire a consultant experienced in river water treatment.

In the meantime, Sue McCormick, director of the Detroit Water and Sewerage Department, earlier this month offered to let Flint rejoin its water system without paying a $4 million reconnection fee, at least until Flint's permanent system comes online. So far, Ambrose has rebuffed the offer.

In the meantime, Rev. Moore said the minister's group was planning a meeting to galvanize church congregations and the community's response to the state's perceived indifference.

"There are rumblings about a class-action suit," he said. "The very first time we get validation from the medical community that there was an illness – or God forbid a death – that can be attributed to this water, I cannot tell you how bad it's going to be.

"The dam is going to burst at that point."

How lead got into Flint's drinking water

INTAKE
Water is pumped from the Flint River into the water treatment plant

DISTRIBUTION
Treated water is pumped to homes, businesses, schools and other customers in Flint.

DISINFECTION
Chlorine is used to treat organic material in the water before distribution

FLINT WATER PLANT

SERVICE LINES

WATER MAINS
Contain little or no lead

SERVICE LINES
Pipes connecting water mains to homes or businesses can be made of lead or have lead solder on iron pipes.

BEFORE THE SWITCH - water from Detroit Water & Sewerage Dept.

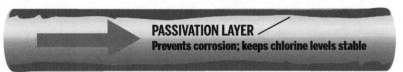

PASSIVATION LAYER
Prevents corrosion; keeps chlorine levels stable

After it drew water from Lake Huron, DWSD treated the water with a phosphate corrosion inhibitor. The treated water reacted with the lead to form a compound on the inner surface of the pipes called a passivation layer. The layer prevents the lead from leaching into the water.

AFTER THE SWITCH - water is drawn from the Flint River

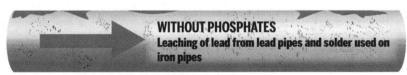

WITHOUT PHOSPHATES
Leaching of lead from lead pipes and solder used on iron pipes

Lack of a corrosion inhibitor combined with high chloride levels caused the passivation layer to flake off. This led to increased corrosion of Flint's leaded water pipes and lead solder connections, ultimately causing lead to leach into the water and flow from customers' taps.

Orthophosphates are often added to corrosive source water (high pH) such as the Flint River to prevent lead leaching. Flint switched from the DWSD water to the Flint River as its source in April 2014. On Oct. 16, 2015, Flint returned to Detroit's treated water. But rebuilding the passivation layer will take time.

CHAPTER 5

FEBRUARY 2015

'WOW! DID HE FIND THE LEAD!'

A FLINT MOTHER SPURS A SINGLE EPA REGULATOR TO INVESTIGATE

Editor's summary: As a state representative warns the governor's office that Flint is "on the verge of civil unrest," one Flint resident takes matters into her own hands. That one mother, Lee-Ann Walters, strikes a nerve deep within the U.S. Environmental Protection Agency and essentially launches a months-long debate between EPA and the Michigan Department of Environmental Quality about lead risk, corrosion control, and other problems with Flint drinking water.

In February, and for months more, key MDEQ water safety regulators cling to wrong-headed reasoning that Flint's water didn't require corrosion control and there was no serious lead danger.

MDEQ admits to little more than 'hiccups' with the city's water. But anxiety begins to rise high up in chain of command in the governor's office, with chief of staff Dennis Muchmore proclaiming, "After all, if GM refuses to use the water in their plant and our own agencies are warning people not to drink it... we look pretty stupid hiding behind some financial statement." But state inaction and denials will continue for months more.

> "I AM NOT AWARE OF ANY SOURCE WATER ASSESSMENT CONDUCTED FOR THE FLINT RIVER WATERSHED."
>
> — MIKE PRYSBY

TIMELINE: FEBRUARY 2015

By John Bebow
Bridge Magazine

2015

FEBRUARY: Key aides to Gov. Rick Snyder briefly pursue a switch from the Flint River back to Detroit drinking water for a second time. Snyder Chief of Staff Dennis Muchmore writes to colleagues:

"Since we're in charge we can hardly ignore the people of Flint," Muchmore tells state treasury and public affairs officials in an email not copied to Snyder. "After all, if GM refuses to use the water in their plant and our own agencies are warning people not to drink it... we look pretty stupid hiding behind some financial statement."

Both Treasury and Flint's Emergency Manager Jerry Ambrose say the switch would be costly and likely require a 30 percent increase in Flint's already high water rates.

FEB. 3: Snyder administration announces $2 million in infrastructure funding for Flint for water system enhancement through improved waste management, leak detection and pipe assessments.

FEB. 6: Email exchange between Liz Murphy, assistant to the emergency manager for the City of Flint and Mike Prysby of MDEQ:

Murphy: "Could you tell me which municipal systems in Michigan treat river water? I would like to get a contact for their labs to see if they could sample and test Flint's water production. This would be an independent source of testing, in addition to our own. I'm also wondering if MDEQ did a source water assessment of the Flint River? Could you direct me to where I might find that report?"

Prysby responds: "I am not aware of any source water assessment conducted for the Flint River watershed," but he adds that he wants to confirm his information.

Later the same day, Prysby emails Murphy a copy of the 2004 "Source Water Assessment Report for the City of Flint Water Supply – Flint River Emergency Intake."

> **TRUTH SQUAD ANALYSIS:** In email records, a colleague describes Mike Prysby as "our most knowledgeable staff member on the Flint and Genesee County water-supply issues.... He has knowledge of the history surrounding the var-

ious alternatives that have been considered and has access to the files where the various reports and studies are kept." Yet, Prysby is initially unaware of the 2004 report when asked for it. The report itself notes that the Flint River is a highly sensitive drinking water source susceptible to contamination. Prysby's failure to recall the report in January 2015 raises questions whether it was considered as state and local officials prepared to switch to Flint River water in April 2014.

EARLY FEBRUARY: Emails the governor's office wrote in preparation for announcing $2 million in state aid to Flint discuss a bipartisan briefing in Flint at which MDEQ Director Dan Wyant "will address ongoing efforts with his agency to test Flint water and explain why the city is facing some of its problems." There is no mention of lead concerns.

Flint Mayor Dayne Walling and State Sen. Jim Ananich, D-Flint, offer remarks and appreciation for state support. A briefing memo to Snyder and other administration officials makes clear that the water situation is growing more dire.

The memo cites several developments, including:

1) Many resident complaining about color, taste and smell of tap water since the switch to the Flint River;

2) U.S. Rep. Dan Kildee distributing bottled water;

3) Mayor Walling seeking state and federal assistance for $20 million in debt forgiveness to upgrade water treatment and calling for the governor to come to Flint (a telephone conference between the two then ensued and they pledged cooperation on solutions);

4) State Rep. Sheldon Neeley, D-Flint, sending a letter to the governor stating his constituents "are on the verge of civil unrest."

FEB. 10: The Detroit Free Press reports that Shurooq Hasan, a Genesee County Health Department epidemiologist, emailed an "outside expert" about the county's 47 Legionnaires' disease cases diagnosed in 2014, saying it almost quadrupled cases in 2013. "We have investigated a hospital as a potential source for the disease, but have expanded our investigation to include the city water supply."

FEBRUARY: MDEQ issues a backgrounder to Snyder on the Flint water situation:

"Following the formal approval of Flint into the KWA in 2012, DWSD sent Flint a letter saying their contract was thereby terminated (by early 2013). Genesee County has been using DWSD water without a contract since May 2014. But Flint took the letter to imply a water cutoff, and promptly turned to DEQ with a proposal to use Flint River (their historic backup system).

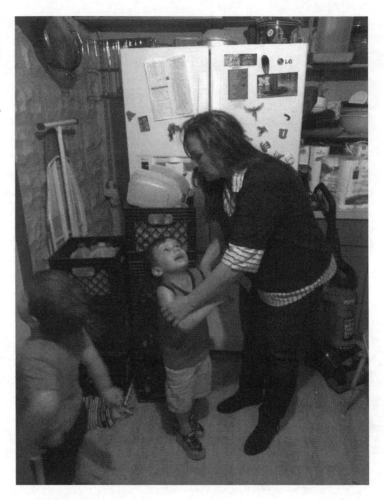

Lee-Anne Walters, the Flint mom with high lead levels in her home's tap water.

Photo courtesy of Michigan Radio

"This proposed shift was pitched primarily as a money saver. But it put the city in the business of water production, where they historically had been in the business of water transmission. DEQ approved the use of river as a source, based on the treatment plant's past performance as a standby facility and the improvements we outlined prior to a switchover."

MDEQ explains "hiccups" ranging from the boil-water advisories, to the side effects of potentially higher trihalomethanes (a potential health threat) because of chlorine treatment: "But it's not like an imminent threat to public health." MDEQ states, "The City of Flint has a tremendous need to address its water delivery system." Regarding the trihalomethanes issue, MDEQ says it's a key thing "to remember that, once the city connects to the new KWA system in 2016, this issue will fade into the rearview."

TRUTH SQUAD NOTE: This is an early example of a reoccurring theme in written communication between state and federal regulators: Flint is enduring issues from Flint River water only until KWA water comes online in late 2016. MDEQ briefing does not mention any lead concern.

FEB. 26: "The EPA discusses a resident's water sample testing results with DEQ (high levels of lead found in water)" A day later, MDEQ responds to an inquiry from EPA saying the Flint Water Treatment Plant has optimized corrosion control program.

TRUTH SQUAD ANALYSIS: This February 2015 MDEQ claim of optimized corrosion control is a complete fabrication, as additional documents soon make clear. Corrosion control is a common water treatment strategy to prevent corrosive water from corroding water lines and causing numerous problems, most notably the leaching of lead from old pipes into public water supplies.

The U.S. Environmental Protection Agency will conclude in a January 2016 order that MDEQ should have ordered and supervised optimized corrosion control as soon as Flint switched to Flint River water. Experts later found MDEQ's failure to insist on corrosion mitigation was a critical mistake in Flint's water crisis. In his flintwaterstudy.org blog, Virginia Tech professor and water expert Marc Edwards wrote in September 2015: "Effective July 1998, the federal Lead and Copper Rule (LCR) has required that all large public water systems maintain a program to control levels of lead in drinking water from corrosion. Moreover, the law also requires the City of Flint to have a state-approved plan, with enforceable regulatory limits for 'Water Quality Parameters' including pH, alkalinity and/or corrosion inhibitor dose measured in the water distribution system. MDEQ never required Flint to have a corrosion control program, nor did it set water quality parameters for the new Flint River source water."

FEB. 26: Email from Jennifer Crooks (EPA) to Stephen Busch and Mike Prysby (MDEQ) with copies to Thomas Poy and Miguel Del Toral (EPA):

"… (T)he main purpose of my emails is to alert you to the high lead levels reported to a citizen yesterday by Flint Water Dept. I have been discussing the water situation with Lee-Anne Walters since January, and she has been talking to Mike Glasgow at the plant about the black sediment in her water.… (Glasgow did test it to find that the iron levels were greater than his test would go.… But, because the iron levels were so high, he suggested testing for lead and copper. WOW!!! Did he find LEAD! 104 parts per billion.) She has two children under the age of three.… Big worries here."

"So, Steve, this goes back to what you and I were talking about yesterday. That the different chemistry water is leaching out contaminants from the insides of the biofilms inside the pipes. I think Lead is a good indication that other contaminants are also present in the tap water that obviously were not present in the compliance samples taken at the plant... And since Ms. Walters' drinking water is showing the high lead levels, her tap water would be a good place to start, I think."

Crooks further suggests, "Dept. of Community Health would want to get involved and look at this from an epidemiological perspective. (Walters) and her family are also exhibiting the rashes when exposed to the water, and her daughter's hair is falling out in clumps."

FEB. 26: Prysby responds to Crooks, with Shekter Smith and Brad Wurfel (MDEQ) copied, among others: "I recall Adam showing me a high lead/copper sample result (perhaps it was this one) ... as part of the city's routine lead-copper monitoring. Adam mentioned that all other samples were below the allowable limit ... and the city will not exceed the lead allowable limit. I will confirm this. The city, however, needs to take further action to help address Ms. Walters' concern. The type of plumbing needs to be identified and sample tap location within the premise plumbing. They should offer to re-sample for PB (lead) after flushing the tap to demonstrate that flushing the tap will reduce the lead concentration. The city also needs to provide other lead reduction strategies to Mrs. Walters."

FEB. 26: Email from Stephen Busch (MDEQ) to Liane Shekter Smith and Richard Benzie at MDEQ, in response to Crooks' email less than an hour earlier:

"As indicated by Mike and Adam the city is meeting 90th percentile. Not sure why region 5 [EPA] sees this one sample as such a big deal."

> **TRUTH SQUAD ANALYSIS:** Months later, after the Flint lead-in-water crisis had exploded, an EPA technical report would conclude that "this one sample," as Busch described it, was a very big deal, indeed: "As indicated by the results from the Walters' home and previous EPA work, the presence of lead pipes over many years has likely resulted in the accumulation of lead in the scales within non-lead pipes downstream of the lead pipe."

FEB. 27: MDEQ emails provide additional context to the Feb. 26 discussions between EPA water officials in Chicago and MDEQ water officials in Lansing about lead in Flint water. Miguel Del Toral, the EPA Region 5 Ground Water and Drinking Water Regulations Manager, emerges as the only key state or federal drinking water regulator to consistently sound the alarm about a potentially serious lead problem in Flint water.

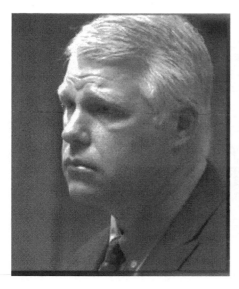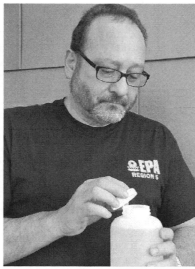

Left, MDEQ district supervisor Stephen Busch.

Photo courtesy of Michigan Radio

Right, Miguel Del Toral, EPA drinking supply regulator.

Photo courtesy of U.S. EPA

Details from the email from Del Toral to Mike Prysby (an engineer in the MDEQ Community Water Supply Program) and Jennifer Crooks (the Michigan program manager for the EPA Region 5 Ground Water and Drinking Water office):

"What I was saying is that where you find lead values that high, it is usually due to particulate lead."

"Particulate lead is released sporadically from lead service lines, leaded solder and leaded brass…. If systems are pre-flushing the tap the night before collection (of Lead and Copper Rule) compliance samples (MDEQ still provides these instructions to public water systems) this clears particulate lead out of the plumbing and biases the results low by eliminating the highest lead values. If systems are pre-flushing and still finding particulate lead, the amount of particulate lead in the system can be higher than what is being detected using these 'pre-flushed' first-draw samples. My point on that was that people are exposed to the particulate lead on a daily basis, but the particulate lead is being flushed away before collecting compliance samples, which provides false assurance to residents about the true lead levels in water."

"… I was wondering what (Flint's) optimized corrosion control treatment was. They are required to have optimized corrosion control treatment in place which is why I was asking what they were using."

TRUTH SQUAD ANALYSIS: Similarly, an email from Crooks to Prysby the day before could have caused alarm, but didn't appear to do so. By now, it is clear that Flint residents are concerned about discolored water, possibly due to high levels of iron caused by corrosion. Quoting Del Toral, Crooks reports to Prysby, "high levels of iron usually bring high levels of lead."

CHAPTER 6

MARCH 2015

'RUNNING OUT OF IDEAS'

LEAD CONCERNS QUIETLY MOUNT;
EMERGENCY MANAGER STICKS WITH RIVER.

Editor's summary: The Flint City Council prods Gov. Rick Snyder's Flint Emergency Manager Jerry Ambrose to switch back to Detroit water, but he stands firm – citing MDEQ assurances that the drinking water meets state and federal standards and switching would be costly for citizens. Independent consulting firm Veolia makes recommendations to improve drinking water aesthetics but doesn't mention lead. A second round of tests of Lee-Anne Walters' tap water shows lead levels about triple what were found in February. Genesee County health officials press concerns on Legionnaires' disease, leading to many exchanges of emails among city, county, state and federal agencies.

"THE OFT-REPEATED SUGGESTION THAT THE CITY SHOULD RETURN TO DWSD, EVEN FOR A SHORT PERIOD OF TIME, WOULD, IN MY JUDGMENT, HAVE EXTREMELY NEGATIVE FINANCIAL CONSEQUENCES TO THE WATER SYSTEM, AND CONSEQUENTLY TO RATE PAYERS."

— JERRY AMBROSE

TIMELINE: MARCH 2015

By John Bebow
Bridge Magazine

2015

MARCH 3: Flint Emergency Manager Jerry Ambrose sends a memo to the Michigan Department of Treasury stating that reconnecting to Detroit Water would be too costly. Key points:

"The current controversy surrounding the provision of water, and the path for resolution, has a potentially significant impact on the progress that is being made. I am satisfied that the water provided to Flint users today is within all MDEQ and EPA guidelines, as evidenced by the most recent water quality tests conducted by MDEQ. We have a continuing commitment to maintain water safety and to improve water quality, and have dedicated resources to assure this commitment will be made."

"The oft-repeated suggestion that the City should return to DWSD, even for a short period of time, would, in my judgment, have extremely negative financial consequences to the water system, and consequently to rate payers. By the most conservative estimates, such a move would increase costs by at least $12 million annually, with that amount achieved only by eliminating virtually all budgeted improvements in the system. For a system with Unrestricted Assets of only $740,745 … the only recourse within the City's control would be to increase revenues significantly. And, in my judgment, that would come from raising rates for water by 30 percent or more. Further, changing the source of the city's water would not necessarily change any of the aesthetics of the water, including odor and discoloration, since those appear to be directly related to the aging pipes and other infrastructure that carry water from the treatment facility to our customers…. At an average of $149 per month for water and sewer service for a residential user, the cost is extremely high in comparison to surrounding areas."

MARCH 3: Gov. Snyder's aides begin working on an idea to provide bottled water in Flint, although it will be more than half a year more before the administration fully acknowledges the depth of the Flint water crisis. Dennis Muchmore emails many other Snyder aides and Treasury officials:

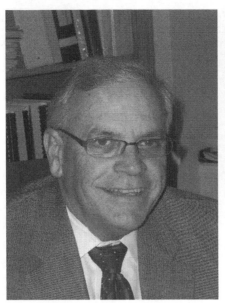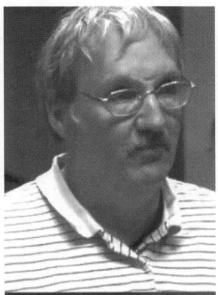

Left: Jerry Ambrose, Flint's Emergency Manager Jan.-April 2015.

Photo courtesy State of Michigan

Right: Mike Prysby, MDEQ district engineer.

Photo courtesy of Michigan Radio

"It's in the city's long term interest to make the KWA work and we can make the river water safe, but we need to work with the ministers this week to help them out. It's tough for everyday people to listen to financial issues and water mumbo jumbo when all they see is problems. You can't expect the ministers to hold the tide on this problem… If we procrastinate much longer in doing something direct we'll have real trouble."

In an email, Deputy State Treasurer Wayne Workman notes a significant contradiction:

"If this does happen, we need to figure out who should hand out the water. It should not be the City. It would undercut every point they are making." Presumably, because Flint and MDEQ officials still were saying Flint drinking water was safe to drink.

At the same time, the Snyder administration pursues water filters for Flint residents. Over the several months, the administration provides 1,500 donated filters to ministers for distribution in the city.

Months later, Snyder aide Harvey Hollins observes in an email to Muchmore a similarly sticky contradiction about the filters that Workman noted about the bottled water. Ministers passed out the filters because City Administrator Natasha Henderson "is the one who told me in late July that the city did not have any part in delivering the 1,500 filters that we secured because their position was that the water was safe to drink."

MARCH 10: Email from EPA's Jennifer Crooks to Busch, Prysby and Benzie at MDEQ. Crooks says she has been "inundated" with citizen email complaints referred to her from the White House about Flint water quality.

MARCH 10: Email from James Henry of the Genesee County Health Department to Flint Public Works Department director Howard Croft, MDEQ's Prysby, Mayor Walling, and many others. Henry raises serious concerns about his department's inability to get information from the City of the Flint for an ongoing investigation into the Legionnaires outbreak. "The increase in illnesses closely corresponds with the timeframe of the switch to Flint River water," he writes. "This is rather glaring information and it needs to be looked into now, prior to the warmer summer months when Legionella is at its peak and we are potentially faced with a crisis. This situation has been explicitly explained to MDEQ and many of the city's officials."

MARCH 11: Email from Benzie at MDEQ to colleagues Shekter Smith, Busch and Prysby about the inquiry from Genesee County. "As I see it, we need a plan of action fast," Benzie writes.

MARCH 11: Email from Busch to Prysby and Benzie: "… there is no evidence or confirmation of legionella coming directly from the Water Treatment Plant or in the community water supply distribution system at this time." And in numerous other emails numerous MDEQ officials, including Busch, say they've received no request to meet from Genesee County.

MARCH 12: Email from Benzie to Poy and Crooks at EPA. The mail is marked "high importance" and regards Genesee County Health Department concerns. "Please treat this information as confidential at this point as I am not sure when and who will bring this matter forward for public knowledge."

MARCH 12: Email from Shekter Smith to many MDEQ colleagues on the Legionnaires' issue: "While the change in source may have created water quality conditions that could provide additional organic nutrient source to support legionella growth, there is no evidence or confirmation of legionella coming directly from the Water Treatment Plant or in the community water supply distribution system at this time.… Seems like the next step is to communicate with DCH and possibly develop a joint strategy/response. Not sure who in Exec wants to take the lead on this. Steve Busch and Mike Prysby will continue to be lead for us on this. They have been in contact with DCH recently but only to learn that little progress has been made in identifying a source or sources for the illnesses."

MARCH 13: Email from Brad Wurfel, MDEQ communications director, to Harvey Hollins:

"In December, our staff became peripherally aware that the hospitals in Genesee were seeing an uptick in Legionnaires cases.… More than 40 cases reported since last April. That's a significant uptick – more than all the cases in the last five years or more combined.… County Health Departments are supposed to perform epidemiological tracebacks on all confirmed cases of this disease, locate the source and address it. Genesee County Halth has not done this work as of November. At a January meeting with area hospitals, MDCH, DEQ and others, [MDCH Director] Nick Lyon reportedly directed the county health folks, in terms not uncertain, to get this done as a priority. As I'm sitting here today, it still is not done to my knowledge.… My counterparts at MDCH informed me today that they cannot step in unless they are invited or unless the outbreak is multi-county. They've not been invited until, I believe, today. That may be in part because of the email string and letter I've enclosed here, which was unknown to MDCH until I shared it over to them.…

"Essentially, Jim Henry with Genesee County Health is putting up the flare. He's made the leap formally in his email that the uptick in cases is directly attributable to the river as a drinking water source – this is beyond irresponsible, given that it is his department that has failed to do the necessary traceback work to provide any conclusive evidence of where the outbreak is sourced, and it also flies in the face of the very thing a drinking water system is designed to do."

MARCH 13: Email from MDEQ's Busch to Jim Henry of Genesee health department, with copies to Mike Prysby and Lianne Shekter Smith at MDEQ: "The DEQ fully recognizes the public health threat posed to individuals that contract Legionnaires' disease with the understanding that the disease is not contracted by ingestion of potable water and therefore not regulated under the federal Safe Drinking Water Act.… (C)onclusions that legionella is coming from the public water system without the presentation of any substantiating evidence from your epidemiologic investigation appears premature and prejudice toward that end… It is highly unlikely that legionella would be present in treated water coming from the City of Flint water treatment plant.… Our office agrees that water main breaks, water leaks, and system repairs are possible vectors for legionella to enter the public water system. These should be investigated as part of your epidemiology."

MARCH 13: MDEQ Communications Director Brad Wurfel once again clues in the governor's top two spokespeople on the Legionnaires' issue and urges action:

"Political flank cover out of the City of Flint today regarding the spike in Legionnaires cases. See enclosed. Also, area ministers put a shot over the bow last night … with a call for Snyder to declare state of emergency there and somehow 'fix' the water situation. It may be very advantageous to get Treasury, Gov's office, DCH, DEQ, and Flint EM around a table Monday to do the following:

1. Update on what the city is doing

2. Update on what County Health Department is working on

3. Discussion of what we might all do next

4. Coordination of communication/messages.

"Did not want to reach out to Dennis without your approval/support. Please advise."

TRUTH SQUAD NOTE: The Legionnaires' issue doesn't become public until the governor announces it nine months later.

MARCH: Engineering firm Veolia makes recommendations to improve Flint River water, including revisions in chemical treatment. Regarding corrosion control, the firm suggests adding a polyphosphate chemical to help deal with discolored drinking water. The report says nothing about lead. Veolia estimated total cost to implement its recommendations at $4 million or less.

MARCH 16: Snyder Communications Director Jarrod Agen gets an email about the Legionnaires' disease. MDEQ Communications Director Brad Wurfel copies Snyder Communications Director Jarrod Agen on a three-day old message Wurfel first wrote to Snyder's urban affairs aide Harvey Hollins and MDEQ Director Dan Wyant about the Legionnaires' concerns. "In December, our staff became peripherally aware that hospitals in Genesee were seeing an uptick in Legionnaires cases," Wurfel writes.

TRUTH SQUAD ANALYSIS: Nine months later, in January 2016, Snyder publicly announces the Legionnaires' outbreak and tells the public nine people have died from it. The governor says that he hadn't personally heard about the problem until days before. (Agen told reporters in February 2016 that he did not open the email at the time.)

MARCH 17: MDEQ's Busch emails Flint's DPW director Howard Croft. Key point on Legionnaires' concerns: "Conduct routine monitoring for legionella bacteria at the water treatment plant tap and at locations within the distribution system. Note: sample locations must take water directly off the main and not be from premise plumbing systems. Distribution locations could include storage tank inlets or pumping stations. Monitoring at the WTP plant tap would demonstrate removal of any legionella present in raw source water. A private laboratory that specializes in water sample analysis for legionella would need to be used."

MARCH 18: Email from EPA's Jennifer Crooks to Busch, Prysby, Benzie at MDEQ and Poy and Del Toral at EPA regarding lead testing follow up with Lee-Anne Walters: "I just received a call from Lee-Anne Walters' home in Flint. She had her water tested again – this time the lead levels came back at 397 parts per billion. I will ask her to fax me the official lab results she has. Are you aware if the City flushed her system after the last test? Any thoughts on how to respond to her? I'm running out of ideas."

MARCH 19: Email from Henry at Genesee's health department to MDEQ's Busch about Legionnaires':

"There have not been any conclusions regarding the source of the illnesses. Our team is gathering information and we suspect there may be several sources. It has been made clear that the Flint municipal water system is in compliance with the Safe Water Drinking Act. It seems reasonable that your office would be involved regardless if a potential health risk from municipal water is related to consumption, inhalation or dermal exposure. Perhaps the legislation should be revisited to better address risks….

"(W)e had communications with your office in October 2014, regarding Legionella, but I also had three telephone conversations with Mr. Michael Prysby, from your office between January 21, 2015 and January 23, 2015. These conversations occurred around the same time that your office participated with the TTHM presentation in Flint. I 'explicitly explained' the details of the Legionella concerns and the possible associations with the Flint municipal water system and I specifically requested to meet with your office for further discussions. Mr. Prysby informed me that the concerns were discussed with you. I was informed there was no reason to meet because the municipal water system is in compliance with the Safe Water Drinking Act." The Genesee County Health Department "has been working closely with MDCH and has consulted with the (Centers for Disease Control) on several occasions regarding the epidemiological investigation. Also, we have been working with Legionella and municipal water experts, and recently with the USEPA. Based upon these discussions we have been informed that it is likely that a small amount of Legionella will survive the water treatment process at the plant and enter into the distribution system."

MARCH 23-24: The Flint City Council votes 7-1 to recommend ending Flint River use and return to Detroit water service. Flint Emergency Manager Jerry Ambrose declares the vote "incomprehensible," as reported by MLive.com: "'Flint water today is safe by all (U.S. Environmental Protection Agency) and (Michigan Department of Environmental Quality) standards, and the city is working daily to improve its quality,' Ambrose's statement says. DWSD 'users also pay some of the highest rates in the state because of the decreased numbers of users and the age of the system.... It is incomprehensible to me that (seven) members of the Flint City Council would want to send more than $12 million a year to the system serving Southeast Michigan, even if Flint rate payers could afford it. (Lake Huron) water from Detroit is no safer than water from Flint.'"

MARCH 30: MDEQ notifies the Flint Water Treatment Plant of the first six-month lead copper monitoring period showing 90th percentile lead results at 6 parts per billion.

MARCH 31: Email from EPA's Crooks to Prysby, Busch and Shekter Smith, all at MDEQ. Others at MDEQ and EPA are copied. Crooks indicates that Darren Lytle, Acting Chief of the Treatment Technology Evaluation Branch of the EPA in Cincinnati, was asked to consult Legionella. "Darren said anytime there is a treatment change, issues arise with the drinking water quality. Thus, what does this do to the transport of organisms like Legionella? Does this cause organisms to desorb and go into solution? The changes in water chemistry change these organisms electrostatically, and the biofilms with the distribution system pipe are disrupted and de-stabilized. Thus, different contaminants can be released. So maybe this isn't happening in people's homes; but it is happening in the distribution system pipes."

CHAPTER 7

APRIL-JUNE 2015

'I'M WORRIED THE WHOLE TOWN MAY HAVE MUCH HIGHER LEAD LEVELS'

A LONE EPA WATER SAFETY REGULATOR ACCELERATES HIS CRUSADE.

Editor's summary: On the one-year anniversary of the switch to Flint River for the city's drinking water, MDEQ makes a big admission. It isn't using any corrosion control as part of its treatment for the highly corrosive Flint River source water. EPA's Miguel Del Toral presses his case that without corrosion control, the water Flint River-sourced water is likely causing lead to leach from old pipes in the city into the water and out the taps of citizens. But it also is clear from emails that MDEQ's drinking water regulators are digging in with a legalistic – and ultimately wrong – interpretation of what they are required to mandate the Flint water treatment plant operators to do.

EMAIL FROM PAT COOK, A WATER TREATMENT SPECIALIST IN THE MDEQ COMMUNITY DRINKING WATER UNIT IN LANSING TO HIS COLLEAGUE PRYSBY: "WHAT IS FLINT DOING NOW (POST DETROIT) FOR CORROSION CONTROL TREATMENT."

PRYSBY'S RESPONSE: "AS WE DISCUSSED, FLINT IS NOT PRACTICING CORROSION CONTROL TREATMENT."

Walters gets good and bad news: Her home's lead levels dropped dramatically after a long lead city service line was removed but one of her children is showing signs of lead poisoning. In late June, Del Toral writes an 8-page memo to his boss that raises his strongest alarms yet about lead in Flint's water and MDEQ's resistance to deal with his concerns. He gives a copy of his memo to Lee-Anne Walters, whose home provided much of the evidence in his report. Walters, in turn, shares the memo with a reporter.

TIMELINE: APRIL – JUNE 2015

By John Bebow
Bridge Magazine

2015

APRIL 24: Two months after telling EPA that Flint had optimized corrosion control in place, MDEQ now tells EPA that no corrosion control is in place. The March 2015 Veolia engineering report also recommended corrosion control. The issue is discussed in MDEQ emails:

Email from Pat Cook, a water treatment specialist in the MDEQ Community Drinking Water Unit in Lansing to his colleague Prysby: "What is Flint doing now (post Detroit) for corrosion control treatment."

Prysby's response: "As we discussed, Flint is not practicing corrosion control treatment."

From MDEQ's Busch to colleagues Prysby and Cook: "… (T)here are no additional requirements for the City of Flint based on the levels of lead and copper in the current source water and the results of the lead and copper distribution monitoring….I believe this condition has been met."

Cook back to Busch: "I agree. I'll forward this to Miguel (Del Toral at EPA). However, don't be surprised if you get a call from him disagreeing with our position."

Prysby back to Cook: "You are correct. I received a call from Miguel regarding his concerns with the lead/copper sampling procedure from lead services and how he believes it is skewing down the lead level results from sites with lead services."

> **TRUTH SQUAD ANALYSIS:** At this point, at least three MDEQ drinking water specialists are fully aware of Del Toral's concerns about lead in Flint water, questions about the state's pre-flushing procedure for accurately measuring lead content and the need for corrosion control. These email records show MDEQ takes no action. Multiple MDEQ regulators discount Del Toral's concerns. MDEQ begin a months-long, legalistic interpretation that no additional corrosion control or anti-lead strategies are required under the law in the Flint drinking water system.

A close-up of the first lead service line removed in Flint on March 3, 2016. Brian Damon, a foreman for Waldorf & Sons Excavating, displays the pipe after his crew spent hours digging.

Photo by Jake May/MLive.com

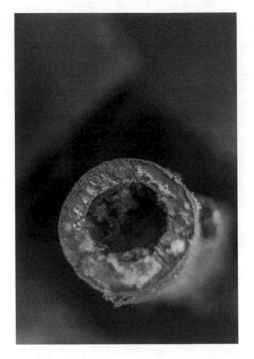

LATE APRIL: Del Toral issues a memo to MDEQ staff: "I wanted to follow up on this because Flint has essentially not been using any corrosion control treatment since April 30, 2014, and they have (lead service lines). Given the very high lead levels found at one home and the pre-flushing happening in Flint, I'm worried that the whole town may have much higher lead levels than the compliance results indicated, since they are using pre-flushing ahead of their compliance sampling."

APRIL 27: In an email, Laurel Garrison of the U.S. Centers for Disease Control and Prevention expresses concerns to Genesee County health officials about the county's Legionnaires' disease outbreak, as well as concern about the responses to the problem, according to the Detroit Free Press. "We are very concerned about this Legionnaires' disease outbreak," she wrote. "It's very large, one of the largest we know of in the past decade, and community-wide, and in our opinion and experience it needs a comprehensive investigation." Garrison's email suggested city and state officials allegedly were not supplying information the county needed for its investigation.

APRIL 27: MDEQ's Busch emails colleague Pat Cook regarding the EPA's Del Toral: "If he continues to persist, we may need Liane or Director Wyant to make a call to EPA to help address his over-reaches." Cook responds: "Hi Steve – I agree, the constant second guessing of how we interpret and implement our rules is getting tiresome.... Any ways, when you have a minute please give me a call so we can figure out how to respond to Miguel."

MAY 1: DEQ's Pat Cook sends email to Del Toral, with copies to Del Toral's EPA colleagues Jennifer Crooks and Thomas Poy and DEQ's Richard Benzie and Stephen Busch.

"The rules you stated below allow large systems to be considered having optimal corrosion control if they have data from two consecutive 6 month monitoring periods that meet specific criteria. (MDEQ's drinking water staff) has not made a formal decision as to whether or not the City of Flint meets the exemption criteria or will be required to do a corrosion control study since Flint has only completed one round of 6-month monitoring. The City of Flint's second round of monitoring will be completed by June 30, 2015, and we will make a formal decision at that time."

"As Flint will be switching raw water sources in just over one year from now, raw water quality will be completely different than what they currently use. Requiring a study at the current time will be of little to no value in the long term control of these chronic contaminants."

"Finally, the City of Flint's sampling protocols for lead and copper monitoring comply with all current state and federal requirements. Any required modifications will be implemented at a time when such future regulatory requirements take effect."

> **TRUTH SQUAD ANALYSIS:** By this point, at least four technical MDEQ drinking water staff members (Cook, Busch, Prysby, and Benzie), are in some way involved in the MDEQ's reasoning that no further corrosion control to stop lead leaching is required in Flint. They have reached this conclusion and ignored Del Toral's warnings. Meanwhile, at least two EPA drinking water officials (Poy and Crooks) are made aware of MDEQ's position. And there's evidence in Cook's emails that regulators are willing to endure the Flint River's quality issues, regardless of risks, until the Karegnondi Water Authority comes online in late 2016.

MAY 11: Jon Allan, director of the Michigan Office of the Great Lakes, emails Liane Shekter Smith at MDEQ to get her reactions to proposed language in a report and recommendations Allan is preparing.

"By 2020, 98 percent of population served by community water systems is provided drinking water that meets all health-based standards…. By 2020, 90 percent of the non-community water systems provide drinking water that meets all health-based standards."

MDEQ Water Resources Division Chief William Creal responds same day, as he, too, has been copied on Allan's proposal: "I think you are nuts if you go with a goal less than 100 percent for (drinking water) compliance in the strategy. How many Flints to you intend to allow???"

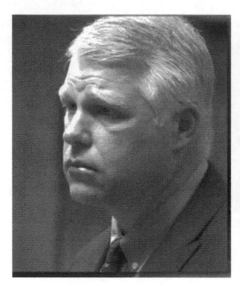
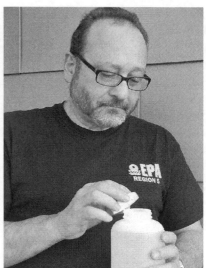

Left: Stephen Busch, MDEQ district supervisor.

Photo courtesy of Michigan Radio

Right: Miguel Del Toral, EPA drinking supply regulator.

Photo courtesy of U.S. EPA

Shekter Smith responds a day later, with a completely different reaction: "The balance here is between what is realistic and what is ideal. Of course, everyone wants 100 percent compliance. The reality, however, is that it's impossible. It's not that we 'allow' a Flint to occur; circumstances happen. Water mains break, systems lose pressure, bacteria gets into the system, regulations change and systems that were in compliance no longer are, etc. Do we want to put a goal in black and white that cannot be met but sounds good? Or do we want to establish a goal that challenges us but can actually be accomplished? Perhaps there's a middle ground?"

TRUTH SQUAD QUESTION TO READERS: Do you want a "middle ground" on the safety of drinking water for your family?

MAY 28: New samples show improved water quality at a residence on Browning Avenue in Flint. This is the home that sparked Del Toral's concerns as first experessed in February to MDEQ. Lead levels are improved after a city water main is replaced. But there's damage. Mother Lee-Anne Walters eventually sees evidence of lead poisoning in her child.

JUNE: A federal lawsuit asks a judge to order Flint to order a reconnection to the Detroit water system. The judge denies the request and the suit is later dismissed, MLive.com reported in a timeline.

JUNE 4: MDHHS sends a "Final Legionellosis outbreak report" to the Genesee County Health Department and discusses the report with the U.S. Centers for Disease Control and Prevention. The report confirms 45 cases of the disease and says more than half of the patients had a "healthcare facility exposure" shortly before developing the illness. Others were exposed to Flint water in their homes – others were not.

JUNE 8: Jim Collins of the MDHHS chastises Genesee health officials for communicating with the U.S. Centers for Disease Control and Prevention about investigating the Legionnaires' outbreak without getting state approval, according to emails obtained by the Detroit Free Press. "I believe that CDC is in agreement that their involvement really should be at the request of the state, rather than the local health department," Collins wrote.

JUNE 24: EPA's Del Toral sounds his loudest alarm to date in an eight-page memo to his supervisor, Thomas Poy. His key points:

The Flint water system has no corrosion control. "Recent drinking water sample results indicate the presence of high lead results in the drinking water, which is to be expected in a public water system that is not providing corrosion control treatment. The lack of any mitigating treatment for lead is of serious concern for residents that live in homes with lead service lines or partial lead service lines, which are common throughout the City of Flint."

Flint's use of ferric chloride to treat organic matter in Flint River water is likely to accelerate corrosion of leaded water pipes and exacerbate the lead problem.

Flint should have continued corrosion control as soon as it switched from Detroit to Flint River water. "In the absence of any corrosion control treatment, lead levels in drinking water can be expected to increase."

MDEQ-allowed sampling procedures for Flint water officials are masking high lead levels in the water. "The practice of pre-flushing before collecting compliance samples has been shown to result in the minimization of lead capture and significant underestimation of lead levels in the drinking water. Although this practice is not specifically prohibited by the LCR, it negates the intent of the rule to collect compliance samples under 'worst case' conditions which is necessary for statistical validity given the small number of samples collected for lead and copper under the LCR. This is a serious concern as the compliance sampling results which are reported by the City of Flint to residents could provide a false sense of security to the residents of Flint regarding lead levels in the water and may result in residents not taking necessary precautions to protect their families from lead in the drinking water." MDEQ was advised of EPA's pre-flushing concerns and responded that the federal lead and copper rule doesn't prohibit it. MDEQ recommends that all Michigan public water systems pre-flush before taking samples.

Samples from the home of Lee-Anne Walters found lead levels as high as 397 parts per billion. Upon investigation, the extreme levels were linked to an old and distant city of Flint lead service line, which was subsequently replaced. Walters' lead water levels subsequently decreased.

Technical reports regarding Flint's water quality to date hadn't addressed lead issues. A report by Lockwood, Andrews and Newman dealt with high trihalomethanes in city water. The Veolia report from March focused mainly on trihalomethane and other operational issues (though it also discussed corrosion control).

Corrosion control experts at EPA in Cincinnati should get involved in Flint.

A full EPA review of MDEQ enforcement in Flint is needed to determine whether the "state has abused its discretion."

JUNE 30: EPA Region 5 Water Division Director Tinka Hyde makes Liane Shekter Smith, the MDEQ Office of Drinking Water and Municipal Assistance chief, aware of Del Toral's memo but doesn't share it. Hyde writes in an email:

"Once Miguel addresses our comments, we will provide you a copy of that report. In most cases, an internal EPA memo would not be distributed outside the agency, but given his interaction with the homeowner for one of the sampling locations, Miguel has shared a copy of the draft interim report as a courtesy with this Flint resident. Based on Miguel's initial analysis, elevated lead levels were found at this residence. In addition, it appears that the source of the lead may be from outside the home (note: plumbing in the home is largely plastic.) Please know that Region 5 management is still being briefed on the lead issues in Flint and we look forward to the opportunity to discuss the situation with you in more detail so we can better characterize what MDEQ is already doing in Flint and how public health protection can best be provided to the citizens of Flint."

Shekter Smith responds in a July 1 email: "We'll need to discuss this after we receive Miguel's report, but before the call later this month."

> **TRUTH SQUAD ANALYSIS:** We can now add two senior water-quality officials at EPA in Chicago and MDEQ in Lansing to the growing list of state and federal regulators aware that Del Toral is sounding a loud alarm about potential lead problems in Flint water. Shekter Smith doesn't get the benefit of the full context of Del Toral's report, as EPA doesn't share. But Shekter Smith's response to Hyde's emails doesn't suggest any great concern. Indeed, emails that subsequently became public made clear that no one at EPA or MDEQ fully shared Del Toral's sense of urgency, or had – as of June 30 – any plan to address Del Toral's concerns. EPA ultimately and officially shares a redacted and final copy of Del Toral's report with MDEQ four months later.

CHAPTER 8

JULY 2015

'THEY ARE BASICALLY GETTING BLOWN OFF BY US'

PRESSURE RISES OVER LEAD IN THE WATER, BUT GOVERNMENT WHIFFS ON ACTION

Editor's summary: ACLU investigative reporter Curt Guyette makes lead concerns public by publishing the damning conclusions of EPA's Miguel Del Toral. In response to the media pressure, EPA's top administrator in the Great Lakes region tells Flint's mayor that Del Toral's conclusions should not have been released outside the agency and apologizes "for the manner in which this matter was handled."

A state government spokesman declares, "Anyone who is concerned about lead in the drinking water in Flint can relax."

The governor's chief of staff privately urges a fresh review by two state agencies and writes that Flint is "basically getting blown off by us." But one agency – the Michigan Department of Environmental Quality – hews to its longstanding line that Flint's water doesn't need corrosion control and meets drinking water standards even as lead levels are clearly rising.

Under MDEQ supervision, lead sampling tests of Flint's water actually decrease and testing procedures are flawed. The other agency – the Michigan Department of Health and Human Services – analyzes its data on lead in human bloodstreams and wrongly concludes there's no lead problem related to the drinking water in Flint – an assertion they will be forced to retract weeks later.

> **"THE DEQ HAS NOT SEEN A CHANGE IN THE CITY'S COMPLIANCE WITH THE LEAD RULE SINCE SWITCHING TO THE FLINT RIVER SOURCE."**
>
> **— LINDA DYKEMA**

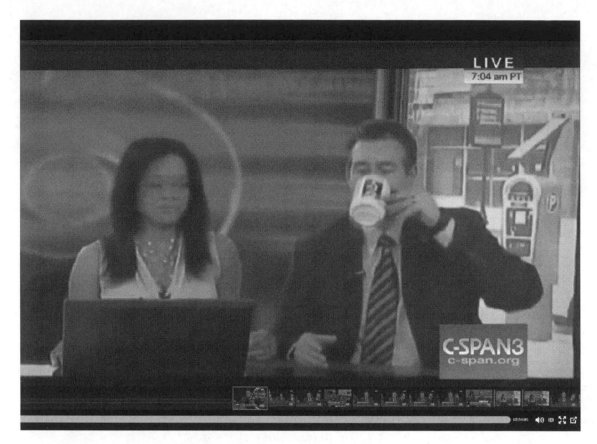

Feeling sufficiently reassured about Flint's water safety, city Mayor Dayne Walling appeared on WNEM and took an on-camera drink of water. A week before, EPA Region 5 Administrator Susan Hedman told him that an EPA draft report raising concerns about Flint water shouldn't have been released. The video was entered into evidence at a March 15, 2016, congressional committee meeting.

TIMELINE: JULY 2015

By John Bebow
Bridge Magazine

2015

JULY 1: EPA's Jennifer Crooks sends an email to 18 people to present draft notes of what appears to be a "semi-annual" regulatory overview call on June 10, 2015, between EPA and MDEQ drinking-water staff. Not all of the recipients' affiliations are noted in Crooks' emails. But recipients include Shekter Smith, Benzie, Prysby, Cook and Busch (all from MDEQ) as well as Poy and Del Toral from EPA. Several other MDEQ staffers not previously included in the now-public email correspondence regarding Flint are also copied. They include: Carrie Monosmith, supervisor of the MDEQ Drinking Water and Municipal Assistance Environmental Health Section; and Dana DeBruyn, Dan Dettweiler and Kevin Holdwick of MDEQ's Noncommunity and Private Drinking Water Supplies Unit. The draft notes of the June 10 conference call detail covered topics, with emphasis on Flint. Key points, as written by Crooks, include:

"Our discussions with MDEQ indicate that no phosphates/corrosion control has been added to the system since April 2014 when the source of drinking water changed to the Flint River. We understand that the City is just finishing up its second set of 6-month initial monitoring for lead where the results will probably warrant a Corrosion Control Study to be conducted. Since Flint has lead service lines, we understand some citizen-requested lead sampling is exceeding the Action Level, and the source of drinking water will be changing again in 2016, so to start a Corrosion Control Study now doesn't make sense."

"Miguel (Del Toral) believes that lead levels in Flint are being affected by the lack of corrosion control being conducted by the City.... Steve Busch stated that in the Lead sampling pool, almost all of the lead sample sites are lead service lines and the State is not seeing large increases in lead levels at the tap."

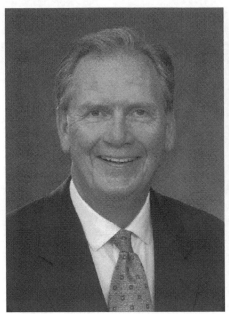 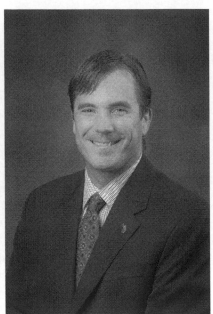

Left, Dennis Muchmore, Gov. Rick Snyder's chief of staff.

Right, Nick Lyon, director, Michigan Department of Health and Human Services.

Photos courtesy State of Michigan

TRUTH SQUAD NOTE: The Michigan Auditor General, outside researchers and reporters soon debunk the assertion that all lead sample sites in Flint have lead service lines.

Del Toral wants EPA technical experts to help in Flint, but Busch says the city is following federal lead copper rule already. Del Toral said that's not good enough, but there's no evidence in the email record that others at the meeting backed him up. Crooks summary says: "Miguel's point is that since the LCR was promulgated 20+ years ago, that research and different situations, like Washington, D.C., have educated scientists, experts, and regulators that the existing requirements in the LCR may not be as protective as previously thought. Thus, he can only make recommendations as to how to revise sampling protocols. And Miguel acknowledges that it may be another year before these regulation changes are promulgated."

TRUTH SQUAD ANALYSIS: In January 2016, EPA issued its well-publicized "Emergency Order" regarding Flint Water. The order accused Michigan of "a lack of transparency" and stated "During May and June 2015, EPA Region 5 staff at all levels expressed concern to MDEQ and the City about increasing concentrations of lead in Flint drinking water and conveyed their concern about lack of corrosion control and recommended that the expertise of EPA's Office of Research and Development should be used to avoid further water quality problems moving forward."

The truth is that only one EPA official, Del Toral, conveyed urgent concern. The portion of the January 2016 EPA order quoted above lacks in any transparency. The above draft notes of the June 10 EPA/MDEQ meeting makes Del Toral's concerns clear. But there is no sense in this record that anyone else at the state or federal agencies share that degree of concern or urgency. EPA issues no orders to MDEQ. MDEQ stands firm in its defense of its interpretation of the Lead and Copper Rule. And the meeting notes, written by an EPA supervisor, imply agreement with the MDEQ contention that "the source of drinking water will be changing again in 2016, so to start a Corrosion Control Study now doesn't make sense."

Again, there's a suggestion of regulators at both the state and federal levels playing a waiting game to endure the Flint River situation until the Karegnondi Water Authority comes online in 2016.

JULY 1: EPA Region 5 Director Susan Hedman significantly downplays – and even apologizes for – Del Toral's June 24 memo in an email to Flint Mayor Dayne Walling. Walling wrote to Hedman on June 30, requesting a copy of Del Toral's memo. Walling heard about the memo from Curt Guyette, a reporter at the Michigan branch of the American Civil Liberties Union. Guyette would soon publicly break the story of Del Toral's memo and his grave concerns about the safety of the Flint drinking water. Hedman writes to Walling:

"The EPA staffer mentioned in your email prepared a draft report and apparently shared it with the citizen as a courtesy because her name and children's blood lead levels were mentioned in the report before sending the draft report up the EPA management chain for review…. The preliminary draft report should not have been released outside the agency. When the report has been revised and fully vetted by EPA management, the findings and recommendations will be shared with the City and MDEQ and MDEQ will be responsible for following up with the city…. Again I apologize for taking all day to get back to you and for the manner in which this matter was handled."

TRUTH SQUAD ANALYSIS: Add the EPA's top official in the Great Lakes region to the growing list of state and federal regulators who know about, but are not urgently acting upon, Del Toral's concerns. Also add Flint's mayor at the time to those at least partially in the know, but Walling tries and can't get the Del Toral memo. Instead, EPA Region 5 Director Susan Hedman apologizes "for the manner in which this matter was handled."

JULY 7: MDEQ Public Information Officer Karen Tommasulo emails MDEQ Communications Director Brad Wurfel: "I got a weird call from a 'reporter' with the ACLU asking about Flint drinking water. His name is Curt Guyette, and I'm 98 percent sure it's the same guy who used to work at the Metro Times. He said he heard from someone at EPA that we use a 'flawed methodology' to collect our water samples…. Additionally, he claimed Flint is not adding corrosion control to their water, and said a city of their size should be doing so by law. But apparently we told Flint they didn't have to. I didn't offer any comment, just took the message from him. Do you want to talk to him, or does this one need to go to Liane's shop?"

Two days later, Tommasulo emails Wurfel again as Michigan Public Radio begins picking up on the ACLU reports. "Apparently, it is going to be a thing now."

JULY 9: ACLU's Guyette breaks the story of serious concerns about lead in Flint's drinking water by detailing the June 24 EPA-Del Toral memo. He reports the high lead levels in Lee-Anne Walters' water and the lack of ongoing corrosion control in Flint drinking water treatment.

JULY 9: MDEQ's Brad Wurfel emails colleague Stephen Busch as Guyette is breaking his story of the June 24 Del Toral memo and Michigan Radio reporter Lindsey Smith is sending related inquiries to Wurfel. At this point MDEQ officials have clearly heard Del Toral's concerns many times. They still don't have Del Toral's memo.

Wurfel writes: "The ACLU has saved us the trouble of waiting on the EPA for the report… it's online at the link below.… Miguel apparently asserts that the DEQ and EPA are at odds on proper protocol. Which seems weird."

Busch responds 27 minutes later: "Obviously we are not going to comment on an interim draft report." Busch then cites federal regulations to defend MDEQ's ongoing lead sampling procedures in Flint under the Lead and Copper Rule.

JULY 10: EPA Region 5 Director Hedman shares EPA's public comment on the ACLU report with Flint Mayor Walling via email: "EPA continues to work closely with the Michigan Department of Environmental Quality and the City of Flint to ensure that Flint residents are provided with safe drinking water.… EPA will work with Michigan DEQ and the City of Flint to verify and assess the extent of lead contamination issues and to ensure that Flint's drinking water meets federal standards."

JULY 13: MDEQ spokesman Brad Wurfel tells Michigan Radio: "Let me start here – anyone who is concerned about lead in the drinking water in Flint can relax." The Michigan Radio story is headlined: "Leaked internal memo shows federal regulator's concerns about lead in Flint's water."

JULY 14: In spite of growing concern and media reports, and Del Toral's alarm, MDEQ allows the City of Flint to decrease the number of homes sampled for lead in its second six-month testing period. This comes to light in an email from Jennifer Crooks (EPA) to Busch, Prysby and Cook at DEQ on July 14: "I understand that Flint didn't get the minimum number of lead samples (100) for the second six-month monitoring period that ended June 30, so I assume Flint is collecting the remaining samples now." Busch responds a day later: "We will provide the 90th percentile when available, but at this point we do not anticipate any violations of the Lead and Copper Rule." MDEQ later explains in written briefings that the number of samples was cut to 60 in the second six-month sampling period because Flint's population had dropped below 100,000. Therefore, a full 100 samples were no longer required by law.

JULY 21: EPA and MDEQ hold a conference call on MDEQ's implementation of the lead and copper rule. There appears to be ongoing disagreement between the agencies. EPA wants optimized corrosion control in Flint. MDEQ believes it is premature.

TRUTH SQUAD NOTE: But the federal agency doesn't take steps to override the state agency until months later. In November, EPA clarifies nationwide policy and says optimized corrosion control should begin at the instant that any such major water source switch begins.

Email from MDEQ's Shekter Smith to EPA's Hyde on the same day in reference to the conference call:

"(W)hile we understand your concerns with the overall implementation of the lead and copper rule(s); we think it is appropriate for EPA to indicate in writing (an email would be sufficient) your concurrence that the city is in compliance with the lead and copper rule as implemented in Michigan.… This would help distinguish between our goals to address important public health issues separately from the compliance requirements of the actual rule which we believe have been and continue to be met in the city of Flint."

TRUTH SQUAD ANALYSIS: Why is Shekter Smith, a top Michigan drinking-water regulator, making this distinction between "our goals to address important public health issues" and "compliance requirements?" Truth Squad is reminded of a key conclusion of the fact-finding body formed in October 2015 by Gov. Snyder – the Flint Water Advisory Task Force. In a December 29 letter to Snyder, this task force said: "We believe that in the Office of Drinking Water and Municipal Assistance at MDEQ (which Shekter Smith headed), a culture exists in which 'technical compliance' is considered sufficient to ensure safe drinking water in Michigan. This minimalist approach to regulatory oversight responsibility is unacceptable and simply insufficient to the task of public protection. It led to MDEQ's failure to recognize a number of indications that switching the water source in Flint would – and did – compromise both water safety and water quality. The MDEQ made a number of decisions that were, and continue to be, justified on the basis that federal rules 'allowed' those decisions to be made."

JULY 22: Snyder Chief of Staff Dennis Muchmore urges state agency directors Nick Lyon of the Michigan Department of Health and Human Services and Dan Wyant, director of MDEQ, to dive deeper:

"I'm frustrated by the water issue in Flint. I really don't think people are getting the benefit of the doubt. Now they are concerned and rightfully so about the lead level studies they are receiving from DEQ samples. Can you take a moment out of your impossible schedule to personally take a look at this? These folks are scared and worried about the health impacts and they are basically getting blown off by us (as a state we're just not sympathizing with their plight)."

The Muchmore email is forwarded by Nancy Grijalva, assistant to the director of the Michigan Department of Health and Human Services (MDHHS), to Paula Anderson, an executive secretary in MDHHS' public health administration division, and Susan Moran, MDHHS deputy director for population health and community services. Anderson also forwards Muchmore's email to another MDHHS employee, Mark Miller, who responds:

"There's an article from the Metro Times I located…. Based on this it sounds like at least one family might have had a child with elevated blood levels, which might or might not have come from the water. Sounds like the issue is old lead service lines…. DEQ has jurisdiction over municipal water supplies, but we do have a program to follow up on children with elevated blood levels, so I think it would be appropriate for the folks above to discuss the situation and recommend any action."

JULY 23: Linda Dykema, director of the MDHHS Division of Environmental Health, gives a more detailed response to Muchmore's questions. She sends an email to colleagues Corrine Miller, State Epidemiologist and director of the MDHHS Bureau of Epidemiology; Nancy Peeler, program director of the MDHHS program for Maternal, Infant, and Early Childhood Home Visiting; Rashmi Travis, MDHHS director for Family, Maternal and Child Health; Nancy Grijalva; Susan Moran; Wesley Priem, manager of the MDHHS Healthy Homes Section; James Bouters, a secretary for MDHHS Zoonotics and Special Projects team; Jacqui Barr, secretary for the MDHHS Division of Environmental Health; Brenda Fink, director of the MDHHS Family and Community Health Division; and Kory Groetsch, manager for the Toxicology and Response Section of the MDHHS Division of Environmental Health.

Dykema's email conveys no urgency after she talked to Busch at MDEQ, summarizing their discussion in her email as "this is what I sent up to my front office" as follows:

"The DEQ has not seen a change in the city's compliance with the lead rule since switching to the Flint River source."

"Regarding the EPA drinking water official quoted in the press articles, the report that he issued was a result of his own research and was not reviewed or approved by EPA management. He has essentially acted outside his authority."

TRUTH SQUAD ANALYSIS: Del Toral, the one regulator who has consistently sounded the alarm about lead in Flint's drinking water, surfaces again. And is ignored – and in this case, discredited – again. The dismissal of Del Toral's warnings now has spread to a second state agency charged with protecting public health.

JULY 24: Evidence that the governor's office is getting more community pressure from Flint. And more deflection and denial from MDEQ staff charged as watchdogs for public drinking water:

Email from MDEQ's Brad Wurfel to colleagues Busch, Prysby, Shekter Smith and MDEQ Director Dan Wyant: "Guys, the Flint Ministers met with the Governor's office again last week. They also brought along some folks from the community – a college prof and GM engineer – who imparted that 80 water tests in Flint have shown high lead levels. Could use an update on the January/June testing results, as well as recap of the December testing numbers, and any overview you can offer to edify this conversation."

MDEQ's Busch responds same day in email to Wurfel, copied to all others on the original note: He says the second round of Flint drinking water testing shows a 90th percentile level of 11 parts per billion.

TRUTH SQUAD NOTE: That's nearly double the level of the first six-month test but apparently no alarm to DEQ as it is below the federal Action Level Standard of 15 parts per billion.

Busch further relates that for the past 20 years Flint's water has never reached the 15 parts per billion level

TRUTH SQUAD NOTE: This seems irrelevant since for those 20 years the source of Flint's drinking water was Lake Huron, which is far less corrosive than Flint River water to start with, and, yet, still was treated with corrosion control.

And Busch states: "Sampling requirements look at the worst case plumbing materials. Samples must be collected in accordance with the regulatory requirements and criteria in order to be used for compliance determinations."

TRUTH SQUAD ANALYSIS: Busch's assertions are very troubling. First, he ignores Del Toral's concerns about MDEQ's sampling protocol. Second, he ignores the fact that the number of samples collected in Flint dropped dramatically in the second sampling period (from 100 to 60). Third, the MDEQ/Flint sampling process is later determined by the State Auditor General to be flawed – the regulators aren't looking at "worst-case" plumbing. In fact, they're not even sure they're sampling from lead service lines.

Busch also relates in this correspondence his version of the latest discussion with EPA over the corrosion control issue: (Flint) now will "complete a study (within 18 months) and are allowed a period of additional time (2 additional years) to install the selected treatment for fully optimized corrosion control.... We are planning to suggest the City directly submit a treatment process to shorten the timeline to achieve full optimization. This letter is currently being drafted but won't be ready to mail out for another week.... Liane and I had a conference call with EPA Region V in Chicago on Tuesday to go over all of this and they are in support or these next steps with the City."

TRUTH SQUAD ANALYSIS: Email correspondence documented considerable disagreement between EPA and MDEQ regulators about the absence of corrosion control for Flint drinking water system – and how, and how quickly, to resolve the situation.

Months later, EPA and the Michigan Auditor General will conclude that Flint never should have switched to Flint River water without corrosion control. And no one on this email chain is reminded of Del Toral's alarms and perspectives, which completely contradict the apparent group-think within MDEQ.

JULY 24: Two days after the governor's chief of staff, Dennis Muchmore, worries that the state is blowing off Flint residents' concerns, MDEQ's Brad Wurfel urges Muchmore, MDEQ Director Wyant and Tom Saxton at the Michigan Department of Treasury not to worry:

"Guys, here's an update and some clarification on the lead situation in Flint. Please limit this information to internal for now."

"By the tenants of the federal statute, the city is in compliance for lead and copper. That aside, they have not optimized their water treatment.... Compliance with the standard started with testing.... Everything checks out in terms of compliance, but now the next step is optimizing the water supply. So, in about two weeks, DEQ will be sending a formal communication about the optimizing issue. The federal program has long timelines for action. A community water supplier gets 18 months to study the options, and two years thereafter to implement water system optimization measures. My point: Conceivably, by the time we're halfway through the first timeline, the city will begin using a new water source with KWA… and conceivably, the whole process starts all over again. In terms of near-future issues, the bottom line is that residents of Flint do not need to worry about lead in their water supply, and DEQ's recent sampling does not indicate an eminent (sic) health threat from lead or copper."

Muchmore sends back a one-word reply: "Thanks."

TRUTH SQUAD ANALYSIS: Wurfel's assertion here that "the residents of Flint do not need to worry" may go down as one of the biggest blow-offs in the entire Flint water saga.

In his defense, Wurfel is a communications director, not a scientist. He's clearly getting his information from the front-line MDEQ drinking-water-regulations team. Even so, there is no sense of urgency from anyone at MDEQ.

It's also worth noting that Muchmore is now being told explicitly that the water flowing through the faucets of Flint residents has not been "optimized" (i.e., treated to prevent lead from leaching into the water) by the state agency charged with keeping the water safe, this on top of the lead concerns raised by the leaked EPA memo. At this point, what is the Snyder Administration to do? At this point, who should the governor and his top advisers trust? Should they trust the many months of public concerns coming directly from Flint? Should they trust the media? Should they trust two state agencies directly charged with protecting public health and drinking water safety – agencies that are providing no sense of alarm but are acknowledging a lack of "optimization" in Flint's water but mitigate any concern by saying the river won't be the source much longer?

Should the Snyder Administration now open an independent investigation that would be outside the norms and boundaries of public health oversight and drinking water regulation? Should Snyder's office, at this point, have reached the same "common sense" conclusion that a serious lead danger existed in Flint that Snyder would later accuse front-line state regulators of failing to reach?

Available public records suggest that the governor's office appeared to choose to continue to weigh options and ask more questions. It would be many weeks before the most important questions would be met with forthright and accurate answers. And only from the work of independent expert researchers outside state government would the full scope of the Flint disaster be revealed to the people of Flint, and the rest of Michigan, the nation and world.

JULY 28, 9:25 A.M.: Cristin Larder, a MDHHS epidemiologist, is among many staffers who begin to analyze state data on childhood lead blood tests in apparent response to Muchmore's July 22 inquiry. Larder emails MDHHS's Nancy Peeler, and Patricia McKane, manager of the MDHHS Maternal and Child Health Epidemiology Section, to report preliminary conclusions from checking the data on Flint children. She notes a spike in blood-lead levels in Flint in the summer 2014 just after the switch to Flint River drinking water:

"Basically, I used the monthly data from 2013-14 to create upper and lower control limits, then plotted the 2014-15 data in a run chart. It shows that the three months in question are the only ones that lie outside the control limit: in fact, they are the only points that lie well above the mean at all. This doesn't say anything about causality, but it does warrant further investigation."

JULY 28, 1:48 P.M.: Robert L. Scott, data manager for the MDHHS Healthy Homes and Lead Prevention program, also is analyzing state data. He also sees the summer 2014 spike in child blood lead levels but doesn't think it's serious.

"I said this morning I'd look to see if the distribution of (elevated blood lead levels) in the July-September 2014 'spike' was any different from the typical distribution of (elevated blood lead levels) in Flint. I compared totals by zip code vs. totals by zip code from 2010 (in micrograms per deciliter). The pattern is very similar and is further evidence, I think, that the water was not a major factor here."

JULY 28, 2:57 P.M.: Nancy Peeler, director of the MDHHS program for Maternal, Infant, and Early Childhood Home Visiting, responds in detail to the July 22 departmental inquiry precipitated by Muchmore's email. The recipients of Peeler's email are unclear. She reports efforts to "review our Childhood Lead Poisoning Prevention program data to see if it might contribute to the understanding of the situation in Flint with their water supply." Key points in her email:

"We compared lead testing rates and lead testing results to the same time frame for the previous 3 years, to see if there were any patterns that suggested that there were increased rates of lead poisoning after water supply was switched…. There was a spike in elevated blood lead tests from July-September 2014 (chart on left, gold line)…. However that pattern is not terribly different than what we saw in the previous three years…. (W)e are working with our epidemiologist to statistically verify any significant differences…. We commonly see a seasonal effect with lead, related to people opening and closing windows more often in the summer, which disturbed old deteriorating paint on the windows…. We suspect that the summer spike may be related to this effect…. If the home water supply lines and/or river water were contributing to elevated blood lead tests, we expected that the increased rates would extend beyond summer, but they drop quite a bit from September to October, stayed low over the winter, and are just starting to tail up again in the spring of 2015…."

"So, upon review, we don't believe our data demonstrates an increase in lead poisoning rates that might be attributable to the change in water for Flint."

A chart in Peeler's email clearly states, "Based on the results ... positive tests for elevated blood lead levels were higher than usual for children under age 16 living in the City of Flint during the months of July, August and September, 2014.... However, it's important to note that the purpose of control charts is to monitor data for quick detection of abnormal variation – not to construct a case for causality."

Brenda Fink, director of the MDHHS Family and Community Health Division at DCH, responds by email: "Really nice job... Great data, great language helping folks understand what the data says."

> **TRUTH SQUAD ANALYSIS:** In fact, additional third-party research will eventually demonstrate that – at this point and for several more weeks – MDHHS does not understand what its own data says. Only after a separate and crucial Flint-specific lead study released in September by Hurley Medical Center in Flint will MDHHS revisit its data and eventually, and painfully, come to the realization that blood lead levels in Flint children are, indeed, rising – and that the increase points toward lead in the drinking water.

On Dec. 22, 2015, Gov. Snyder's new director of communications, Meegan Holland, declares in email talking points prepared to respond to ongoing criticism: "It wasn't until the Hurley report came out that our epidemiologists took a more in-depth look at the data by zip code, controlling for seasonal variation, and confirmed an increase outside of normal trends. As a result of this process, we have determined that the way we analyze data... needs to be thoroughly reviewed."

MDHHS's failure to see warning signs in child lead-testing data is the second punch in a one-two combination of state government incompetence in the Flint water crisis. First comes many months of ignorance, missed warnings, denial, and inaction in the MDEQ regarding the lack of corrosion control in the Flint water pipes, even after alarms are repeatedly raised by EPA. Then comes weeks of ignorance, missed warnings, denial and inaction in MDHHS regarding elevated lead levels in Flint children.

CHAPTER 9

AUGUST 2015

MARC EDWARDS TO THE RESCUE

A NATIONALLY RECOGNIZED WATER SAFETY EXPERT BEGINS TO CRACK THE CASE

Editor's summary: As state and federal regulators continue a byzantine debate over corrosion control, Virginia Tech water safety expert Marc Edwards rides into Flint with vigilance and testing equipment in hand. By the end of August, Edwards gathers 72 water samples from Flint homes and announces publicly that 20 percent exceed the safe drinking water standard of 15 parts per billion for lead.

Yet Michigan Department of Environmental Quality deflections continue. MDEQ's chief spokesman tells a governor's aide that agitators are "raising hell with the locals" and there's "a steady parade of community groups keeping everyone hopped-up and misinformed." In fact, MDEQ is the master of misinformation.

"(I)T'S BEEN ROUGH SLEDDING WITH A STEADY PARADE OF COMMUNITY GROUPS KEEPING EVERYONE HOPPED-UP AND MISINFORMED."

— BRAD WURFEL

TIMELINE: AUGUST 2015

By John Bebow
Bridge Magazine

2015

AUG. 3: Key points in an email from EPA's Tinka Hyde to DEQ's Liane Shekter Smith regarding notes taken during a July 21 conference call between the agencies about Flint:

The first question at the top of the document: "Is there a public health concern regarding lead in Flint or other regulatory requirements?"

The document notes that the second six-month monitoring period for lead in water (January-June) found levels had nearly doubled from the first test period. The 90th percentile was 11 parts per billion. On the first round, it was 6 parts per billion. The meeting notes suggest no serious concern about the increase.

Much of the rest of the safety discussion is about long-anticipated timelines for corrosion control studies and the anticipated 2016 Flint switch from Flint River water to Karegnondi Water Authority service.

"MDEQ explained that they did not treat the switch to Flint River water as a 'new system,' but as a new source.... Region 5 (EPA) noted that under 141.81b3iii that any system that has been deemed optimized must notify the State of any long-term change in treatment or the addition of a new source. The state must review and approve the change.... Region 5 explained that they have talked to HQ about the interpretation of regulations and believes that systems that have been deemed optimized need to "maintain corrosion control".... MDEQ mentioned that other communities may leave the Detroit system or connect to the new Lake Huron pipeline, but many of those either don't need to treat for corrosion control or will be building new treatment plants."

"MDEQ is not interested in changing its position on pre-flushing until new regulations come out. They also pointed out that the pre-flushing instructions are not requirements, but suggestions."

"MDEQ and the Region were in agreement that it is important to get phosphate addition going in Flint as soon as possible."

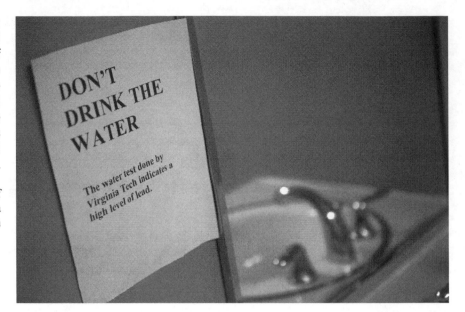

Flintwaterstudy.org retested for lead in the tap water of many Flint homes in early March. The volunteers posted "Don't Drink The Water" signs at sinks where they found high lead levels.

Photo courtesy of Logan Wallace/Virginia Tech

TRUTH SQUAD NOTE: It is clear now for the first time that EPA believes the MDEQ accepts that corrosion control is needed and will begin soon, even as MDEQ regulators continue to disagree whether it is required under the regulations. But as events will unfold, this step obviously was not only way too little and too late, but sidestepped by MDEQ's Busch in the letter he soon sent to Flint water plant officials.

"Region 5 commented that we now have a path forward for Flint despite a difference of opinion on whether the regulations required Flint to 'maintain' corrosion control when they started serving treated water from the Flint River."

And an admission from MDEQ, that despite not requiring corrosion control in the switch to Flint River water, they are going to require corrosion control from the start when the switch back to KWA/Lake Huron water eventually happens. "MDEQ and Region 5 agreed that after Flint implements corrosion control treatment, when they switch back to Lake Huron water, they will need to continue the corrosion control treatment while conducting monitoring to determine if this treatment is optimized with the new Lake Huron water quality."

"Region 5 will get back to MDEQ once it gets HQ/OGS's opinion on the need to 'maintain' corrosion control treatment once a system is deemed optimized."

TRUTH SQUAD NOTE: The opinion is released in November in a new nationwide order that corrosion control must occur from the start of any major water source switch.

AUG. 10: EPA pushes MDEQ to move faster on corrosion control. Email from Thomas Poy (EPA) to Shekter Smith, Busch and others at MDEQ:

"Liane: Any news on Flint since our call a couple weeks ago? Has the letter been sent to inform (Flint) that they are not optimized for lead based on their monitoring? Have they been approached about starting corrosion control sooner rather than later?" The next MDEQ action documented in publicly-released emails takes another week.

AUG. 17: MDEQ advises Flint of the second six-month lead/copper monitoring results and orders optimized corrosion control. But the timeline outlined by MDEQ gives Flint two years to implement the corrosion measures. And an email from MDEQ's Stephen Busch to Brad Wurfel (MDEQ) seems to continue to downplay the urgency and instead favor a long grind of hewing to interpretation of government regulations:

"As there has been much interest regarding lead related to Flint drinking water, I have attached our latest letter which covers the most recent January-June 2015 monitoring period. The City is in compliance with the 15 part per billion action level for lead. Yet based on these results, the treatment cannot be deemed to provide fully optimized corrosion control treatment, and the City will need to recommend additional treatment to achieve this optimization under the Lead and Copper rule requirements established under the Michigan Safe Drinking Water Act."

AUG. 23: Virginia Tech professor Marc Edwards notifies MDEQ that he will begin an independent study of Flint water quality. The Virginia Tech study will prove to be a major breakthrough to fully and scientifically document a serious public health threat from lead in Flint's drinking water. Very soon, the fears of EPA's Miguel Del Toral will be fully realized.

AUG. 24: MDEQ's Shekter Smith sends an email to MDEQ's Brad Wurfel outlining a draft email to Flint resident Lee-Anne Walters, whose high drinking-water lead levels earlier in the year sparked Del Toral's sounding of alarm bells at the EPA. The Shekter Smith email says Walters was in the governor's office for a meeting on August 4. Shekter Smith indicates she intends to make these points to Walters:

"As indicated during the meeting, the City's sampling for lead complies with the Action Level standard of 15 parts per billion, but … the City will need to make a recommendation to the MDEQ on how they will fully optimize their corrosion control treatment."

"Samples collected at your residence of 212 Browning Avenue were not included in this compliance determination as you utilize a whole home filter." But DEQ confirmed very high lead levels, up to 707 parts per billion in the spring, before the water main serving that residence was replaced and lead levels dropped.

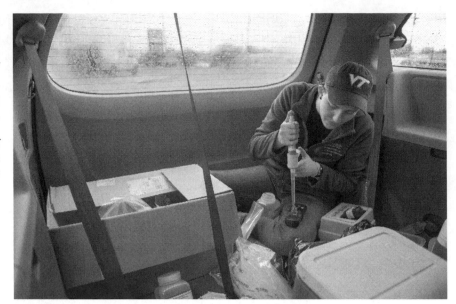

One of the Virginia Tech students working with Marc Edwards' Flintwaterstudy.org water-sampling project.

Photo courtesy of Logan Wallace/Virginia Tech

"… (O)ur office has been in contact with the Department of Health and Human Services…. And had some preliminary discussions about a public education and assistance campaign regarding household lead issues, guidance and abatement."

TRUTH SQUAD NOTE: State email records indicate the memo from Shekter Smith to Walters is emailed in late August. Virginia Tech University professor and water expert Marc Edwards later says Walters never received the email.

AUG. 27: Virginia Tech's Edwards releases his first preliminary analysis of Flint tap water test results and deems those results "worrisome." More than half of the first 48 samples exceed 5 parts per billion lead; 30 percent exceeded 15 ppb.

AUG. 27: More deflection from MDEQ after more questions from the governor's office. Mike Brown, the governor's senior federal policy representative, emails MDEQ's Wurfel after apparently an inquiry from U.S. Sen. Gary Peters' office. Wurfel appears to share the Shekter Smith report of Lee-Anne Walters. Wurfel appears to refer to Walters as "a very vocal resident." Brown inquires: "So this resident's lead levels are much higher than the 90th percentile mentioned in the previous email. What is the discrepancy?"

Wurfel responds: "Don't know what it is, but I know what it's not. The key to lead and copper in drinking water is that it's not the source water, or even the transmission lines (most of which are cast iron). It's in the premise plumbing (people's homes)."

TRUTH SQUAD ANALYSIS: This assertion proves to be very wrong a few weeks later, in early October, when Flint Department of Public Works officials tell MLive.com that many city pipes have the possibility of leaching lead, but the city can't immediately get its finger on the issue because the info is stored on 45,000 paper index cards. And Dr. Mona Hanna-Attisha eventually asserts in a peer-reviewed and published medical journal article that between 10 and 80 percent of city lines leach lead. In Walters' case, the lead source in her water was clearly a lead city-owned service line.

Wurfel also then cites federal regulations for the slow pace of response as MDEQ orders Flint to finally attain, over the next couple of years, optimized corrosion control. "Such is the wisdom and flexibility of the federal statute."

Wurfel then appears to refer to EPA's Del Toral, without mentioning him by name, to Brown: "This person is the one who had EPA lead specialist come to her home and do tests, then released an unvetted draft of his report (that EPA apologized to us profusely for) to the resident, who shared it with ACLU, who promptly used it to continue raising hell with the locals."

TRUTH SQUAD ANALYSIS: In other words, the inquiring Snyder aide, Mike Brown, can be left with the misguided impression that Del Toral is wrong, Lee-Anne Walters is wrong, ACLU is wrong, they're all a bunch of hell-raisers, MDEQ is right, and there's no reason to worry.

Wurfel continues: "Bottom line is that folks in Flint are upset – because they pay a ton for water and many of them don't trust the water they're getting – and they're confused, in no small part because various groups have worked hard at keeping them confused and upset. We get it. The state is trying like mad (to) get the word out that we're working on every aspect of the health safety of local water that we can manage, and the system needs a lot of work…. (I)t's been rough sledding with a steady parade of community groups keeping everyone hopped-up and misinformed."

TRUTH SQUAD ANALYSIS: As would become tragically clear by year's end, the real and worst confusion was not among local Flint residents. It was within MDEQ and MDHHS. Over the next few months, it wasn't the state agencies that brought urgent action to protect Flint's public, it was the "outside agitators" whom Wurfel scorns.

AUG. 28: Email from EPA's Thomas Poy to MDEQ's Shekter Smith and others at MDEQ: "Marc Edwards is working with some of the citizens in Flint and they are finding lead at levels above five parts per billion and some above 15 parts per billion. There's no indication of whether any of these homes were also sampled and analyzed by Flint and will now be part of their compliance calculations. Virginia Tech sent out 300 bottles and have gotten 48 back. We are not involved in this effort by Dr. Edwards."

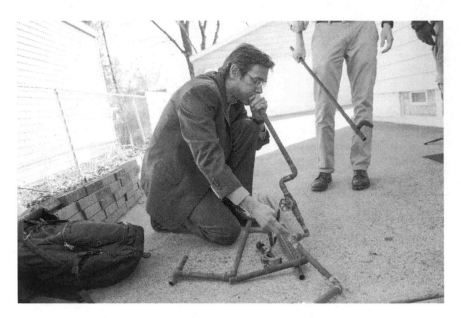

Professor Marc Edwards, Virginia Tech water supply expert.

Photo courtesy of Logan Wallace/Virginia Tech

AUG. 31: Virginia Tech is up to 72 lead samples tested, with 42 percent above 5 parts per billion and 20 percent exceeding 15 parts per billion.

AUG. 31: Email from MDEQ's Brad Wurfel to colleagues Stephen Busch, Liane Shekter Smith, Mike Prysby and director Dan Wyant. With the following five key Snyder aides copied: Chief of staff Dennis Muchmore; Harvey Hollins, director of the Office of Urban Initiatives); Dave Murray, deputy press secretary; Eric Brown, senior federal policy representative, and Sara Wurfel, press secretary and Brad Wurfel's wife.

Brad Wurfel writes: "… just got this from the ACLU. Call me if you have questions/counsel."

The rest is an email forwarded from Curt Guyette at ACLU-Michigan asking Brad Wurfel to respond to Virginia Tech's growing evidence of lead in Flint tap water.

Busch responds: "Brad, we are aware of the VT professor. I can bring you up to speed this afternoon or whenever you are available."

Busch forwards another email to Wurfel marked "High" priority and comes from Jennifer Crooks at EPA to Shekter Smith, Busch and others at MDEQ:

"Today's updates on Marc Edwards' site. His staff is phone calling and emailing results to citizens. Talk at 2."

CHAPTER 10

SEPT. 1-15 2015

EDWARDS: DON'T DRINK THE WATER WITHOUT FILTERS

BUT THE MDEQ CONTINUES TO DEFLECT

Editor's summary: After six months with EPA's Manuel Del Toral as the chief antagonist to state agencies' defense of the safety of Flint water, the professor and national drinking-water expert from Virginia Tech takes center stage. Marc Edwards' testing in Flint shows plenty of elevated lead levels in Flint drinking water, including some samples with more than 100 parts per billion (nearly ten times the federal action limit). He urges residents not to drink or cook with tap water unless it's filtered and the water has been flushed through the tap for several minutes. He says MDEQ's resistance to Del Toral's findings caused residents months of added exposure to high lead levels in their water. MDEQ questions Edwards' findings in media interviews.

> **"I AM PLEASED TO REPORT THAT THE CITY OF FLINT HAS OFFICIALLY RETURNED TO COMPLIANCE WITH THE MICHIGAN SAFE DRINKING WATER ACT AND WE HAVE RECEIVED CONFIRMING DOCUMENTATION FROM THE DEQ TODAY."**
>
> **— SEPT. 3: EMAIL FROM FLINT DEPARTMENT OF PUBLIC WORKS DIRECTOR HOWARD CROFT TO NUMEROUS STATE AND LOCAL OFFICIALS, INCLUDING FLINT MAYOR DAYNE WALLING.**

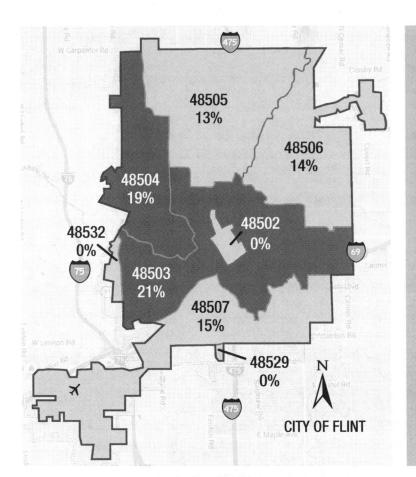

Lead levels in water of Flint zip codes

In August 2015, new tests detected much higher levels of lead in Flint's drinking water than city-conducted tests had found. Virginia Tech's Flintwaterstudy.org testing project was led by Marc Edwards who received help from researchers, students and volunteers. As the map shows, more than 10 percent of the homes in all the largest zip codes had lead in water above the 15 parts per billion trigger for regulatory action. The map highlights in dark the two zip codes with the most lead in the water.

Source: Flintwaterstudy.org

Professor Marc Edwards' team of researchers came to Flint to test water samples.

Photo courtesy of Logan Wallace/ Virginia Tech

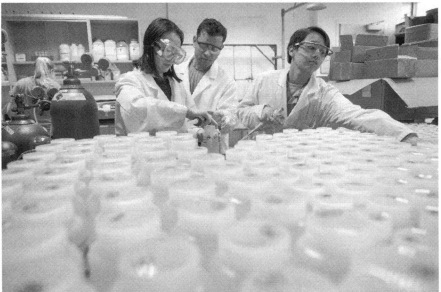

TIMELINE: SEPT. 1 – 15, 2015

By John Bebow
Bridge Magazine

2015

SEPT. 2: Marc Edwards publicly releases a report that changes the narrative in the bureaucratic fight among regulators over whether Flint's water is safe to drink. Edwards, a Virginia Tech professor, researcher and nationally known expert on public water supplies, asserts that the corrosiveness of the Flint River water is causing lead to leach into residents' water. With a team of volunteers and students, he showed that lead is clearly leaching into the water of Flint residents. The full report, published on FlintWaterStudy.org on Sept. 11, declares:

On average, the Detroit water Flint used before the switch (sourced from Lake Huron) is 19 times less corrosive than Flint River water.

Phosphate treatment of Flint's water only produces a slight improvement.

> **TRUTH SQUAD ANALYSIS:** In other words, even with common anti-corrosion treatments, Edwards concludes that Flint River water would be a potentially dangerous source for drinking. This begs two fundamental questions: Why did it take a Virginia Tech researcher to run these tests a year and a half after the switch to Flint River water? Why didn't the Flint Department of Public Works, MDEQ, or third-party engineers who studied the Flint water system connect the corrosion dots before the switch?

In January 2016, Gov. Snyder would apologize to the people of Flint. He would take responsibility for what he acknowledged were failures of government at all levels. His political legacy is undoubtedly and deeply stained forever by the crisis. He and his administration now face numerous forms of official investigation and surely many legal claims that will take years to adjudicate. The extent of the governor's personal culpability – and the pace of response by the governor and his key aides – will surely be key questions.

Yet Edwards' fairly basic Flint corrosion and lead discoveries, MDEQ's many failures, and MDHHS's delays in seeing a lead connection in Flint children also bring legitimacy to questions the governor himself raised about front-line state-agency incompetence in a January 2016 interview on MSNBC's Morning Joe show.

Snyder asserted the department heads he appointed "were not being given the right information by quote-unquote experts.... I use that word with great trial and tribulation because they were considered experts in terms of their backgrounds." At many turns, those state experts failed.

Another fundamental question going forward: Can other Michigan residents trust state experts, and elected officials, to protect statewide public drinking water supplies?

SEPT. 2: Snyder adviser Harvey Hollins emails the governor to inform that 1,500 kitchen water filters were donated, and coordinated by the administration, to the Flint Concerned Pastors for Social Action organization "as a way of providing added comfort amid concerns about Flint's water quality."

SEPT. 2: MDEQ's Brad Wurfel responds to Virginia Tech revelations with more deflection and denials in a press release emailed to MLive.com reporter Ron Fonger. Key points:

"(W)e want to be very clear that the lead levels being detected in Flint drinking water are not coming from the treatment plant or the city's transmission lines.... The issue is how, or whether, and to what extent the drinking water is interacting with lead plumbing in people's homes."

"The results reported so far fail to track with any of the lead sampling conducted by the city. In addition, Virginia Tech results are not reflected by the blood lead-level testing regularly conducted by the state department of community health that have not shown any change since Flint switched sources."

SEPT. 3: Email from Flint Department of Public Works Director Howard Croft to numerous state and local officials, including Flint Mayor Dayne Walling:

"I am pleased to report that the City of Flint has officially returned to compliance with the Michigan Safe Drinking Water Act and we have received confirming documentation from the DEQ today."

"Recent testing has raised questions regarding the amount of lead that is being found in the water and I wanted to report to you our current status. At the onset of our plant design, optimization for lead was addressed and discussed with the engineering firm and with the DEQ. It was determined that having more data was advisable prior to the commitment of a specific optimization method. Most chemicals used in this process are phosphate based and phosphate can be a 'food' for bacteria. We have performed over one hundred and sixty lead tests throughout the city since switching over to the Flint River and remain within EPA standards."

TRUTH SQUAD ANALYSIS: Croft may not know what will soon become public, including these revelations: 1) Investigators will determine that the city's sampling methods were flawed – the city couldn't confirm it was testing high-risk lead homes; 2) EPA would ultimately, but slowly, reach the forceful conclusion that MDEQ's decision to not use corrosion control when the water source was switched was completely wrong; and 3) Controversy had long brewed between MDEQ and EPA over the state's practice of pre-flushing home water lines before Flint lead samples were taken.

SEPT. 6: MDEQ's spokesman Brad Wurfel tells Michigan Radio regarding the Virginia Tech lead test results: "The samples don't match the testing that we've been doing in the same kind of neighborhoods all over the city for the past year. With these kinds of numbers, we would have expected to be seeing a spike somewhere else in the other lead monitoring that goes on in the community."

TRUTH SQUAD NOTE: Hurley Medical Center's Dr. Mona Hanna-Attisha would soon prove the kind of lead-in-blood spike that MDHHS and MDEQ continue to deny is real.

SEPT. 8: Virginia Tech's Marc Edwards publishes the full results to date of his Flint water testing. Key points:

"FLINT HAS A VERY SERIOUS LEAD IN WATER PROBLEM." (No Truth Squad emphasis added.)

"Forty percent of the first draw samples are over five parts per billion. That is, 101 out of 252 water samples from Flint homes had first draw lead more than 5 ppb."

"Flint's 90th percentile lead value is 25 parts per billion in our survey.... This is over the EPA allowed level of 15 ppb that is applied to high risk homes. This is a serious concern indeed.... Another mystery which must be examined very carefully in the days and weeks ahead: How is it possible that Flint 'passed' the official EPA Lead and Copper Rule sampling overseen by MDEQ?"

"Several samples exceeded 100 ppb and one sample collected after 45 seconds of flushing exceeded 1,000 ppb."

"Until further notice, we recommend that Flint tap water be only used for cooking or drinking if one of the following steps are implemented...." Those recommended steps included filtering and/or five-minute flushing at a high flow rate every time a Flint water tap is used.

SEPT. 8: Virginia Tech's Marc Edwards sounds yet another alarm in email to Mayor Dayne Walling, who had requested a meeting.

Edwards writes: "Had MDEQ studied the scientific validity of the points Mr. Del Toral was making months ago, and acted on that information, Flint residents would have been informed about the high lead in water risk at that time. Months of harmful exposures to this neurotoxin could have been avoided. Instead, MDEQ openly attempted to discredit and smear Mr. Del Toral to Flint residents – the residents told me this directly…..

"Frankly, I feel that MDEQ's action in this regard, is not consistent with its mission of upholding the public welfare. In large part because it was clear that MDEQ was behaving in an unscientific and regretful manner in relation to Mr. Del Toral's work, a 16-person team at Virginia Tech decided to launch the Flint water study, to take an unbiased look at this urgent public health issue on behalf of Flint consumers."

Walling responds in an email a day later, and tells Edwards he thought the July apology to him by EPA Region 5 Administrator Susan Hedman and ongoing internal review of Del Toral's June 24 draft memo at EPA was "part of the customary organizational process."

Edwards responds: "I understand how you could have been misled. All I can tell you, is that from a scientific and engineering perspective, everything in Mr. Del Toral's memo was 100 percent accurate…. I am sorry that MDEQ did not take his memo seriously, and that they did not cause the City of Flint to consider corrosion control from the start of this process. It was their job to do so. I have no idea what MDEQ's agenda is, but based on their press releases and actions to date, protecting the public and following Federal laws, does not seem to be a priority…. If you want to protect consumers in your city, you should start listening directly to Mr. Del Toral."

SEPT. 9: Email from MDEQ's Brad Wurfel to Ron Fonger as MLive.com questions Edwards' conclusions:

"(T)he state DEQ is just as perplexed by Edwards' results as he seems to be by the city's test results, which are done according to state and federal sampling guidelines and analyzed by certified labs."

> **TRUTH SQUAD ANALYSIS:** This reasoning does not include such important things as: 1) Del Toral's longstanding concerns about the sampling methods in Flint, and, 2) The fact that the number of lead samples in Flint actually decreased after Del Toral first made his lead concerns known to MDEQ, with state approval, from 100 in the first six-month test to 60 in the second six-month test. Later, investigators conclude that the city's sampling procedures were flawed. Ultimately, in January 2016, the EPA announces it will take over lead sampling and monitoring in Flint.

Wurfel further reasons that the Virginia Tech researchers "only just arrived in town and (have) quickly proven the theory they set out to prove, and while the state appreciates academic participation in this discussion, offering broad, dire public health advice based on some quick testing could be seen as fanning political flames irresponsibly."

"The state and the EPA are working together in Flint...."

> **TRUTH SQUAD ANALYSIS:** Of course, this assertion completely ignores the controversy and explicit Del Toral warnings over corrosion control and sampling methods between EPA and MDEQ.

SEPT. 9: An email from Michelle Bruneau, a health educator in the MDHHS Toxicology and Response Section, to Kory Groetsch, MDHHS manager for Toxicology and Response, has the subject line: "Flint Lead is blowing up – may want to push meeting if we're going to do something." The email links to Michigan Radio coverage and MLive.com coverage of Virginia Tech's testing results.

SEPT. 10 THRU SEPT. 25: Some moments of seeming disbelief on the part of a national lead and copper rule expert connected with EPA as she seeks details from MDEQ about Flint's water quality parameters.

Sept. 10 email from Dr. Yanna Lambrinidou to MDEQ's Brad Wurfel and Stephen Busch: "As a member of the EPA National Drinking Water Advisory Council Lead and Copper Rule workgroup that just completed its recommendations to EPA about the agency's upcoming revisions to the LCR, I am watching with great interest and concern the developments in Flint in relation to lead. I am looking for information on the optimal water quality parameter ranges that MDEQ has set for Flint's water. Are those posted online? If so, could you send me the link? If not, could you let me know where they are?"

Sept. 14 response from MDEQ's Busch: "Dr. Lambrinidou, All previous water quality parameter ranges would have been established for the City of Flint's wholesale finished water supplier, the Detroit Water and Sewerage Department, not the City of Flint itself. As the City of Flint has not yet established optimized corrosion control treatment, the MDEQ is not yet at the point of regulatory requirements where the range of water quality parameters would be set."

> **TRUTH SQUAD ANALYSIS:** Busch's response is a clear admission the MDEQ let Flint switch drinking water sources to the Flint River without establishing water quality parameters.

CHAPTER 11

SEPT. 16-23, 2015

THE DAWNING REALIZATION

AS PRESSURE MOUNTS, STATE HEALTH OFFICIALS SECOND-GUESS THEMSELVES

Editor's summary: Professor Marc Edwards says water sampling by the City of Flint has been biased, intentionally or not, to produce lower numbers. In an email to EPA, he cites the city water plant operator's comments in an ACLU video: "We threw bottles out everywhere just to collect as many as we can, just to hit our number, and just turn in every result we get in." Clearly, federal-testing protocols weren't met. Meanwhile, state public health officials are starting to second-guess themselves after Flint pediatrician Dr. Mona Hanna-Attisha requests the state's test results of lead levels in blood and hints that her early findings show a sharp spike.

ELEVEN DAYS AFTER VIRGINIA TECH'S EDWARDS PUBLISHES HIS FULL FLINT LEAD SAMPLING RESULTS, MDHHS OFFICIALS ARE FINALLY GRAPPLING WITH HIS FINDINGS IN EMAIL CORRESPONDENCE.

— TRUTH SQUAD ANALYSIS

TIMELINE: SEPT. 16 – 23, 2015

By John Bebow
Bridge Magazine

2015

SEPT. 17: Email from Susan Moran to numerous MDHHS colleagues: "FYI Front office also is asking about Flint water, let's make sure we are communicating consistently. Copying Linda and Corrinne. While this is a public health concern, this is largely DEQ/local jurisdiction." Corrinne Miller at MDHHS responds later same day: "Per the MDEQ, the compliance monitoring for lead within the city has never exceeded the EPA action level for lead."

SEPT. 20: Virginia Tech's Marc Edwards alleges in email to EPA officials that Flint's lead sampling techniques are seriously flawed. Key points:

"They do not have an approved lead sampling pool. Only 13 of the lowest lead sampled homes from 2014 were resampled in 2015. The homes sampling high in 2014 were not asked to be resampled. At best, their program is sending out sampling bottles at random across the city."

"This message exemplifies the type of site selection that they are doing to satisfy their high risk LCR monitoring pool site. That is, none. They are not even trying to hide it. This link reveals this June alert from the Flint Department of Public Works:

"Good Afternoon,

"I am writing everyone in regards to drinking water testing for lead & copper. The City needs assistance from residents to collect samples from their home. I believe I bothered everyone with a correspondence regarding this matter last year for our first sample round, but we are trying to finish up our second 6 month round of testing before the end of this month. If you live in the City or have family/friends who live in the city that would like to be part of the sampling group please contact me via email or call the water plant at (810) 787-6537. Please forward this email to anyone who might be willing to participate.

"Collecting a sample consists of letting the water sit stagnant in the pipes for 6 – 8 hours (usually overnight, or while at work/school/etc during the day) then filling a sample bottle and recording sampling and contact information on a form that is provided. Water Plant staff will deliver and pick up the sample bottle and accompanying form.

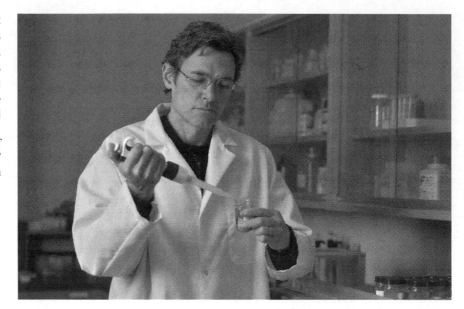

Virginia Tech's Marc Edwards alleges in email to EPA officials that Flint's lead sampling techniques are seriously flawed

Photo courtesy of Logan Wallace/ Virginia Tech

"Thank you,

"Mike Glasgow
"Utilities Administrator
"City of Flint"

Edwards's email to EPA officials continues: "Furthermore, in a video now on the ACLU website, at the end of the interview, Mike Glasgow notes what is perfectly obvious from looking at the MDEQ FOIA materials. 'We threw bottles out everywhere just to collect as many as we can, just to hit our number, and we just turn in every result we get in.'…. On top of that, according to my count, MDEQ covered up no fewer than 5 violations in the 2015 sample round." Edwards also included allegations of late reports, 87 sites from 2014 being not resampled, no written justification for site changes and … "In video Mike admits he has no knowledge of what sites actually have lead pipe or not."

SEPT. 22: Email from MDHHS Environmental Public Health Director Lynda Dykema to MDHHS colleagues Geralyn Lasher, MDHHS deputy director for external relations and communications, Nancy Peeler, and many others: "Here is a link to the VA Tech study re city of Flint drinking water. … It appears that the researchers have completed testing of a lot of water samples and the results are significantly different than the city and DEQ data. It also appears that they've held public meetings in Flint, resulting in concerns about the safety of the water that have arisen in the last few days."

TRUTH SQUAD ANALYSIS: Eleven days after Virginia Tech's Edwards publishes his full Flint lead sampling results, MDHHS officials are finally grappling with his findings in email correspondence.

SEPT. 22: Flint pediatrician Dr. Mona Hanna-Attisha requests from Robert Scott and others at MDHHS full state records on blood tests to supplement her own Flint blood lead research. The doctor says: "… since we have been unable to obtain recent MCIR blood lead data for Flint kids in response to the lead in water concerns, we looked at all the blood lead levels that were processed through Hurley Medical Center …" and she describes "striking results."

TRUTH SQUAD NOTE: Hurley is a major hospital in Flint.

SEPT. 22: Email meeting notice from Kory Groetsch at MDHHS regarding a lead-related conference call among MDHHS, MDEQ and Genesee County health officials. One agenda item for the meeting is: "Current status of resources to put toward desired efforts (i.e., Who has time to do what? AKA – reality check.")

SEPT. 23: A day before Dr. Mona Hanna-Attisha releases her study concluding the levels of lead in blood of young children rose sharply since the water-source switch, the ongoing questions prompt Nancy Peeler, program director of the MDHHS program for Maternal, Infant, and Early Childhood Home Visiting, to reconsider the department's conclusions in July. Then, MDHHS had noted elevated lead levels in blood in Flint in the summer of 2014, but also concluded there was no relation to Flint water.

Now Peeler's email says: "Based on questions coming through, I do think we need to run our Flint charts for the same population group that the Flint docs ran (as close as we can approximate the sample) but I'd look at it across the five years again. Depending on what our charts show, we may want to consider having (state epidemiologists) help us run an analysis more like the docs ran. …"

SEPT. 23: Email from Mikelle Robinson at MDHHS to colleagues describing a planned briefing for the governor's office on Flint: "The DEQ … gave a long summary about the Flint water issues ... bottom line is that the water itself is safe but they have an old water treatment plan and old cast iron pipes that haven't been upgraded in more than 40 years.... Flint is not in violation of the lead standards.... DEQ briefed the mayor and some legislators on Monday.... Flint's water supply is not an imminent public health problem but a public confidence problem due to the many groups getting involved and controversial reports/ media coverage."

CHAPTER 12

SEPT. 24-30

THE DOCTOR CHANGES EVERYTHING

PRESSURE PROMPTS GOVERNOR TO ACT ON ELEVATED LEAD LEVELS IN CHILDREN

Editor's summary: For six months, EPA and MDEQ water regulators have argued whether there's a lead problem in Flint's drinking water. But in one fell swoop, a Flint pediatrician, Dr, Mona Hanna-Attisha, turns the debate from theoretical to personal. Her study, released on Sept. 24, finds that since the Flint River became the source of drinking water in April 2014, blood-lead levels of young children (5 and under) have nearly tripled in one high risk zip code and doubled in another. In wake of the study's release, it's become abundantly clear that MDEQ and MDHHS errors have put Flint's citizens, especially young children, most vulnerable to lead exposure, at great risk.

> **"IT'S BAD ENOUGH TO HAVE A DATA WAR WITH OUTSIDE ENTITIES, WE ABSOLUTELY CANNOT ENGAGE IN COMPETING DATA ANALYSES WITHIN THE DEPARTMENT, OR, HEAVEN FORBID, IN PUBLIC RELEASES."**
>
> **— LINDA DYKEMA**

TIMELINE: SEPT. 24 – 30, 2015

By John Bebow
Bridge Magazine

2015

SEPT. 24, 10:26 A.M.: MDHHS Deputy Director Geralyn Lasher emails MDHHS Director Nick Lyon and many other MDHHS staffers and managers. She had "just gotten off the phone with Nancy Peeler and Bob Scott and are putting together talking points about this 'study' that the physicians will be discussing that claims an increase in elevated blood levels in children since the change to the water system source."

SEPT. 24, 1:16 P.M.: Angela Minicuci at MDHSS distributes "Flint Talking Points" in advance of a planned press conference by Hurley Medical Center and Dr. Mona Hanna-Attisha. Key points:

Hurley results are "under review" by MDHHS.

Hurley's analysis is "different" than the way MDHHS does it.

The state's methodology is better. "Looking at the past five years as a whole provides a much more accurate look at the seasonal trends of lead in the area … MDHHS data provides a much more robust picture of the entire blood lead levels for the Flint area."

> **TRUTH SQUAD ANALYSIS:** As we noted during MDHHS's internal analysis of lead data earlier in July, by year's end the governor's office would acknowledge significant weaknesses in MDHHS's data analysis. Again, as the governor's communications director, Meegan Holland, stated in Dec. 22, 2015, talking points for the governor: "It wasn't until the Hurley report came out that our epidemiologists took a more in-depth look at the data by zip code, controlling for seasonal variation, and confirmed an increase outside of normal trends. As a result of this process, we have determined that the way we analyze data collected needs to be thoroughly reviewed."

SEPT. 24, 1:56 P.M.: Snyder Deputy Press Secretary Dave Murray emails more than a dozen state officials, including chief of staff Muchmore, future chief of staff Jerrod Agen, Lasher at MDHHS and Brad Wurfel at MDEQ: "Team, Here's the data that will be presented at the Hurley Hospital press conference at 3 p.m. As you'll see, they are pointing to individual children, a very emotional approach. Our challenge will be to show how our state data is different from what the hospital and the coalition members are presenting today."

SEPT. 24: Hanna-Attisha releases her study of elevated blood lead levels in Flint children at a press conference. MLive.com posts a story at 2:09 p.m. Key points:

"The data show that the percentage of Flint infants and children with above average lead levels has nearly doubled citywide, and has nearly tripled among children in 'high risk' areas of lead exposure."

The study recommends ending Flint River water as its drinking source "as soon as possible."

The study recommends that the city declare a health advisory that could trigger additional federal resources.

SEPT. 24, 3:14 P.M.: As Hanna-Attisha releases her results, a MDHHS staffer scoffs. Email from Wesley Priem, manager of the MDHHS Healthy Homes Section, to colleague Kory Groetsch: "Yes, the issue is moving … at the speed of rushing water … I am trying to keep everyone updated.… I am also trying at this minute to watch the teleconference on MLive.… But not having much success.… This is definitely being driven by a little science and a lot of politics."

Three minutes later, Groetsch responds: "Best of luck."

SEPT. 24, 3:45 P.M.: MDHHS lead data manager Robert Scott emails colleague Nancy Peeler with a new discovery. He attaches a spreadsheet to the email, says he has attempted to "recreate Hurley's numbers," and says he sees "a difference between the two years (presumably pre- and post-water switch), but not as much difference as (Hurley) did." In other words, in attempting to replicate Hanna-Attisha's methodology, he's seeing something similar to what she found. Scott notes in his email to Peeler: "I'm sure this one is not for the public."

SEPT. 24: Virginia Tech's Marc Edwards presses hard on Robert Scott at MDHHS for state blood-lead records. In an email to Scott, Edwards says Hurley researchers have been unable to get access to state records. Edwards asks: "Can you tell me why it is so difficult to get this data, and why your agency is raising so many obstacles to sharing it with everyone who asks?... I have to say, it is very disturbing that the state keeps issuing these blood lead reports and statements in their press releases, and refuses to share the data backing them up with outside researchers.… I note that I have been asking to see your data since MDEQ first sent it to reporters back in August, and I count 10 emails that I sent responding to all your questions. As of yet, you have given me nothing in response."

Scott drafts an email response a day later:

"As you well know, the data you and Dr. Hanna-Attisha are requesting are derived from personal health data, which of course is confidential.... I worked with you earlier this month to get data to you relatively quickly but did not manage to complete the process before I went on annual leave for several days. I neglected to inform you that I'd be away, and I apologize for not informing you."

But Scott doesn't send the email. He sends it to colleague Peeler for review. Peeler tells Scott to "apologize less" in his letter, and is further focused on image protection: "The email you received could be read as an intent to escalate and spin things, and I don't think you need to get caught up in that."

Scott writes back to Peeler: "I agree that his statements are inappropriate; there are plenty of things I'd LIKE to say in response, but won't."

SEPT. 25: A day after Hanna-Attisha releases her study, the City of Flint issues a health advisory, telling residents to flush pipes and install filters to prevent lead poisoning.

SEPT. 25, 2015, 1:19 P.M.: MDHHS's Robert Scott responds to email from colleagues about Detroit Free Press interest in doing a lead story. At 12:16 p.m., Free Press reporter Kristi Tanner sends an email to Angela Minicuci at MDHHS saying Tanner had looked at the lead increase in Flint as shown in DHS records between 2013-2014 and 2014-2015 and Tanner is concluding that the increase "is statistically significant." MDHHS's Peeler tasks Robert Scott with responding.

Scott writes to Minicuci: "The best I could say is something like this: 'While the trend for Michigan as a whole has shown a steady decrease in lead poisoning year by year, smaller areas such as the city of Flint have their bumps from year to year while still trending downward overall.'"

Peeler appears to be looking for a positive media spin, too. She writes back to Scott and Minicuci: "My secret hope is that we can work in the fact that this pattern is similar to the recent past."

TRUTH SQUAD ANALYSIS: This attempted media spin completely ignores what Scott had told Peeler by email the previous afternoon. He'd crunched numbers and replicated something somewhat similar to the results of the Hurley lead study. Then again, as Scott had opined in his email to Peeler the previous afternoon, "I'm sure this one is not for the public."

SEPT. 25: Again, a day after telling Nancy Peeler he has begun to roughly approximate Hanna-Attisha's Flint lead test results, Robert Scott makes no such acknowledgement in an email exchange directly with Hanna-Attisha:

At 3:12 p.m. on the 25th, Hanna-Attisha writes to Scott: "Bob, did you ever look at your data that was released for kids less than 5, rather than 16? 16 seems so strange – we rarely do lead levels in kids over the age of 5."

At 3:45 Scott responds: "No, I didn't run the data for kids 0-5. We normally would use that age range, and I don't completely recall the conversation that led to using 0-15 – possibly trying to cast as wide a nest as possible?" In Scott's email to Peeler the day before, he asked Peeler to "Let me know if you think it's worth pursuing any farther." Publicly available emails do not suggest he asked the same question of the lead researcher on the Hurley study just one day later.

SEPT. 25: Email from Snyder Chief of Staff Dennis Muchmore to Snyder and others on the governor's staff. Rather than rallying full resources to the rising crisis, the email is mainly a political analysis:

"The issue of Flint water and its quality continues to be a challenging topic. The switch over to use Flint River water has spurred most of the controversy and contention. The DEQ and (MDHHS) feel that some in Flint are taking the very sensitive issue of children's exposure to lead and trying to turn it into a political football claiming the departments are underestimating the impacts on the populations and are particularly trying to shift responsibility to the state. We have put an incredible amount of time and effort into this issue because of the impacted neighborhoods and their children, and the KWA/DWSD controversy and Dillon's involvement in the final decision.

"(U.S. Rep. Dan) Kildee is asking for a call with you. That's tricky because he's sure to use it publicly, but if you don't talk with him it will just fan the narrative that the state is ducking responsibility. I can't figure out why the state is responsible except that Dillon did make the ultimate decision so we're not able to avoid the subject. The real responsibility rests with the County, city, and KWA, but since the issue is the health of citizens and their children we're taking a pro-active approach putting (MDHHS) out there as an educator.

"I'm not sure how much background you need on all this so I don't want to flood you with stuff. Jarrod and Dave have a lot of info that we can supplement your understanding and we can put a briefing or face to face with (DEQ Director Dan) Wyant and (MDHHS Director Nick) Lyon if you want to go there."

SEPT. 25: Detroit Free Press publishes a report about Hanna-Attisha's revelations and quotes MDEQ's Brad Wurfel with yet another deflection: "We're confident with what we've done, but we know there are concerns."

SEPT. 25: "High Importance" emails are now circulating within MDHHS. Rashmi Travis forwards a PowerPoint related to Hanna-Attisha's study to Marc Miller. Miller forwards it to Linda Dykema and Wesley Priem and cautions: "FYI … Don't distribute too broadly." Dykema responds, "It would appear that the Hurley physicians are looking just at younger children, rather than 0-16" as did previous MDHHS analyses of the Flint lead situation.

SEPT. 25: Allison Scott, executive director to Gov. Snyder, sends an email to the governor and key staff. The email suggests the governor's concerns are heightening. Key points:

"Governor spoke with (State Sen. Jim) Ananich this afternoon. He would like to do a call Monday morning with Dennis (Muchmore) and Dan Wyant to get latest and greatest information on this topic. After that will be some combination of he and Wyant speaking with Ananich. Any material on this topic please share over the weekend."

SEPT. 25: Flint issues a lead advisory. "The City of Flint is issuing a Lead Advisory for residents to be aware of lead levels in drinking water after hearing concerns from the medical community. While the city is in full compliance with the Federal Safe Drinking Water Act, this information is being shared as part of a public awareness campaign to ensure that everyone takes note that no level of lead is considered safe."

SEPT. 25: Email from MDHHS Deputy Director Geralyn Lasher to Muchmore, Wyant, MDEQ Spokesman Brad Wurfel and others. The email offers continued state agency skepticism of increased lead levels due to Flint water. Key points:

"MDHHS epidemiologists continue to review the 'data' provided by a Hurley Hospital physician that showed an increase in lead activity following the change in water supply. While we continue to review this data, we have stated publicly that Hurley conducted their analysis in a much different way than we do at the department. Hurley used two partial years of data, MDHHS looked at five comprehensive years and saw no increase outside the normal seasonal increases. The Hurley review was also a much smaller sample than MDHHS data as ours includes all hospital systems in Flint as well as outside laboratories."

"We have also provided the attached data chart that outlines if the elevated blood lead levels were being driven by change in water, we would have seen the elevated levels remain high after the change in water source."

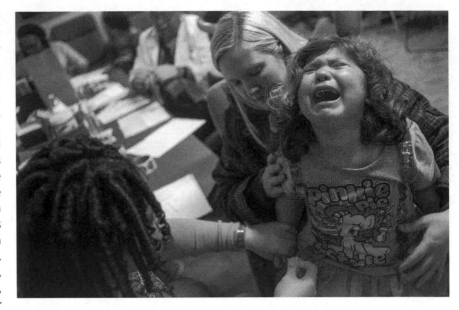

Getting her finger pricked was a scary experience for 5-year-old Gabriella Venegas. Her blood was taken for a lead test on Feb. 8, 2016. Dr. Mona Hanna-Attisha used blood-test results like these to prove that the percentage of children with elevated lead levels had more than doubled in Flint. Gabriella's mother, Sarah Truesdail, said her daughter had been having stomachaches. "I'm thinking she doesn't have lead poisoning, but it's just worrying me."

Jake May/MLive.com

The MDHHS charts further question the assertion of elevated lead levels being due to the Flint water change. Lead paint is another cause of elevated lead levels, with data suggesting routine elevations in warmer months due to more lead paint chips/dust being in the air. The charts suggested lead levels "remained fairly steady" over the past five years, including before and after the water shift.… "If elevated blood levels were being driven by the change in water, we would expect to see the elevated levels remain high after the change in water source, rather than follow the seasonal pattern as they did by decreasing in the fall months."

SEPT. 25: While Lasher tells the governor's chief of staff and other top officials that MDHHS continues to review the Flint doctor's "data," there's a flurry of emails the same day within the MDHHS with several people seemingly not sure what to do:

MDHHS's Sarah Lyon-Callo emails the coverage of Hanna-Attisha's announcement to several colleagues.

Linda Dykema responds: "Do we have a copy of the doctor's Flint study?"

Lyon-Callo responds: "Just the powerpoint online, which I can't download."

Despite growing media attention and many Flint residents bordering on panic, there's not an apparent sense of urgency among MDHHS employees now involved. At 5:33 p.m. on that Friday afternoon, MDHHS employee Cristin Larder emails colleagues Angela Minicuci, Sara Lyon-Callo and Patricia McKane: "After looking at the data Kristi sent you and talking with Sarah, I realize I do not have access to the data I need to answer her specific question about significance. I won't be able to get access before Monday. Sorry I wasn't able to be helpful right now." Angela Minicuci responds. "Not a problem. Let's connect on Monday."

SEPT. 26: Email from Muchmore to the governor and other key staffers. More politics.

"(U.S. Rep. Dale) Kildee is engaged in his normal press hound routine, which is unfortunate because he's a really smart, talented guy who needs to roll up his sleeves while (State Sen. Jim) Ananich is looking for relief but doesn't know where it would come from and is as usual a positive force. Frankly, I think both know that (Flint Mayor Dayne) Walling went out on CYA effort due to the election, but of course can't say so. Neither has any idea where his $30M figure came from, or where we would get it even if you were so inclined."

"The water certainly has occasional less than savory aspects like color because of the apparently more corrosive aspects of the hard water coming from the river, but that has died down with the additional main filters. Taste and smell have been problems also and substantial money has been extended to work on those issues."

"Now we have the anti everything group turning to the lead content which is a concern for everyone, but DEQ and DHHS and EPA can't find evidence of a major change per Geralyn's memo below. Of course, some of the Flint people respond by looking for someone to blame instead of working to reduce anxiety. We can't tolerate increased lead levels in any event, but it's really the city's water system that needs to deal with it. We're throwing as much assistance as possible at the lead problem as regardless of what the levels, explanations or proposed solutions, the residents and particularly the poor need help to deal with it."

TRUTH SQUAD ANALYSIS: The governor's chief of staff is clearly hearing the explanations of the state agencies (MDEQ and MDHHS) charged with protecting drinking water and public health. But he's apparently not hearing Virginia Tech's Marc Edwards and Dr. Hanna-Attisha. As events unfold in coming weeks, it will become clear that Muchmore is hearing the wrong people when he writes these words in late September:

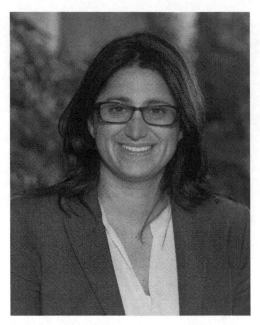

Dr. Mona Hanna-Attisha,
Hurley Medical Center
pediatrician

Photo courtesy Michigan
State University College of
Medicine

"It seems that continuing to find funds to buy local residents home filters is really a viable option and Harvey and all are pursuing more assistance in that work. Almost all the 'experts' I've talked to are convinced the problem is in the old lines leading to homes and short of a massive replacement CSO type bond that wouldn't resolve the issue for a couple of years, nature (temp reductions), filters and a final connect seem to be the best courses of action. The residents are caught in a swirl of misinformation and long term distrust of local government unlikely to be resolved."

SEPT. 28: Associated Press publishes another quote attributed to MDEQ's Brad Wurfel, who contends the water controversy is turning into "near hysteria." And, "I wouldn't call them irresponsible. I would call them unfortunate," Wurfel said of the Hurley doctors' comments. "Flint's drinking water is safe in that it's meeting state and federal standards. The system has an aging portion that needs to be addressed. They haven't had meaningful maintenance for four decades or more."

SEPT. 28: Letter from State Sen. Ananich to Snyder: "It is completely unacceptable that respected scientific experts and our trusted local physicians have verified that the City of Flint's drinking water is dangerous for our citizens, especially our most vulnerable young people." Ananich calls for: 1) Switching water back to DWSD until KWA is ready; 2) Corrosion control; 3) Filters and bottled water assistance; 4) A long-term commitment to address outdated infrastructure.

Pediatrician's study links water switch to lead in children's blood

Dr. Mona Hanna-Attisha's study of lead exposure among Flint children showed the percentage of children under five years old with elevated blood-lead levels (more than five micrograms per deciliter) more than doubled after the water source switch. Hanna-Attisha's study released in September 2015, found the highest percentage of children with elevated blood-lead levels and the most dramatic increase after the water switch were in zip codes 48503 and 48504 in southwestern Flint. Those findings correspond with the study of lead in tap water by professor Marc Edwards of Virginia Tech. The two zip codes have among the highest concentrations of poverty and African-American residents.

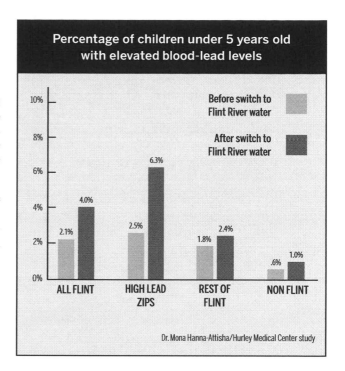

Percentage of children under 5 years old with elevated blood-lead levels

Before switch to Flint River water

After switch to Flint River water

Dr. Mona Hanna-Attisha/Hurley Medical Center study

SEPT. 28: While Ananich is demanding answers from the governor, MDHHS Director Nick Lyon is seeking help within his department to seemingly fight the Hurley/Virginia Tech research. He writes in a 7:52 a.m. email: "I need an analysis of the Virginia Tech/Hurley data and their conclusions. I would like to make a strong statement with a demonstration of proof that the lead blood levels seen are not out of the ordinary and are attributable to seasonal fluctuations. Geralyn (Lasher) is working on this for me but she needs someone in public health who can work directly with her on immediate concerns/questions."

SEPT. 28: Genesee County Health Officer Mark Valacak demands answers via email to Mark Miller and Rashmi Travis at MDHHS: "I want to know whether you have confirmed with the lead program staff at MDHHS that the state results that purport that lead levels have not shown a significant increase since the changeover of the water supply for the city of Flint indeed represent Flint city zip codes only and not Flint mailing addresses. As I mentioned to you both this morning, Flint mailing addresses include outlying areas like Flint and Mundy Townships which obtain their water from the Detroit water authority." Valacak presses the next morning … "Any results yet?" Twenty minutes later Miller responds, says he's checking on it, but no, there are no results yet.

SEPT. 28: Another staff briefing email on which the governor is copied. How does the state decide if the water is creating a lead problem? "Compliance with the federal lead rule is based on a 90th percentile calculation. If more than 10 percent of samples report lead above the federal action level of 15 parts per billion, a water supply has an 'action level exceedance.' An exceedance is not a violation. It triggers other requirements which could include public notification, additional water quality sampling, and possibly further treatment. While some of Flint's individual samples exceeded 15 parts per billion lead action level, compliance is based on the 90th percentile of samples. The City of Flint's 90th percentile level has ranged from 0 parts per billion in 2008 and 2011 and 15 parts per billion in 1992, but never exceeded the action level. The two most recent sampling periods, in 2014 and 2015, were 6 parts per billion and 11 parts per billion, respectively."

The memo further states that it would take 15 years to replace more than 15,000 lead service lines in the Flint water system at a cost of $60 million or more, plus up to $8,000 more per homeowner to replace lead connections on private property from city lines to residential taps.

> **TRUTH SQUAD ANALYSIS:** The governor is still getting guidance from his administration that Flint's lead levels are not out of compliance with drinking water standards. This is seven months after EPA's Del Toral first raises alarms, weeks after Virginia Tech's Edwards reports deeply troubling independent lead test results in Flint, four days after Hurley Dr. Hanna-Attisha releases research concluding major increases in Flint children's blood lead levels after the Flint River switch, and three days after the City of Flint has issued its own lead advisory to the public.

SEPT. 29: Kristi Tanner and Nancy Kaffer at the Detroit Free Press publish their own analysis of the state's blood-lead data in Flint: "Data that the State of Michigan released last week to refute a hospital researcher's claim that an increasing number of Flint children have been lead-poisoned since the city switched its water supply actually supports the hospital's findings, a Free Press analysis has shown. Worse, prior to the water supply change, the number of lead-poisoned kids in Flint, and across the state, had been dropping; the reversal of that trend should prompt state public health officials to examine a brewing public health crisis."

> **TRUTH SQUAD ANALYSIS:** The Free Press report comes the morning after MDHHS Director Nick Lyon issues his directive that he wants an analysis that makes "a strong statement with a demonstration of proof that the lead blood levels seen are not out of the ordinary and are attributable to seasonal fluctuations."

SEPT. 29, 10:45 A.M.: Email from Executive Director to the Governor Allison Scott to top Snyder aides Dennis Muchmore, Jarrod Agen, Beth Clement, Dan Wyant and Nick Lyon. The email shows the governor may now finally be rising above months of state agency deflections, shifting his focus to the Hurley results, and beginning to use the term "emergency." Key points:

"You will be receiving a meeting notice from Beth Emmit for a meeting with the Governor this afternoon. Listed below are areas that we should provide him an update on engagement; if not yet engaged, then we need to engage asap.

"1. Emergency management – similar to disasters, is there some form of action we can engage for this situation to help manage.

"2. Chief Medical officer – should be speaking with Hurley

"3. WIC – re water and formula – status update

"4. Drain commissioner – how do we expedite KWA."

SEPT. 29: Genesee County Health Supervisor Jim Henry emails Michelle Bruneau at MDHHS regarding ongoing lead education plans and the growing street-level despair in Flint:

"Today, I talked to a 46-year-old man who told me that he and his dog have not drank water or anything else, since he ran out of bottled water two days ago…. In general, the most immediate concern seems to be the unknown lead levels and the cost to reduce or eliminate the risk."

Bruneau forwards the email to colleague Kory Groetsch with commentary: "Wow … this is just sad. It sounds like third world country, but it's here and in our backyard. At what point can EPA/ATSDR step in and provide resources?"

SEPT. 29, 12:06 P.M.: MDHHS Deputy Director Geralyn Lasher circulates to department colleagues an advisory from Genesee County indicating that the locals are taking matters in their own hands, demanding fresh analysis of state blood-level data from DCH, and threatening to seek third-party analysis of the state data DCH has consistently used to suggest no elevated blood-lead levels due to the Flint water.

"The county is prepared to take further action if the State fails to provide the requested data by September 30, 2015. Further action could include a request for outside independent evaluation of the data and to declare a Public Health Emergency in Flint."

Lasher writes: "I uderstand that we are still reviewing the data – but the county has basically issued a ransom date that they want this information by tomorrow.… Eden – please coordinate an answer so Nick can walk into the 1 p.m. (meeting with the governor) prepared on this."

SEPT. 29: Gov. Snyder receives a detailed timeline by email on all Flint water events from 2012 forward. It is prepared by the Michigan Department of Treasury and its findings are fully represented throughout this Truth Squad timeline.

SEPT. 29: Email from MDHHS Deputy Director Lasher to Nancy Peeler, Eden Wells (the state's chief medical officer), Robert Scott, and others at MDHHS:

"Is it possible to get the same type of data for just children under the age of six? So basically, the city of Flint kids ages six and under with the same type of approach as the attached chart you gave us last week?"

A response, less than an hour later, from Linda Dykema to Corinne Miller, Sara Lyon-Callo and Eden Wells:

"It's bad enough to have a data war with outside entities, we absolutely cannot engage in competing data analyses within the Department, or, heaven forbid, in public releases."

Moments later, Eden Wells responds: "Agree."

SEPT. 29, 12:25 P.M.: On the same day there's worry in MDHHS about a "data war," Dr. Hanna-Attisha emails MDHHS Chief Medical Officer Eden Wells with clear, updated findings of the Hurley study. Using geographic information system software, Hurley has isolated blood-level results just in the city of Flint, especially in high-risk areas of the city (something the state analysis has not yet done).

In the two highest-risk wards, Hanna-Attisha reports in this email, "the elevated blood-lead level percentage more than tripled." Wells responds in an email two hours later and says the state is working on replicating the analysis, and wants to know when Hurley is going public with its results.

Hanna-Attisha responds: "Our intent has never been to go public with anything. However, when we noticed our findings and the glaring correlation to elevated water lead levels in the same locations and learned that corrosion control was never added to the water treatment, we ethically could not stay silent. In addition, your annual elevated blood level percentage supports our findings – annual decrease (as seen nationally) and then an increase post-water switch. We also knew that releasing our data would only incite a data war; however, the more we dig, the more alarming the results. (Do you know GM stopped using Flint River water because it was too corrosive on their parts??? That should have alerted us to its effect on lead pipes.)"

TRUTH SQUAD ANALYSIS: In other words, this Flint physician (with groundwork by Virginia Tech) put all the pieces together – in contrast to months of inaction and denial by the two state agencies charged with protecting public health and drinking water.

That same evening, Wells responds again: "I certainly understand your role and the need to address the problem you identified; as physicians, our ethical and professional vows to care for and prevent harm to our patients is paramount. No need for data wars – I think we are all just trying to be sure, as you and I said earlier, that we are comparing the same data the same way – 'apples to apples.'"

SEPT. 29: Genesee County issues a health advisory for Flint water.

SEPT. 30: Mayor Dayne Walling receives fierce criticism for his repeated declarations that Flint River water was safe. Fr. Phil Schmitter, one of several concerned religious figures in Flint, writes: "You delayed your action on this issue for an inordinate amount of time. People were told over and over that it was all fine.... I no longer trust the city on this issue. And that we have now a lead problem for babies and children is unconscionable."

Walling forwards the email directly to MDEQ Director Dan Wyant and says, "I have searched myself over and over on this. I don't know what more I could have done given the guidance coming from EPA and DEQ and subsequently city staff but this major health issue did come up anyway and our community is paying a huge price. As the press conference is put together, it is necessary in my mind that we provide an explanation for how this happened and outline the steps that ensure it will never happen again."

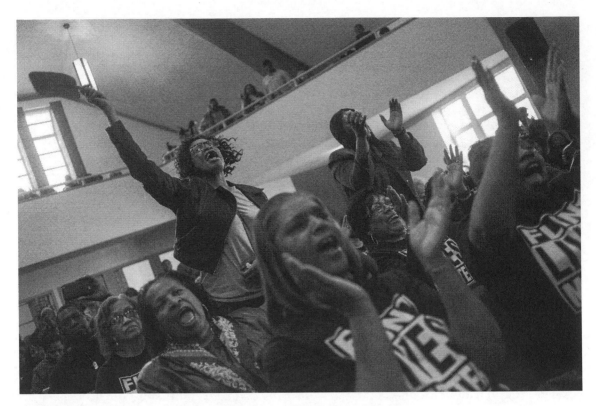

The Flint Water Advisory Task Force cited the protests of Flint's residents as important in forcing state regulators and the Snyder administration to acknowledge the water disaster. In the photograph, Flint resident Sharon Moore, back left, leaps in support as pastor David Bullock speaks during a town hall meeting on Feb. 1, 2016, at First Trinity Missionary Baptist Church.

Photo credit: Jake May/MLive.com

CHAPTER 13

THE PERSISTENT, HEROIC FOUR ... AND OTHERS

THEY CHANGED THE FLINT NARRATIVE

By Bob Campbell
"Poison on Tap" Editor

"The Flint water crisis is also a story, however, of something that did work: the critical role played by engaged Flint citizens, by individuals both inside and outside of government who had the expertise and willingness to question and challenge government leadership, and by members of a free press who used the tools that enable investigative journalism. Without their courage and persistence, this crisis likely never would have been brought to light and mitigation efforts never begun."

This observation in the Flint Water Advisory Task Force's final report is a brilliant summary of the role citizens, scientists, a pediatrician, at least one bureaucrat, many journalists and others played in resisting the official pronouncements that Flint's water was safe.

That's why we pause from our analysis of the crisis to recognize those who stepped up and pushed back because they knew the stained, smelly, awful-tasting water coming from Flint taps was wrong. And maybe dangerous. They were right.

We highlight:

LEE-ANNE WALTERS, the mother of four, who insisted on lead tests of her tap water that ultimately began a process that confirmed suspicions that something sinister was happening inside the pipes carrying the treated Flint River water to thousands of homes like hers.

MIGUEL DEL TORAL, the U.S. Environmental Protection Agency drinking-water regulations manager in Chicago. He got wind of the lead results from Walters' home and began pressing Michigan's Department of Environmental Quality for answers on what measures it required of Flint water plant operators to prevent lead from leaching from the city's old pipes after the switch to Flint River water.

MARC EDWARDS, a Virginia Tech professor and nationally recognized expert on lead issues in public water systems. Del Toral put Walters in touch with Edwards, who soon began community-wide water sampling that revealed lead contamination in tap water far greater than the city's flawed testing.

DR. MONA HANNA-ATTISHA, a Flint pediatrician. Even after Del Toral's questioning and Edwards' results, MDEQ officials remained dismissive of lead concerns until Hanna-Attisha's study showed lead in the blood of vulnerable young children had more than doubled in two zip codes after the switch to Flint River-sourced drinking water. Within days of her study's release, the state accepted the crisis and Gov. Rick Snyder ordered Flint to return to Lake Huron water.

THE HUNDREDS OF CITIZENS, PASTORS, COMMUNITY ACTIVISTS, NON-PROFIT AGENCIES AND OTHERS who carried jugs of yellow- and brown-stained water to the streets and public meetings and demanded action, and those who coordinated and led efforts to provide bottled water and filters, medical screenings and other help for residents.

JOURNALISTS who shined the light of attention on Flint. Of special note: Reporter Ron Fonger and photographer Jake May of the Flint Journal/MLive.com, who pressed the issue before others noticed; Curt Guyette, an ACLU investigative reporter who broke the lead story; Detroit Free Press columnist Nancy Kaffer, who was the clear opinion leader on the Flint story with eloquent, tough, solidly-reported pieces; and Lindsey Smith of Michigan Radio for her documentary "Not Safe to Drink" and other stories.

A TENACIOUS FLINT MOM WARNED, RALLIED A PUBLIC

By Ted Roelofs
Bridge Magazine Contributor

Until a few years ago, Lee-Anne Walters was your classic stay-at-home mom.

With four children, Walters split her time between home-schooling her young twin sons, cooking lasagna or mozzarella chicken dinners and scurrying to football and basketball games or choir concerts for her older kids. In spare moments, she'd sneak in a TV crime show or some scrap-booking.

Things changed one night in late December 2014, when she and her husband, Dennis, loaded the dishwasher. She turned on the tap and watched a stream of orange-brown water spill out.

"'I'm like, 'What is going on here?'" Walters recalled.

Walters wasn't deterred as she waited months for an answer. That came as no surprise to Darrick Puffer, Walters' former teacher at a high school bordering Flint.

"She was tenacious," said Darrick Puffer, who had Walters in English literature and journalism classes. "It was her personality to say, 'You're not going to pull the wool over my eyes.'" Her attitude helped her as news editor of the school paper her senior year and again as the Flint water crisis unfolded.

"She would stand up for the little guy. If someone was being bullied and maybe that person was a little shy, she would say, 'Cut that out. We don't treat people that way,'" Puffer said.

Walters and her husband, a career Navy enlistee, worried before the tap water turned brown. The previous summer, every time she bathed her twins, Garrett and Gavin, their skin erupted with small red bumps. At times, a scale of red skin formed on Gavin's chest as he soaked in the tub.

Flint officials insisted nothing was amiss. In April 2014, Flint had switched from the Detroit water system, which draws water from Lake Huron, to the Flint River to save money while waiting for completion of a new pipeline to

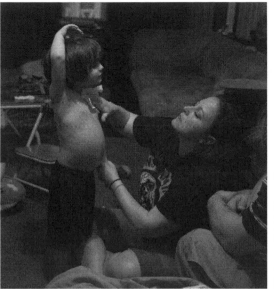

Photo credit: Brittany Greeson

LEE-ANNE WALTERS BATHES HER SON GAVIN WITH BOTTLED WATER.

Lake Huron. Unknown to most Flint citizens, state Department of Environmental Quality regulators failed to mandate corrosion controls that experts say was needed to prevent lead from leaching from the city's water service lines.

"The city water is safe to drink," Flint Mayor Dayne Walling said at a press conference. "My family and I drink it and use it every day."

After that December day when the water color changed, her family drank only bottled water. She protested outside city hall. At a January public hearing, she held up a bottle of her discolored tap water.

A month later, after Walters complained, the city sent an employee to test her water. A few days later, she had a voice message from the water department. "Please, whatever you do, don't let your kids drink the water," she recalled it saying.

Federal water standards require intervention when testing shows at least 10 percent of homes with known lead delivery pipes have at least 15 parts per billion lead in tap water. There is no safe level for lead in children, and the Centers for Disease Control calls for intervention at blood-lead levels above five micrograms per deciliter.

Lead is a neurotoxin, linked to lower test scores. The first city test in Walters' home found lead at 104 ppb. A few weeks later, a water sample found 397 ppb – a whopping 26 times the standard.

Walters went door-to-door, warning neighbors and others.

"Some of them called me crazy," she said.

By then, Walters had immersed herself in researching the hazards of lead in water – and what it could mean for her children. She had them tested and Gavin's lead blood level was 6.5 micrograms per deciliter. During the height of the water crisis, Gavin stopped gaining weight and developed anemia, conditions Walters attributes to lead poisoning.

As Walters tried to rally public concern, officials maintained all was right. Then emergency manager Jerry Ambrose expressed concern in a March 2015 memo to a state Treasury department official that switching back to the Detroit water system could cost $12 million a year, stating: "I am satisfied that the water provided to Flint users today is within all MDEQ and EPA guidelines, as evidenced by the most recent water quality tests conducted by MDEQ."

Walters contacted a U.S. Environmental Protection Agency official in Chicago – Miguel Del Toral – who proved to be a singular voice of alarm within that agency over lead in Flint's water.

Del Toral suggested she contact Virginia Tech professor Marc Edwards, a leading national expert on lead and drinking water. Edwards was a key figure in uncovering treatment failures in the Washington, D.C. water system that led to widespread lead contamination from 2001 to 2004.

Walters said she already knew the name from her online research.

"I stumbled across Marc Edwards online. He was the only person I could find who did anything about lead in water," Walters said.

In April 2015, she called Edwards. She was frantic.

"We knew our family had been exposed to lead. We needed help," she said.

It was a pivotal moment, as Edwards assembled researchers and headed to Flint to conduct their own water tests. Edwards, like Del Toral, feared the MDEQ had skewed test results downward by allowing Flint officials to flush water lines before collecting samples.

His team's results, released in early September, showed much higher lead levels in water samples, including an April result from Walters' tap exceeding 13,000 ppb. It turned out that the lead service line to the home connected to another street instead of the water main in front of her home. The April sample was collected about three weeks after the city cut water to the home – as a safety precaution.

Edwards' bombshell was followed about three weeks later by a Flint pediatrician's release of a study that showed levels of lead in the blood of young children had more than doubled in some Flint zip codes since the Flint River became the city's drinking water source.

Finally, the push back that began with Walters' demands for answers had overcome state resistance. On Oct. 2, Gov. Rick Snyder announced a "comprehensive plan" to address Flint's water crisis. A couple of weeks later, Flint reconnected to the Detroit water system.

Later that month, Walters moved with her family to Virginia after her husband received a transfer.

But she was far from finished with the battle in Flint or her broader advocacy for children facing lead poisoning. She now splits time between her new home, Flint and other battlegrounds. She has consulted this year with Philadelphians concerned about lead in their water. She's also testified before congressional and legislative committees investigating the Flint crisis.

"The only regret I have is that people didn't listen sooner. People say this is such a victory. This is never a victory. Too many people were hurt."

As the saga of Flint's poisoned water first crept into headlines, high school teacher Puffer remembered hearing Lee-Anne Walters' name and not being surprised.

"I realized that her water problems were sort of the epicenter of this issue. I thought, if it's going to happen to somebody, at least when it happens to her, she's going to push for answers.

"That's Lee-Anne."

'ROGUE' EPA EMPLOYEE PUT HIS CAREER AT RISK

By Ted Roelofs
Bridge Magazine Contributor

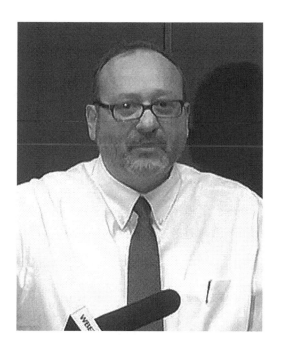

"Rogue employee" was how the chief spokesman for Michigan's Department of Environmental Quality described Miguel Del Toral in September 2015.

Del Toral might accept the label with pride.

In the Flint water crisis, Del Toral, a public water-supply regulations manager for the Great Lakes office of the U.S. Environmental Protection Agency, emerged as the only hero who is also a government bureaucrat.

He may be a reluctant hero (he declined requests for an interview), but others have been singing his praises.

"Miguel Del Toral called it right from the beginning," said Ken Sikkema, who co-chaired a Michigan task force on Flint's water crisis. The task force's final report in March 2016 described Flint's story as one of "government failure, intransigence, unpreparedness, delay, inaction and environmental injustice."

Del Toral, by contrast, "had this very clear vision about what was wrong and what needed to be done," said Sikkema, a former Michigan legislator.

> "THIS IS NO SURPRISE. LEAD LINES + NO TREATMENT = HIGH LEAD IN WATER = POISONED CHILDREN."
>
> — MIGUEL DEL TORAL

Neither the state DEQ nor his EPA bosses listened to Del Toral, Sikkema said, "but it didn't stop him. In the face of that kind of indifference, he did not go quietly into that good night."

In April 2014, Flint switched as a cost-saving measure from the Detroit water system to the Flint River as its source. Within weeks, residents complained about discolored, smelly and foul-tasting water spilling from their taps.

Del Toral was among the first to raise a red flag. In February 2015, Del Toral warned the MDEQ and EPA that Flint's lead levels were higher than was being reported because local officials were flushing water through pipes before taking samples. He asked whether MDEQ required Flint's water plant to use corrosion control to reduce potential leaching of lead from lead service lines.

He was assured Flint was using corrosion control. Two months later, MDEQ admitted there was no corrosion control.

In June, Del Toral wrote an eight-page memo to his supervisor at EPA, noting Flint still had no corrosion control, calling it a "serious concern for residents that live in homes with lead service lines or partial lead service lines, which are common throughout the City of Flint." He reiterated that pre-flushing pipes caused "significant underestimation of lead levels in the drinking water."

Del Toral knew that lead is a neurotoxin especially hazardous to brain and nervous-system development in young children. At one point, the Detroit News reported, he offered to pay his own expenses to travel to Flint and conduct water tests without pre-flushing.

He jeopardized his career when he gave a copy of his draft memo to Lee-Anne Walters, because it included details about her home and children. Her water lead levels were off the scale and, at that time, lead in the blood of one her children had tripled since the switch to Flint River water. Walters, in turn, leaked the memo to a reporter. The lead levels measured in Walters' water, Del Toral told an NPR reporter in January 2015, were "the absolute highest I've ever seen.... Those numbers blew my mind."

A few days after Del Toral wrote the memo, EPA Region 5 chief Susan Hedman told Flint Mayor Dayne Walling, who had received an interview request from the reporter, that: "The preliminary draft report should not have been released outside the agency." She added that it would be vetted and edited. Walling, apparently feeling reassured, went on a local television station the following week and drank Flint water at the dare of a reporter.

Meanwhile, Brad Wurfel, the MDEQ spokesman who would later call Del Toral a "rogue employee," dismissed Del Toral's report, telling a Michigan Radio reporter: "Anyone who is concerned about lead in the drinking water in Flint can relax." Wurfel later resigned in disgrace.

In an interview with Michigan Radio in January, Del Toral said he first learned that the city wasn't using corrosion control from Walters. He couldn't believe it. "It's inconceivable that someone would not require the treatment in the first place."

Del Toral did not respond to interview requests from Bridge Magazine. Julia Valentine, a spokesperson for EPA, said: "His preference is to return to his primary focus of fixing the problem in Flint and ensuring that the upcoming switch to the new water source is done properly."

The words Del Toral wrote in a September 2015 memo confirmed what he saw coming: "This is no surprise. Lead lines + no treatment = high lead in water = poisoned children."

VIRGINIA TECH PROFESSOR AND HIS TEAM FORCED THE HAND OF STATE OFFICIALS

By Ted Roelofs
Bridge Magazine Contributor

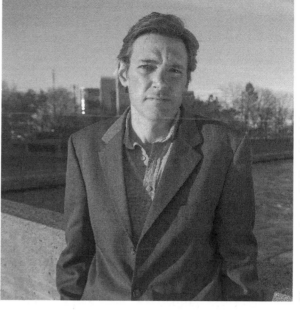

Photo courtesy Logan Wallace/Virginia Tech

With tousled brown hair and glasses, at times soft-spoken, Marc Edwards seems like a mild-mannered professor.

Don't be fooled. As bureaucrats in Michigan and with the U.S. Environmental Protection Agency know, Edwards' actions and words pack a punch.

In early 2015, Edwards, a professor of civil engineering at Virginia Tech, heard from a friend at the EPA about a "problem in Flint" regarding its water. Then he got a frantic phone call from a Flint mother who was worried about brown water coming from her tap.

Edwards had been through water wars before, when he tackled the EPA, the Centers for Disease Control and the local water authority over lead contamination in the Washington D.C. water system. Edwards eventually proved that a change in chemical treatments led to dangerous lead levels in the water, contradicting initial findings of the CDC. A U.S. House committee concluded in 2010 that the CDC had made "scientifically indefensible" claims about the safety of the water.

After what happened there, Edwards told Bridge Magazine: "I knew another water lead crisis was inevitable."

It could have been in Flint, or any older city carrying drinking water through old lead mains.

Over the phone, Edwards carefully instructed the Flint mom, Lee-Anne Walters, on how to draw her water samples. She mailed them to him the next day.

The findings were among the highest he'd ever seen.

> "SOMEONE HAS TO DO SOMETHING TO STOP THESE INJUSTICES. PROFESSORS COULD DO A LOT MORE. REPORTERS COULD DO A BETTER JOB TAKING ON AUTHORITY AND SCIENTIFIC CONTROVERSIES. WE ALL NEED TO HOLD THESE AGENCIES ACCOUNTABLE."
>
> **— MARC EDWARDS**

Though he shared his findings with the EPA, Edwards sensed another brush-off. In July 2015, Flint Mayor Dayne Walling drank from a cup of city water in front of TV cameras and proclaimed it safe. Officials with the Michigan Department of Environmental Quality insisted lead was not an issue.

Edwards assembled a team of two dozen scientists and students to conduct independent tests of Flint's water. He was concerned the city's switch in April 2014 from Lake Huron to the corrosive Flint River as a water source was endangering residents, especially vulnerable young children, by leaching lead from pipes into the system.

He also believed the city's lead test results were deceivingly low, in part because officials flushed out water lines before collecting samples. Their results, he said, were "smoke and mirrors."

Federal regulations require water utilities to certify that 90 percent of homes in a community contain 15 parts-per-billion of lead or less in drinking water.

In September, Edwards published results that included samples exceeding 100 ppb and one exceeding 1,000 ppb. An early test of Walters' water found levels exceeding 13,000 ppb. Water with lead levels above 5,000 ppb is considered hazardous waste.

Coupled with the findings of a Flint physician that blood lead levels among Flint children in high-risk zip codes had doubled, even tripled, since the water-source switch, the reports forced the hand of state officials and Gov. Rick Snyder. In October 2015, Snyder ordered a switch back to the Detroit water system, which gets its water from Lake Huron.

Chris Kolb, who co-chaired a task force report on Flint's water crisis, credits Edwards as a key player in uncovering the scale of the problem.

"He was extremely important," said Kolb, president of the Michigan Environmental Council. "The state was putting out this narrative that everything was fine; that there was no problem with lead in the water; that you didn't have to worry. Marc's results said that you did.

"Marc is someone you want on your side. We owe him a debt of gratitude."

As a professor, Edwards insists that words in the classroom must be backed up by real world deeds. Edwards was a 2008 winner of a MacArthur genius grant – $500,000 to use as he saw fit. He poured the cash into his battle over the Washington D.C. water system. As of spring 2016, he was still raising money for his Flint research.

In March, Edwards was named Number 31 on Fortune magazine's list of the World's Greatest Leaders for his efforts in Flint. He also was named on one of the world's 100 most influential people by Time magazine. He appeared twice in 2016 before a congressional committee investigating the Flint crisis and was one of the few panelists whose work was praised by members of both political parties.

His most stinging critique was aimed at EPA leaders, especially resigned Region 5 administrator Susan Hedman and the agency's top administrator Gina McCarthy, for denying any responsibility for failing Flint's citizens. Hedman, he testified, "aided, abetted and emboldened the unethical behavior of civil servants" at the MDEQ.

In an interview with Bridge Magazine, Edwards explained his motivation: "Someone has to do something to stop these injustices. Professors could do a lot more. Reporters could do a better job taking on authority and scientific controversies. We all need to hold these agencies accountable."

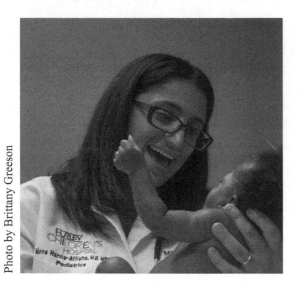

Photo by Brittany Greeson

DOCTOR DID HER OWN TESTS TO PROVE WATER'S DANGER

By Chastity Pratt Dawsey
Bridge Magazine

Since her parents moved to Michigan from England when she was 5 years old, Dr. Mona Hanna-Attisha has always lived within a few hours' ride of Flint.

Her interests in health and social issues inspired Hanna-Attisha to pursue a major in environmental health at the University of Michigan where she conducted research on environmental justice – the concept that people of different race, heritage and financial circumstance deserve fair treatment in the development and enforcement of public environmental policy.

They are issues entrenched in the Flint water crisis.

After medical school at Michigan State University and several years at the Children's Hospital of Michigan in Detroit, Hanna-Attisha became director of the pediatric residency program at the College of Human Medicine at Hurley Medical Center in Flint.

In August 2015, a high school friend came to her house for dinner. Elin Betanzo, a senior policy analyst and source-water expert at the Northeast Midwest Institute, told Hanna-Attisha she had heard the city of Flint didn't use corrosion control when it switched to the Flint River as its water source in 2014.

That meant the city wasn't treating its drinking water to reduce its ability to chemically disintegrate a protective layer inside old lead pipes and allow lead particles to leach into the water and end up in the bodies of vulnerable and unsuspecting Flint citizens.

Hanna-Attisha was seeing patients and their parents at Hurley complaining of rashes and hair loss since the water source switch.

> "IT'S NOT THAT I WAS NAÏVE TO START WITH, BUT YOU'D EXPECT THAT UTILITIES, STATES, FEDERAL AGENCIES WOULD TAKE THEIR JOBS SERIOUSLY AND TRY TO PROTECT PEOPLE RATHER THAN DELIBERATELY MISLEAD, LIE AND MAKE UP EXCUSES NOT TO PROTECT PUBLIC HEALTH."
>
> — DR. MONA HANNA-ATTISHA

Angered at the possibility of widespread lead poisoning, Hanna-Attisha began comparing lead-blood test results in children before and after the switch. She told CNN it was "the easiest research project I've ever done."

She reviewed Hurley's records, which included 1,746 tests from Flint children. The data showed that the number of Flint children with elevated lead levels had nearly doubled from 2.1 percent to 4 percent after the water switch. In one zip code, lead levels exceeding 5 milligrams per deciliter – the federal standard for health intervention – jumped from 2.5 percent of children tested to 6.3 percent.

On Sept. 24, 2015, Hanna-Attisha released her findings. Within days, a spokesman for the Michigan Department of Environmental Quality said the water crisis was becoming "near hysteria" and called Hanna-Attisha's comments on her findings "unfortunate." The doctor second-guessed herself in the face of public criticism.

"I think my heart rate went up to 200. You know, you check and you double-check, and you know your research is right," she told CNN. "The numbers didn't lie, but when the state is telling you you're wrong, it's hard not to second-guess yourself."

The Michigan Department of Health and Human Services initially miscalculated lead-poisoning data and helped delay discovery of the lead crisis in Flint. Their subsequent review of Hanna-Attisha's results concluded she was right.

While EPA's Miguel Del Toral and Virginia Tech's Marc Edwards had pressed for answers and found high lead levels in the tap water that set the stage for proving state regulators wrong, Hanna-Attisha's research was the *coup de grace*.

She proved that real Flint kids undeniably were getting much higher doses of lead, suggesting that harm to their health would follow. The state recanted and changes came rapidly.

In an interview with the Huffington Post in January, Hanna-Attisha said the Flint crisis "has really shattered my trust in government."

"It's not that I was naïve to start with, but you'd expect that utilities, states, federal agencies would take their jobs seriously and try to protect people rather than deliberately mislead, lie and make up excuses not to protect public health."

In its May 2, 2016, issue, Time Magazine cited Hanna-Attisha and Marc Edwards in its annual list of the world's most influential people for their work in Flint. It's clear they had earned the trust of an increasingly skeptical citizenry.

"People say 'Oh, you're a hero, you did amazing work,' and my response is: This is my job – this is the job of a pediatrician," Hanna-Attisha told Medpage Today. "It is our job to be the voice of the voiceless."

A COMMUNITY OF HEROES HELPED REVEAL FLINT'S POISONED WATER

By Chastity Pratt Dawsey
Bridge Magazine

Flint stood up for itself long before anyone else would.

Almost immediately after the city's water source was switched to Flint River water in April 2014, residents began lugging jugs of discolored tap water to public meetings to demand a fix. Over the next two years, they called water experts, government agencies and stormed the capitol building in Lansing. Many wore "Flint Lives Matter" T-shirts that became their unofficial uniform of dissent.

Sincere Smith, 2, scarred from rashes linked to bathing in Flint's tap water, became – literally – the face of the crisis. Eight-year-old Amariyanna (Mari) Copeny, known as Little Miss Flint, wrote a letter that lured President Barack Obama to Flint in May 2016, four months after Gov. Rick Snyder tried to get the Flint water crisis declared a federal disaster. The Coalition for Clean Water emerged as residents well-known and unknown joined forces to demand safe water.

Individuals and groups, some well-connected, others born of the crisis, were among Flint's true heroes. The Flint Water Advisory Task Force, appointed by the governor to investigate what happened and why, cited the residents' protests as critical in finally forcing action from the Snyder administration, even as state regulators balked. Their cooperative work and concerns prodded researchers to investigate and prove the link between the water switch and high lead levels in the water and the blood of Flint's children.

Claire McClinton and Nayyirah Shariff of the Flint Democracy Defense League were among those who stepped to the frontlines to organize residents. Shariff helped Virginia Tech researchers distribute 300 water test kits to citizens. The testing proved a lead problem in the tap water of many Flint homes.

In an online interview with GMO Free News, Shariff listed names of residents she considers heroes for their early activism. They included Lee-Anne Walters, Tony Palladino and City Councilman Eric Mays. He also cited help from Bishop Bernadel Jefferson, City Councilman Scott Kincaid and resident Paul Jordan, plaintiffs in a 2013 federal lawsuit challenging the state's emergency manager law.

"We all just kind of came together because we were dissatisfied with what the city was doing," she said.

Melissa Mays was one of the first residents quoted widely in national media about medical problems she and her family suffered. Mays founded Water You Fighting For, an advocacy group. She said she wants to leave Flint, but can't afford to move and won't leave with the crisis unsolved.

"I don't want to leave the people we're fighting with," she told the New York-based news program, Democracy Now.

Mays, the Concerned Pastors for Social Action, the American Civil Liberties Union and the Natural Resources Defense Council, filed a federal lawsuit in January 2016 asking that the state be compelled to ensure safe drinking water in Flint. The activists didn't ask for money. Instead, they want a rescue plan of services to address medical harm Flint residents have suffered.

The local branch of the NAACP and Flint churches also reacted early, organizing rallies and protests with support from high-profile Detroit pastors. The Concerned Pastors for Social Action, a coalition of Flint church leaders, filed a lawsuit in June of 2015 to force the city to switch back to the Detroit water system, months before the lead contamination was confirmed.

Due to his activism, Alfred Harris, president of the Concerned Pastors, was dropped from consideration for an appointment to the city's Receivership Transition Advisory Board, according to an April 2015 email from Snyder's chief of staff, Dennis Muchmore, to Snyder's urban affairs adviser, Harvey Hollins. Harris was penalized for holding a news conference to complain about the lack of progress in solving Flint's water troubles. (Muchmore would later laud the pastors as key supporters for residents in the crisis).

When the emails were publicized in early 2016, Harris told MLive.com: "If it cost me, it cost me. My interest was strictly for the people."

Editor's note: The White House posted the following on its website on April 27, 2016:

At eight years old, Mari Copeny — known around town as "Little Miss Flint" — wrote to President Obama last month from her home in Flint, Michigan to share how she is working to bring attention to the public health crisis in her community. She also noted that she's headed the President's way, and asked if she could meet him during her trip to Washington, D.C. This week, President Obama wrote back to "Little Miss Flint" with some big news: He's coming to town. On Wednesday, May 4th, the President will travel to Flint, Michigan where he will hear first-hand from Flint residents like Mari about the public health crisis, receive an in-person briefing on the federal efforts in place to help respond to the needs of the people of Flint, and speak directly with members of the Flint community.

Read Mari's letter to President Obama, and then check out his reply:

Mr. President,

Hello my name is Mari Copeny and I'm 8 years old, I live in Flint, Michigan and I'm more commonly known around town as "Little Miss Flint". I am one of the children that is effected by this water, and I've been doing my best to march in protest and to speak out for all the kids that live here in Flint. This Thursday I will be riding a bus to Washington, D.C. to watch the congressional hearings of our Governor Rick Snyder. I know this is probably an odd request but I would love for a chance to meet you or your wife. My mom said chances are you will be too busy with more important things, but there is a lot of people coming on these buses and even just a meeting from you or your wife would really lift people's spirits. Thank you for all that do for our country. I look forward to being able to come to Washington and to be able to see Gov. Snyder in person and to be able to be in the city where you live.

Thank You, Mari Copeny

THE WHITE HOUSE
WASHINGTON

April 25, 2016

Amariyanna Copeny
Flint, Michigan

Dear Mari:

Thank you for writing to me. You're right that Presidents are often busy, but the truth is, in America, there is no more important title than citizen. And I am so proud of you for using your voice to speak out on behalf of the children of Flint.

That's why I want you to be the first to know that I'm coming to visit Flint on May 4th. I want to make sure people like you and your family are receiving the help you need and deserve. Like you, I'll use my voice to call for change and help lift up your community.

Letters from kids like you are what make me so optimistic for the future. I hope to meet you next week, "Little Miss Flint."

Sincerely,

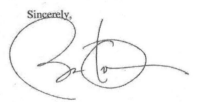

CHAPTER 14

OCTOBER 2015

FLINT STOPS DRINKING FROM THE RIVER

BACK TO DETROIT WATER AS MDEQ BOSS FINALLY ACKNOWLEDGES ERRORS

Editor's summary: In the face of Dr. Mona Hanna-Attisha's study on blood-lead levels since the water switch and professor Marc Edwards' study of lead in tap water, Gov. Rick Snyder moves quickly to order a return to Detroit's far less corrosive Lake Huron-sourced water. Many other steps are taken to help Flint deal with its pain. Later in October, MDEQ Director Dan Wyant acknowledges that his drinking-water staff erred in not requiring corrosion control for Flint River water when the switch was made in April 2014.

AFTER EIGHT MONTHS OF SYSTEMIC DENIAL THROUGHOUT HIS DEPARTMENT, THE MDEQ DIRECTOR FINALLY ADMITS THAT EPA RESEARCHER MIGUEL DEL TORAL WAS RIGHT ALL ALONG.

— TRUTH SQUAD ANALYSIS

TIMELINE: OCTOBER 2015

By John Bebow
Bridge Magazine

2015

OCT. 1: Genesee County Public Health Officials issue an advisory telling Flint residents not to drink the city water.

OCT. 1: MLive.com reports the "city knows which homes in Flint have pipes most likely to leach lead into tap water but can't easily access the information because it's kept on 45,000 index cards." Flint Department of Public Works Director Howard Croft said he can't say how long it will take to put the paper records into an electronic data base to map the lead pipes. "It's on our to-do list," he was quoted.

OCT.1: The Michigan Department of Health and Human Services confirms the results of the Hanna-Attisha/Hurley Medical Center Study (showing greatly increased blood-lead levels in some Flint neighborhoods). A MDHHS "talking points" memo from email records offers more admissions and context, yet the agency is still downplaying the issue in some ways. Key points of the memo:

"Initial analysis of MDHHS data found that blood-lead levels of children in Flint have followed an expected seasonal trend; due to small numbers further analysis was initiated."

"After a comprehensive and detailed review down to the zip code level, we have found that the state analysis is consistent with that presented by Hurley."

"There is an increased proportion of children with elevated blood-lead levels in several zip codes, particularly 03 and 04. These appear to have increased over the past 1.5 years."

Yet more downplaying: "Lead exposure can occur from a number of different sources (such as paint, gasoline, solder, and consumer products) and through different pathways (such as air, food, water, dust and soil.) Although there are several exposure sources, lead-based paint is still the most widespread and dangerous high-dose source of lead exposure for young children."

Finally, more than two months after offering a far-less complete analysis, MDHHS follows Hurley's methodology and discovers the same problem: "We reviewed MDHHS statewide data using the same methodology used by Hurley, looking at our numbers by zip code and age ranges, and filtering out non-Flint

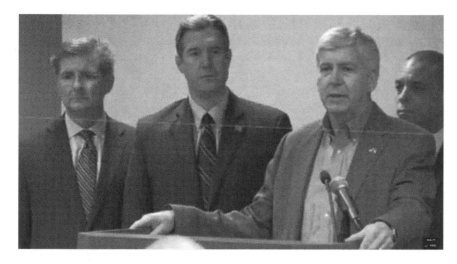

Gov. Rick Snyder, at a press conference, announces plans to help Flint. Standing immediately to the left of him is Flint Mayor Dayne Walling and next to Walling is Michigan Department of Environmental Quality Director Dan Wyant.

Frame capture courtesy Livestream.com

children. Routine surveillance of blood-lead levels does not analyze data down to the zip code level. Detailed analysis like this occurs when there is reason to focus on precise locations or populations."

TRUTH SQUAD ANALYSIS: Here's the bottom line – the state had not previously performed this detailed analysis, despite clear reason to focus on precise locations and populations in the city of Flint for months. It took a Flint doctor to show state government experts the path to the truth. With this admission, state agencies and the Snyder administration finally begin to shift from defense, denial and deflection to action.

More emails that evening, between DHHS Director Nick Lyon and Chief Medical Officer Eden Wells:

Lyon: "I'd like to express my appreciation to the Hurley doctors for bringing this issue to our attention. Is that ok?"

Wells: "Yes, yes, yes, is my vote!!!!"

Lyon: "Can I confidently say that we were not aware before last week?"

Wells: "I was aware only of (Virginia Tech) and DEQ media; until Thursday last week."

TRUTH SQUAD ANALYSIS: Lyon didn't get the MDHHS data defense he'd requested just a few days earlier because the data supported Hanna-Attisha's conclusions. The proof of the true extent of the Flint disaster is brought to light by outside researchers (Virginia Tech and Hurley). They had to overcome the denials and deflections of two state departments in which dozens of state workers – from Snyder appointees and spokespeople, to medical "experts," to technical regulators and other government employees – all whiffed.

OCT. 1: The Snyder administration begins swift action. In an email from chief of staff Dennis Muchmore to the governor and others, Muchmore says: "We have the proposal back" from the Detroit Water and Sewerage Department to reconnect the City of Flint to Detroit water. Details: "Short term reconnect is ok until KWA starts operating.... No reconnect fee and immediate reconnect.... Expenses incurred at actual cost.... Fixed monthly rate of $662,000.... Only extends to Flint.... (Detroit) Mayor (Mike) Duggan is more than willing to lend his support."

OCT. 2: The Snyder administration is making more moves on Flint's behalf, as documented in email from aides to the governor. There are new outlines of info-graphics/posters of planned state action including:

- Testing in Flint schools to ensure that drinking water is safe.

- Expanding health-exposure testing of individual homes.

- Offering free water testing to Flint residents to assure their drinking water is safe.

- Accelerating corrosion controls in the Flint drinking-water system.

- Accelerating water system improvements.

- Expediting completion of the KWA pipeline.

- Providing water filters to Flint residents.

- Creating a comprehensive lead education program.

OCT. 2: Email from Snyder Deputy Press Secretary Dave Murray transmits a release by MDEQ Director Dan Wyant and MDHHS Director Nick Lyon with more admissions:

- "A recent announcement by local doctors that blood lead levels are rising in children residing in Flint's most at-risk ZIP codes added to the state's knowledge and sparked some additional precautionary measures."

- And, despite all the errors, the release makes this claim: "The state takes lead seriously. Although continued analysis is being conducted, the MDHHS analysis is consistent with the local finding."

OCT. 2: Gov. Snyder announces a "comprehensive action plan" to address Flint water issues. Key talking points provided by staff:

"The water leaving Flint's drinking water system is safe to drink, but some families with lead plumbing in their homes or service connections could experience higher levels of lead in the water that comes out of their faucets."

"State health experts said there has been an increase in elevated childhood blood lead levels in some specific communities. Initial analysis of MDHHS data found blood lead levels of children in Flint have followed an expected seasonal trend. While this analysis for Flint as a whole remains true, a comprehensive and detailed review breaking down data by ZIP codes with the city revealed that MDHHS data is consistent with a study presented recently by Hurley Children's Hospital."

"While we cannot conclusively say that the water source change is the sole cause of the increase, this analysis supports our efforts as we take active steps to reduce all potential lead exposures in Flint," MDHHS Director Nick Lyon said.

"This action plan offers concrete steps we will take in a local, state and federal partnership to ensure all Flint residents have safe water to drink," MDEQ Director Dan Wyant said. "The DEQ will work closely with the city to gather further data to ensure the water that leaves Flint's system as well as the water that arrives in Flint homes is safe to drink."

The Detroit Free Press quotes Gov. Snyder suggesting he's now believing the outside researchers and wants state agencies to work closely with them: "This is an important issue and I want to make sure that people are working well together to address this. We all have a concern about Flint's drinking water in terms of what we're seeing on lead."

Wyant tells the Detroit Free Press that Dr. Mona Hanna-Attisha's work is what led to the state acceleration. "There's no doubt that new testing data is justifying these actions," he said.

OCT. 6: Emails indicate MDEQ Director Dan Wyant will update the governor daily on the Flint water action plan announced October 2. Other correspondence says 4,600 water filters are distributed on this day alone.

OCT. 7: State Budget Director John Roberts outlines $10.4 million in state aid to implement the action plan of October 2.

OCT. 8: City of Flint develops its plan to reconnect to Detroit Water and Sewerage Department.

OCT. 15: Snyder signs a bill authorizing $6 million in state aid to move Flint back to Detroit water until the Karegnondi Water Authority pipeline is finished. Several million more dollars authorized for drinking-water sample testing, water filters for Flint residents, follow-up services for children. City of Flint kicks in $2 million and the Charles Stewart Mott Foundation provides $4 million.

OCT. 15: MDEQ's drinking-water chief Liane Shekter Smith sends an email to departmental colleagues Brad Wurfel, Jim Sygo and George Krisztian. Key points:

Before the switch to Flint River water, "Staff believed that it was appropriate to monitor for two 6-month rounds of sampling to determine if additional measures were necessary. Based on the sampling performed, the city is required to install corrosion control treatment (see August 17, 2015 letter)."

"A pilot test was not required or conducted. Staff believed that it was appropriate to monitor for two 6-month rounds to determine if additional measures would be necessary."

OCT. 16: Flint reconnects to the Detroit drinking water sourced from Lake Huron. But, after nearly 18 months without corrosion control in the Flint distribution system, the switch does not immediately solve the lead problem. Bottled water will remain the safest drinking source for Flint residents into 2016.

OCT. 16: EPA establishes the Flint Safe Drinking Water Task Force to ""assist with developing and implementing a plan to secure water quality" in Flint.

OCT. 18 (A SUNDAY): MDEQ Director Dan Wyant admits to the governor that his department has made a huge mistake.

Wyant writes: "… staff made a mistake while working with the city of Flint. Simply stated, staff employed a federal (corrosion control) treatment protocol they believed was appropriate, and it was not."

Wyant continues: "Attached is our response to the Detroit News for a story that they are preparing for tomorrow. Part of that story looks at whether the DEQ staff followed appropriate federal protocols in light of Flint's population size. My responses, enclosed here, are an effort to acknowledge something that has come out in the past week through internal review. Simply said, our staff believed they were constrained by two consecutive six-month tests. We followed and defended that protocol. I believe now we made a mistake. For communities with a population above 50,000, optimized corrosion control should have been required from the beginning. Because of what I have learned, I will be announcing a change in leadership in our drinking water program. I've spoken with Dennis about this, and we will be making that announcement as part of the Detroit News article that likely will be out tomorrow."

TRUTH SQUAD ANALYSIS: After eight months of systemic denial throughout his department, the MDEQ director finally admits that EPA researcher Miguel Del Toral was right all along.

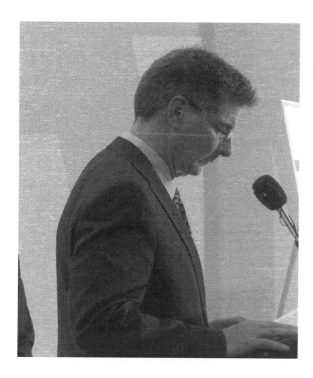

Dan Wyant, MDEQ's director.

Photo courtesy of Michigan Radio

Wyant also responds in writing to a Detroit News inquiry at this time:

"There is substantial controversy over the lead and copper rule – the EPA has been working for years on ways to update it, and Michigan will be an active part of that conversation going forward. The situation in Flint is a snapshot of an issue affecting cities around the state and the nation. More than a dozen states use the same sampling protocol Michigan uses – that's not a defense of the protocol, but rather an indication that even experts on the issue disagree about the most effective testing methods.

"What everyone can agree on is that lead is a serious issue. And I think everyone can agree that when the state came to recognize that there could be a health threat in the city, we took appropriate action. We are now engaged in an unprecedented effort to protect kids and families in Flint, develop more knowledge about what has happened and how people were affected, and take steps to make sure it doesn't happen again – in Michigan, or anywhere else. All the people who brought this issue forward deserve credit for bringing it to us. Our actions reflected inexperience, and our public response to the criticism was the wrong tone early in this conversation. But the best we can do with the situation going forward is represented in our present course – the Governor's plan represents all the suggestions outlined in the draft EPA memo, the Virginia Tech report, and the guidance we've gotten from EPA."

OCT. 19: Detroit News reporter Jim Lynch puts the Wyant admission in clear context in a lengthy published report. Key points:

"Dan Wyant, director of Michigan's Department of Environmental Quality, said late Sunday that staff members applied the wrong standards of the Lead and Copper Rule that governs testing and monitoring for drinking water. The result was that proper controls regarding corrosion were not put in place when the city began drawing its water from the Flint River in spring 2014."

"Our actions reflected inexperience, and our public response to criticism was the wrong tone early in this conversation," Wyant said.

"State officials seemingly failed to heed repeated warnings from the Environmental Protection Agency as far back as February about potential problems with Flint's water system."

"Communications released this week between the federal agency and DEQ also show how an environmental law designed to protect the public allowed the government to utilize questionable water testing practices and move slowly in addressing problems, all while remaining 'in compliance' with regulations."

"Emails and letters released by the state this week show many missed opportunities for health and environmental agencies to identify the lead problems months ago."

OCT. 21: Gov. Snyder announces a Flint Water Advisory Task Force to review state, federal and municipal actions related to the Flint crisis.

OCT. 26: Former Flint Emergency Manager Darnell Earley pens a Detroit News guest column titled, "Don't blame EM for Flint water disaster." Among the assertions: "This was a local decision that was made by local civic leaders. Anyone who says otherwise is being disingenuous."

> **TRUTH SQUAD ANALYSIS:** Earley writes this despite the fact that then-State Treasurer Andy Dillon made the "ultimate decision" to switch from DWSD to the Karegnondi Water Authority, state-appointed emergency manager Ed Kurtz hired an engineering firm to figure out how to use the Flint River as a primary water source, and Earley himself wrote the letter to DWSD saying Flint was switching to the Flint River as its water source.

CHAPTER 15

NOVEMBER 2015

CLEANUP AND PROBES BEGIN

A NEW INVESTIGATIVE TASK FORCE ASKS TOUGH QUESTIONS

Editor's summary: Months after EPA's Miguel Del Toral told Michigan officials they blundered in Flint, EPA clarifies national rules on corrosion controls. Del Toral's interpretation finally gets the agency's full support. Meanwhile, after MDEQ's director Dan Wyant's contrite admission in October that MDEQ erred in its interpretation of the federal rules, agency appears to backtrack in the face of questioning from a new task force investigating the Flint crisis. MDEQ also denies that its district supervisor, Stephen Busch, intentionally misled the EPA on whether it was using corrosion control in Flint water. Six months later, Busch will be charged with various crimes for his role in the Flint disaster, including intentionally misleading the EPA.

> "WHEN GENERAL MOTORS ANNOUNCED ITS INTENT TO TERMINATE WATER SERVICE FROM THE CITY ... SHOULD THIS HAVE BEEN A SIGN THAT THERE WERE CONCERNS WITH THE QUALITY OF THE WATER AFTER THE SWITCH TO THE FLINT RIVER? NO."
>
> — MDEQ MEMO

TIMELINE: NOVEMBER 2015

By John Bebow
Bridge Magazine

1015

NOV. 3: EPA issues clarifying national orders on the Lead and Copper Rule and corrosion control. The EPA acknowledges ambiguity in the LCR in the past regarding corrosion control, but the Nov. 3 letter sets out strong language for change and how to prevent the Flint situation from reoccurring in the future:

"This memorandum clarifies how the LCR applies to this situation and eliminates the uncertainty for water systems and primacy agencies (note: this means state regulators like the MDEQ) that may face these circumstances in the future."

"It is important for large systems and primacy agencies to take the steps necessary to ensure that appropriate corrosion control treatment is maintained at all times, thus ensuring that public health is protected."

"Due to the unique characteristics of each primary water source (e.g., source water, existing treatment processes, distribution system materials) it is critical that public water systems, in conjunction with their primacy agencies and, if necessary, outside technical consultants, evaluate and address potential impacts resulting from treatment and/or source water changes."

"Primacy agencies should work with systems that plan to disconnect from a supplier that had installed corrosion control treatment to determine the optimal corrosion control treatment for the new source and establish water quality parameters for that treatment instead of using the optimal corrosion control treatment and water quality parameters for the previous source."

"This will allow a system to … ensure protection of public health during and after the change in source. "

"(I)t is important to conduct a system-wide assessment prior to any source water and/or treatment modifications and to identify existing or anticipated water quality, treatment or operational issues that may interfere with or limit the effectiveness of corrosion control treatment optimization or re-optimization."

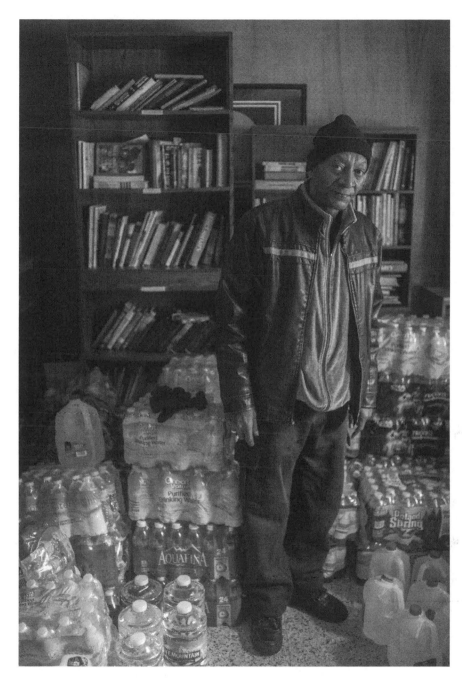

Michael Simmons arrives to pick up donated water from Pastor Bobby Jackson after Detroit-area volunteers dropped off more than 500 cases on Jan. 16.

Photo courtesy of Jake May/Mlive.com

TRUTH SQUAD ANALYSIS: Susan Hedman, EPA's top official in the Great Lakes region, essentially apologized in early July for her water regulator Miguel Del Toral's leaked memo that laid out many of the same points. And MDEQ's staff ignored and discredited him for months. Now, the clarification issued by EPA's national office reinforces virtually all of Del Toral's concerns about Flint's water supply dating back to February.

NOV. 10: EPA publicly announces a full audit of the MDEQ's oversight of public water supplies statewide. The audit will take several months.

NOV. 16: MDEQ briefing paper to the Flint Water Advisory Task Force. Key points:

Two weeks after EPA issues new lead and copper rules, and a month after MDEQ Director Dan Wyant's disclosure to the governor of a big mistake, MDEQ officials in this memo cling anew to their legalistic conclusion that they were not required to call for corrosion control in Flint.

"Did the DEQ require the City to have corrosion control in place when it switched to the Flint River as its source of drinking water? No … The DEQ requested that the City perform two 6-month rounds of monitoring to demonstrate if the City was practicing optimal corrosion control treatment…. Since the City water system had not been the supplier of water before, the DEQ did not require the City to maintain corrosion control for which it was not responsible…. The DEQ's instructions to the City were consistent with past practices afforded to all other large water systems. At the beginning of the (Lead and Copper Rule), all large systems were initially granted the option to demonstrate optimal corrosion control treatment through full-scale monitoring under the applicable rules. For these reasons, two 6-month rounds of monitoring, as required by the LCR, were the required means to determine whether or not optimal corrosion control was being achieved."

"What was the DEQ's response to the USEPA's inquiry in February 2015 regarding optimized corrosion control treatment being implemented by the City under the LCR? The DEQ indicated that the City was complying with the LCR, the lead 90th percentile level was below the action level of 15 ppb, and the City was already conducting the second round of monitoring which would provide for a determination of whether additional treatment needed to be installed. It should be noted that once treatment is designated as optimal, there is no requirement in the LCR that lead results be lower than they were before treatment was installed. The 90th percentile only needs to be lower than the action level in the LCR."

"Did the DEQ attempt to mislead the USEPA in a February 27, 2015, email responding to the USEPA's inquiry regarding Optimal Corrosion Control Treatment? No. There was no attempt by the DEQ to mislead the USEPA. There is an email from Steve Busch, Jackson and Lansing District Supervisor, Office of Drinking Water and Municipal Assistance, indicating that the City was practicing a corrosion control program. What was meant was that the City was performing the required monitoring to determine whether or not they were practicing optimized corrosion control. The DEQ subsequently clarified its position in follow-up emails and telephone conversations with the USEPA."

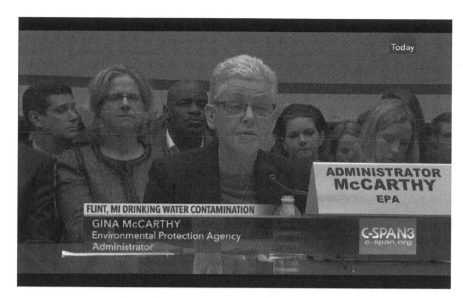

Gina McCarthy, U.S.
EPA administrator.

Screen capture
courtesy of CSPAN

"When General Motors announced its intent to terminate water service from the City … should this have been a sign that there were concerns with the quality of the water after the switch to the Flint River? No. General Motors made a decision regarding the quality of the water for its manufacturing processes. At the time, the company indicated that the chloride levels were above limits acceptable as part of the manufacturing facility's limit for production purposes. The level of chlorides in the water treated by the City was not a human health or aesthetic concern."

TRUTH SQUAD ANALYSIS: This is an amazing statement. Chlorides accelerate corrosion, so much so that the Flint water was no longer suitable for GM's manufacturing processes. Corrosion also accelerates lead leaching from old lead water service lines and solder joints, allowing lead to get into drinking water. Outside experts like Virginia Tech's Marc Edwards and Dr. Mona Hanna-Attisha clearly connected these dots. Yet MDEQ did not react to this General Motors warning sign.

Additional revelations about how lead samples were collected in Flint:

(TRUTH SQUAD NOTE: This was an issue first raised in part by Miguel Del Toral in February 2015 and amplified in September by Virginia Tech's Marc Edwards.)

"DEQ had no reason to question the validity of the City's reports until the DEQ heard City employees revealing to the media that the City did not know for certain if its compliance monitoring was collected from homes with lead service lines.… (T)he DEQ determined from information available that a significant number of these sites that had been listed as having lead service lines either did not have them or the information was unavailable. On November 9, 2015, the

DEQ notified the City in writing that it would be necessary to conduct a complete assessment of its sampling pool and report back its findings by December 30, 2015."

"Do the DEQ's sampling instructions comply with the Lead and Copper Rule? The DEQ continues to seek official clarification from the USEPA regarding the sampling protocols."

> (TRUTH SQUAD NOTE: This is NINE months after EPA's Del Toral raises serious questions about MDEQ's sampling protocols.)

"Early in the implementation of the LCR, the DEQ had encountered too many situations where compliance samples had been collected from kitchen and bathroom taps that had not been used in days and in some cases, even weeks, resulting in excessively stagnated water and correspondingly high lead levels that did not represent typical exposure expected after overnight stagnation.... In order to ensure samples were taken at customer taps representative of typical use, the DEQ devised the current recommendations for ensuring appropriate but not excessive stagnation for LCR monitoring."

NOV. 21: The American Journal for Public Health accepts for publication in its February 2016 edition a peer-reviewed research paper led by Dr. Mona Hanna-Attisha titled, "Elevated Blood Lead Levels in Children Associated With the Flint Drinking Water Crisis: A Spatial Analysis of Risk and Public Health Response." Key conclusions:

"Incidence of elevated blood lead levels increased from 2.4 percent to 4.9 percent after water source change, and neighborhoods with the highest water lead levels experienced (an even larger increase). No significant change was seen outside the city."

"The percentage of children with elevated blood lead levels increased after water source change, particularly in socioeconomically disadvantaged neighborhoods. Water is a growing source of childhood lead exposure because of aging infrastructure."

"Water from the Detroit Water and Sewerage Department had very low corrosivity for lead as indicated by low chloride, low chloride-to-sulfate mass ratio, and presence of an orthophosphate corrosion inhibitor. Flint River water had high chloride, high chloride-to-sulfate mass ratio, and no corrosion inhibitor. Switching from Detroit's Lake Huron to Flint River water created a perfect storm for lead leaching into drinking water."

"The aging Flint water distribution system contains high percentage of lead pipes and lead plumbing, with estimates of lead service lines ranging from 10 percent to 80 percent."

"Experiments by Virginia Tech university show Flint's treated water – drawn from the Flint River – is about 19 times more corrosive than Lake Huron water than had been purchased from the City of Detroit for decades, making the problem much worse than in the past."

"Armed with reports of elevated water lead levels and recognizing the lifelong consequences of lead exposure, our research team sought to analyze blood lead levels before and after the water source switch with a geographic information system to determine lead exposure risk and prioritize responses. This research has immediate public policy, public health, environmental, and socioeconomic implications."

"The declining industrial and residential tax bases strained the city's ability to provide basic city services and reversed public health fortunes of the city and the suburbs. Severely reduced city population densities reduced water demand in the distribution system, exacerbating problems with lead corrosion."

"This retrospective study includes all children younger than 5 years who had a blood lead level processed through Hurley Medical Center's laboratory, which runs blood lead levels for most Genesee County children."

"Our city of Flint sample included 736 children in the pre period and 737 children in the post period." Across all of Flint, the proportion of children under five years old with lead levels above 5 micrograms per deciliter doubled after the Flint River switch, from 2.4 percent to 4.9 percent. In areas of the city identified by Virginia Tech as having high water lead levels, the proportion of children under 5 years old with blood lead above 5 micrograms per deciliter nearly tripled after the water source switch.

"A review of alternative sources of lead exposure reveals no other potential environmental confounders during the same time period."... No corresponding increase in home demolitions that would have spread lead, no new manufacturing sources of lead, no correspondence between the neighborhoods with high blood lead or water lead levels and historical manufacturing, etc.

"Because there was no known alternative source for increased lead exposure during this time period, the geospatial water lead levels results, the innate corrosive properties of the Flint River water, and, most importantly, the lack of corrosion control, our findings strongly implicate the water source change as the probable cause for the dramatic increase in elevated blood lead level percentage."

"Increased lead-poisoning rates have profound implications for the life course potential of an entire cohort of Flint children already rattled with toxic stress contributors (e.g., poverty, violence, unemployment, food insecurity.)"

"More stable neighborhoods in the far north and south of the city may have experienced improved predicted blood lead levels because of prevention efforts taken by the more-often middle-class residents in response to the water source change."

"Lead is a potent neurotoxin, and childhood lead poisoning has an impact on many developmental and biological processes, most notably intelligence, behavior, and overall life achievement. With estimated societal costs in the billions, lead poisoning has a disproportionate impact on low-income and minority children."

"A once-celebrated cost-cutting move for an economically distressed city, the water source change has now wrought untold economic, population health, and geo-political burdens."

"The legal safeguards and regulating bodies designed to protect vulnerable populations from preventable lead exposure failed."

"As our aging water infrastructures continue to decay, and as communities across the nation struggle with finances and water supply sources, the situation in Flint may be a harbinger for future safe drinking-water challenges. Ironically, even when one is surrounded by the Great Lakes, safe drinking water is not a guarantee."

NOV. 23: EPA's Flint Drinking Water Task Force provides comments to MDEQ's revised Lead and Copper Sampling Instructions, and appears to validate Del Toral's early warnings about how the state directed lead sampling in Flint. "The task force agrees with the removal of pre-flushing."

CHAPTER 16

NOV. 19, 2015

DEMOLITION: A FLINT SUCCESS STORY

'IT GIVES PEOPLE ROOM TO BREATHE'

Editor's summary: With all the attention on Flint's water crisis, Chastity Pratt Dawsey of the Bridge team found this good news story about the success Flint is having in demolishing blighted homes. The Genesee County Land Bank Authority spearheads a program that is a model of efficiency in removing abandoned, often dilapidated homes that are a scourge – like lead pipes proved to be – of old inner-city neighborhoods.

By Chastity Pratt Dawsey
Bridge Magazine

With so much focus on the city's water crisis, a Flint success story has had little notice.

The Genesee County Land Bank Authority has demolished more than 1,766 blighted houses in Flint since 2014 with federal grants. That exceeds its stated goal of 1,600 home demolitions when the city received more than $20 million for blight removal in 2013. The Flint program boasts significantly lower average demolitions cost than those in Detroit.

The most visible sign of the city's progress: Hundreds of lots with neglected or abandoned homes have been transformed into fields of clover.

Of five Michigan cities that shared $100 million in Hardest Hit federal grants, Flint is the only one to meet – and exceed – its demolition goals, records show.

Flint has eradicated nearly 30 percent of the city's blighted homes.

To be fair, the blight fight in Detroit is on a huge scale – at least 3,683 houses were demolished in the Motor City with Hardest Hit grant funds, records show. Detroit estimates it needs to knock down 80,000 structures.

Flint's program is its largest blight battle ever, said Lucille James, brownfields and demolition program manager for the land bank.

"We've never worked at this scale," she said.

The federal blight money is intended to stabilize neighborhoods around the city's anchor institutions – "schools, hospitals, churches, main thoroughfares," James said. "So it doesn't address all our needs."

A ride through Flint's neighborhoods offers glimpses of the same sort of poverty Detroit has become known for: streets pocked with wood frame bungalows that now lean in on themselves, empty; brick houses, crumbling.

But absent in Flint are large numbers of gentrifying hipsters to stoke hopes, and no world-renown decay like Detroit to attract attention to its plight. When Antonio Dunn drives through Flint, he hardly recognizes the city of his childhood.

But he sees vestiges of progress – soft carpets of clover grow where rotting houses stood only months ago.

Dunn, an inspector for the Genesee County Land Bank Authority, stood on Mackin Road, on the city's north side, and explained how the north side of the block – save one vacant house – was demolished. An elementary school stands on one end of the block.

"Before, it wasn't safe. It was a hot mess," Dunn said. "Abandoned houses are used for trap houses, stash houses," referring to structures where drugs and money are hidden. "And you get the rodents and pest problems. When we take down the blight, it just gives people room to breathe."

I n 2013, the U.S. Department of Treasury gave Michigan $100 million from its $498 million Hardest Hit Fund grant (for homeowners hurt by the mortgage crisis) to focus on eliminating blighted single family homes in five cities. The big winners: Detroit, which received $57.3 million to demolish 4,000 houses. Flint, which received $22.7 million for 1,604 houses; Saginaw $11.1 million for 100 houses; Pontiac $3.7 million for 200 houses; and Grand Rapids $2.4 million for 100 houses.

At the time of the first infusion of grant funds, about 6,000 houses in Flint needed demolition, James said. So the 1,766 homes demolished as of Nov. 15 represented nearly 30 percent of the city's blighted houses.

In November 2015, more federal light reduction grants were announced. Flint will get another $11 million to tear down 900 vacant houses.

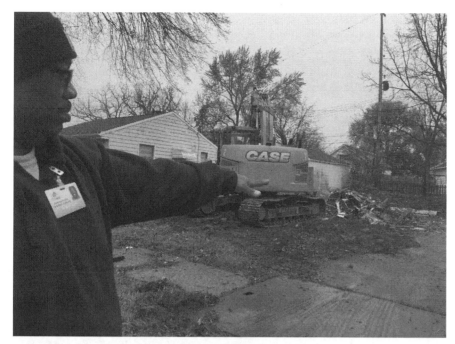

Contractors demolished a frame house in November 2015 on Van Buren Street in Flint. About 30 percent of the city's blighted houses were demolished with federal grant funds. Another round of funding recently announced will take down 900 more vacant Flint houses.

Bridge photos by Chastity Pratt Dawsey

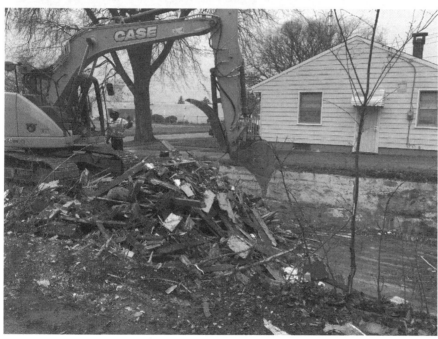

The Genesee County land bank is knocking down Flint's blight for about $11,600 per structure, while Detroit's demolition costs have jumped to about $16,400, up from $10,000 in 2013. Overall, the demolition cost to knock down a house now averages $13,830 for a single-family residence demolition in Detroit, said Craig Fahle, spokesman for the Detroit Land Bank Authority.

Fahle said Detroit house demolitions peaked at nearly 300 structures a week, but that pace "proved to overwhelm the available contractor pool." Currently, Detroit is moving at a clip of 100 to 150 homes a week "within the existing contractor pool."

Like Detroit, Flint saw upticks in costs when the program peaked with about 400 demolitions happening at the same time. Abatement costs, increased oversight requirements from federal and state regulations, and competition for contractors drove up costs across the state, James said.

One reason Flint demolition costs may be lower than in Detroit has to do with better access to clean, safe dirt to fill the hole left by demolition, James said. Flint vendors have access to soil from nearby quarries and stockpiles of dirt, she said.

There's an often-repeated saying in Flint: "People moved, but they didn't take their houses."

The land bank estimates that Flint has about 22,000 vacant properties, representing about a third of the city: 14,500 vacant lots and 7,500 vacant houses and commercial buildings. Of that, the land bank owns 23 percent of the vacant houses and buildings and 55 percent of the vacant lots.

Most of the blighted houses are privately owned, according to the land bank.

"It can be falling down a hole and some individual could still be paying the taxes," James said. "If the land bank doesn't own it, our hands are tied."

That may change soon.

Though the mortgage and housing crisis has ebbed nationally, private owners in Flint are still losing properties to tax foreclosure in big numbers. In the past year, a couple thousand properties went to tax foreclosure and then were handed over to the land bank to demolish or try to sell.

At that rate, the land bank will be the largest owner of Flint's vacant buildings in the next three years or so, said Doug Weiland, executive director for the land bank.

"It's inevitable," he said.

In Michigan's hardest hit cities, more blight springs up every week. A house that is standing today could be a teetering danger by Tuesday.

Maurice Davis, 59, lives in the Civic Park neighborhood, an area populated by historic homes. Of about 1,000 parcels there, more than 200 have been demolished since last year, according to land bank records.

Davis, president of the Historic Civic Park Preservation Association and owner of a commercial strip, has bittersweet feelings about the blight fight.

Blight is wrapped around Civic Park School like a bad rash, and another 200 eyesores need to be demolished in the area, he said. He appreciates the demolition program, but wishes more money was used to preserve homes and help owners stay.

"What the land bank is doing is welcome, we need houses torn down," he said. "But what happens to the residents who are left?"

CHAPTER 17

DECEMBER 2015

TASK FORCE SLAMS MDEQ AS TOP VILLAIN

DIRECTOR AND HIS SPOKESMAN RESIGN

Editor's summary: The Flint Water Advisory Task Force issues its first report Dec. 29 and assigns MDEQ the lion's share of blame for the Flint water crisis. Before the day is out, the department's director, Dan Wyant, and its spokesman, Brad Wurfel, resign. The task force says MDEQ took a "minimalist approach" to its regulatory responsibility that "is unacceptable and insufficient to the task of public protection." The task force also says MDEQ's response to outside questioning "was often one of aggressive dismissal, belittlement and attempts to discredit." Its third key finding is confirmation of MDEQ's wrong interpretation of the federal Lead and Copper Rule that led to decisions not to require corrosion treatment after the switch to the Flint River as the city's water source. That decision resulted in lead leaching from old pipes into the city's drinking water and the poisoning of Flint's children.

"I WANT THE FLINT COMMUNITY TO KNOW HOW VERY SORRY I AM THAT THIS HAS HAPPENED. AND I WANT ALL MICHIGAN CITIZENS TO KNOW THAT WE WILL LEARN FROM THIS EXPERIENCE, BECAUSE FLINT IS NOT THE ONLY CITY THAT HAS AN AGING INFRASTRUCTURE."

— STATEMENT PREPARED FOR GOV. RICK SNYDER

TIMELINE: DECEMBER 2015

By John Bebow
Bridge Magazine

2015

DEC. 3: The staff of State Rep. Adam Zemke, D-Ann Arbor, sends email to MDEQ requesting feedback on a bill he plans to introduce to require drinking water in schools be tested at least once every three years. MDEQ's Liane Shekter Smith responds in email four days later:

"(T)his is a huge expense.... They have to figure there are approximately 30 drinking water faucets on average at each school.... I suspect it's a really big number! This proposal is also disconnected from how water sampling is accomplished. Most parameters are required to be met at the plant tap (at the point the water enters the distribution system). Only a few parameters (lead, copper, disinfection byproducts, bacteria) are monitored out in the system at customer taps. Even if the proposal were to be for only lead and copper, this is a huge expense that would be placed on the supplier of water inappropriately. I understand the desire to have this kind of information, but if the legislature wants to require this monitoring, the burden for this should be on the schools or the board of education."

DEC. 5: A Genesee County Health Department official accuses state officials of attempting to cover up their mishandling of the investigation into the outbreak of Legionnaires' disease that sickened 87 people in 2014 and 2015, and killed 10, according to emails obtained by the Detroit Free Press. "The state is making clear they are not practicing ethical public health practice," Tamara Brickey, Genesee's public health division director, writes to other county health officials. "Now evidence is clearly pointing to a deliberate cover-up.... In my opinion, if we don't act soon, we are going to become guilty by association."

DEC. 14: City of Flint declares emergency.

DEC. 16: EPA Flint Drinking Water Task Force says Flint should not switch to KWA water in 2016 until the treated water meets finished water quality goals, plant operational issues are identified and dealt with, water plant operations staff are proficient in treating the new source, and Flint performs numerous assessments.

   TRUTH SQUAD NOTE: These are the pre-planning and safety checks Flint never performed and MDEQ never required before the switch to Flint River water.

DEC. 22: Email from Snyder Communications Director Meegan Holland to Snyder and other aides regarding new revelations by Virginia Tech's Marc Edwards. Key points:

Holland notes the headline of a new Edwards' blog post: "Michigan Health Department Hid Evidence of Health Harm Due to Lead Contaminated Water. Allowed False Public Assurances by MDEQ and Stonewalled Outside Researchers." The blog post is based on state email records obtained by Edwards under the Freedom of Information Act.

Holland's response: "The Michigan Department of Health and Human Services has been, and continues to be, committed to full disclosure of information regarding the city of Flint and blood lead levels. To suggest otherwise is not consistent with how we have responded."

"It wasn't until the Hurley report came out that our epidemiologists took a more in-depth look at the data by zip code, controlling for seasonal variation, and confirmed an increase outside of normal trends. As a result of this process, we have determined that the way we analyze data collected needs to be thoroughly reviewed."

TRUTH SQUAD ANALYSIS: Here's yet another huge gap in the regulatory framework to protect public health. The concerns of two established outside researchers (from EPA and Virginia Tech) weren't sufficient to prompt state agencies to reconsider their approach to lead detection. It took a local physician to open the state's eyes to the problem they had repeatedly denied.

DEC. 23: The Michigan Auditor General provides an investigative report on Flint water issues as requested by State Sen. Jim Ananich. Key points:

"We did not note any instance of major infractions (i.e., intentional disregard of policies, laws, regulations, or specific directions) committed by DEQ staff during the course of our review.... (O)ur review of DEQ correspondence confirmed the escalation of key issues up the chain of command related to the Flint situation."

"Did DEQ consult with the EPA prior to determining how to apply the Lead and Copper Rule? DEQ did not consult with the EPA on how to apply the LCR prior to implementing two consecutive six-month monitoring periods of the Flint Water Treatment Plant beginning July 1, 2014."

"When Flint switched to the Flint River water source, should corrosion control treatment have been maintained? We believe that corrosion control should have been maintained."

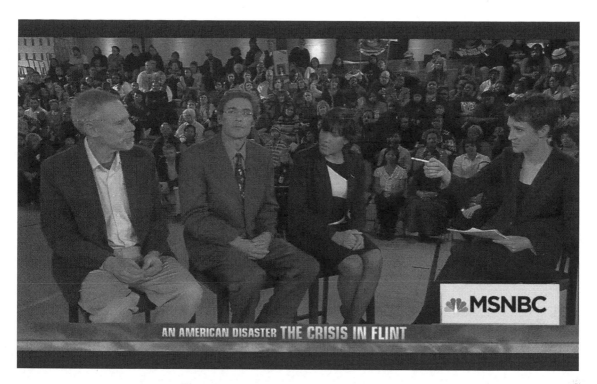

On Dec. 18, MSNBC's Rachel Maddow Show devoted a special segment to the water crisis, the first extensive network presentation about Flint. Maddow, far right above, laid the blame squarely on Gov. Rick Snyder and the state law he championed allowing state-appointed emergency managers to take power from elected officials. "I maintain that it really is the single-most radical policy, the single-most radical piece of legislation put into law by any state in the country in our modern American political history," she said. In January, Maddow held a town hall, pictured above, with Flint residents. (Screen acapture courtesy of MSNBC)

Citing the Nov. 3 EPA memorandum, the AG report concluded, "based on this clarification, it appears that corrosion control treatment should have been maintained."

"Should DEQ have required the Flint Water Treatment Plant to start pursuing optimized corrosion control treatment after the first round of six-month sampling results were above the lead action level of five parts per billion? Yes. The first round of six-month sampling results were received in late March 2015. Because the results were 1 part per billion over the lead action level of 5 parts per billion, DEQ would not be able to achieve two consecutive six-month periods below 5 parts per billion. Therefore, DEQ should have notified the Flint Water Treatment Plant to start pursuing optimized corrosion control treatment. However, DEQ waited until the second round of sampling was completed (June 30, 2015) to assess whether water sample results improved."

"Did DEQ verify that only tier 1 sample sites were selected by the Flint Water Treatment Plant (for the two rounds of six-month lead sampling)? DEQ did not verify that only tier 1 sample sites were selected."

"Was flushing of taps the night before drawing a sample an appropriate sample methodology? Yes. The LCR requires that samples be a first draw of water after six hours of stagnation. The LCR does not indicate whether or not the water line should be flushed prior to collecting the sample. In the sample instructions, DEQ required pre-flushing to ensure that sampled facets were not stagnant for an excessive period of time beyond the targeted six hours…. The LCR requires six hours of stagnation, however it does not preclude DEQ from instructing resident to flush prior to stagnation."

DEC. 28: Email from Jerrod Agen, who is transitioning from communications director to chief of staff, to Gov. Rick Snyder, alerting him to the release coming the next day of the key Flint Water Advisory Task Force conclusions:

"The recommendations in this letter suggest profound change at DEQ and openly criticize Director Wyant. If this is the path that the Task Force is on, it is best to make changes at DEQ sooner rather than later. That likely means accepting Dan's resignation. It also means moving up the termination of the 3 DEQ personnel previously planned for Jan. 4 to tomorrow."

DEC. 29: The Flint Water Advisory Task Force, the investigation team established in October by Gov. Snyder, issues its first conclusions. Key points:

"We believe the primary responsibility for what happened in Flint rests with the Michigan Department of Environmental Quality (MDEQ). Although many individuals and entities at the state and local levels contributed to creating and prolonging the problem, MDEQ is the government agency that has responsibility to ensure safe drinking water in Michigan. It failed in that responsibility and must be held accountable for that failure."

The MDEQ failed in three fundamental ways:

- **REGULATORY FAILURE:** "We believe that in the Office of Drinking Water and Municipal Assistance (ODWMA) at MDEQ, a culture exists in which 'technical compliance' is considered sufficient to ensure safe drinking water in Michigan. This minimalist approach to regulatory and oversight responsibility is unacceptable and simply insufficient to the task of public protection. It led to MDEQ's failure to recognize a number of indications that switching the water source in Flint would – and did – compromise both water safety and water quality.

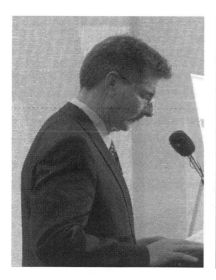 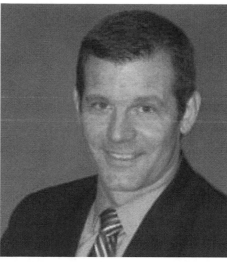

Left, MDEQ Director Dan Wyant resigned on Dec. 29, 2015.

Photo courtesy Steve Carmody/Michigan Radio

Right, MDEQ spokesman Brad Wurfel, resigned on Dec. 29, 2015.

Photo from Linkedin page

- **FAILURE IN SUBSTANCE AND TONE OF MDEQ RESPONSE TO THE PUBLIC:** "Throughout 2015, as the public raised concerns and as independent studies and testing were conducted and brought to the attention of MDEQ, the agency's response was often one of aggressive dismissal, belittlement, and attempts to discredit these efforts and the individuals involved. We find both the tone and substance of many MDEQ public statements to be completely unacceptable.... What is disturbing about MDEQ's responses, however, is their persistent tone of scorn and derision. In fact, the MDEQ seems to have been more determined to discredit the work of others – who ultimately proved to be right – than to pursue its own oversight responsibility."

- **FAILURE IN MDEQ INTERPRETATION OF THE LEAD AND COPPER RULE:** Prior to the Flint River water source switch, "MDEQ staff instructed the City of Flint water treatment staff that corrosion control treatment was not necessary until two six-month monitoring periods had been conducted.... The decision not to require corrosion control treatment, made at the direction of the MDEQ, led directly to the contamination of the Flint water system."

"We are not finished with our work. Other individuals and entities made poor decisions, contributing to and prolonging the contamination of the drinking water supply in Flint. As an example, we are particularly concerned by recent revelations of MDHHS's apparent early knowledge of, yet silence about, elevated blood lead levels detected among Flint's children."

TRUTH SQUAD NOTE: This task force includes: 1) Ken Sikkema, former Republican Senate Majority Leader; 2) Chris Kolb, head of the Michigan Environmental Council and a former Democratic state legislator; 3) Matthew Davis, a University of Michigan pediatrician and professor of public policy; 4) Eric Rothstein, a water consultant; 5) Lawrence Reynolds, a Flint pediatrician and president of the Mott Children's Health Center.

DEC. 29: Communications Director Meegan Holland sent an email to Gov. Snyder detailing the statement the governor would release that afternoon. Details:

"When I became aware that the city of Flint's water showed elevated lead levels and that the state's handling of the situation was being questioned, I requested funding to switch the source back to (Detroit) and appointed an independent task force to identify possible missteps and areas for improvement."

"I want the Flint community to know how very sorry I am that this has happened. And I want all Michigan citizens to know that we will learn from this experience, because Flint is not the only city that has an aging infrastructure."

"I know many Flint citizens are angry and want more than an apology. That's why I'm taking actions today to ensure a culture of openness and trust. We've already allocated $10 million to test the water, distribute water filters, and help in other ways. Last week, I called Flint Mayor Karen Weaver, and we're going to meet soon to discuss other ways the state can offer assistance."

"I understand there can be disagreements within the scientific community. That is why I have directed both the departments of Environmental Quality and Health and Human Services to invite every external scientist who has worked on this issue to be our partners in helping us improve Flint water. Together, we should work to affirm that we're using the very best testing protocols to ensure Flint residents have safe drinking water and that we're taking steps to protect their health over the short term and the long term."

DEC. 29: MDEQ Director Dan Wyant and MDEQ chief spokesman Brad Wurfel resign.

DETROIT

ZIP CODE	TOTAL TESTED	# OF ELEVATED LEVELS	PERCENT ELEVATED
48206	651	132	20.3%
48211	253	43	17.0%
48214	618	102	16.5%
48204	808	132	16.3%
48202	393	60	15.3%
48238	1002	125	12.5%
48213	812	100	12.3%
48203	742	87	11.7%
48205	1553	156	10.0%
48215	431	43	10.0%
48216	136	13	9.6%
48208	302	27	8.9%
48210	1569	137	8.7%
48224	1599	130	8.1%
48212	1597	128	8.0%
48209	1508	116	7.7%
48207	565	38	6.7%
48227	1447	97	6.7%

REST OF MICHIGAN

ZIP CODE	TOTAL TESTED	# OF ELEVATED LEVELS	PERCENT ELEVATED
49073 - Nashville	51	9	17.6%
49247 - Hudson	87	13	14.9%
49256 - Morenci	54	7	13.0%
49221 - Adrian	640	78	12.2%
49507 - Gd. Rapids	1309	145	11.1%
49224 - Albion	153	14	9.2%
49504 - Gd. Rapids	813	73	9.0%
49442 - Muskegon	818	74	9.0%
49506 - E. Gd. Rapids	433	38	8.8%
49203 - Jackson	859	75	8.7%
49007 - Kalamazoo	242	19	7.9%
49858 - Menominee	140	11	7.9%
49503 - Gd. Rapids	830	64	7.7%
49454 - Scottville	79	6	7.6%
48335 - Farm. Hills	477	33	6.9%
49441 - Muskegon	489	33	6.7%
48602 - Saginaw	776	51	6.6%
49431 - Ludington	256	17	6.6%

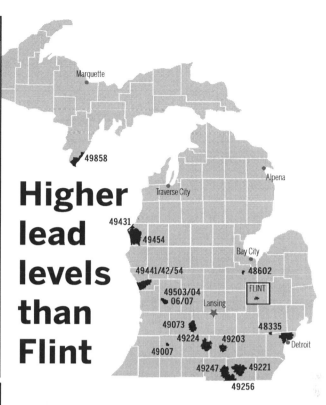

Higher lead levels than Flint

The man-made disaster that unfolded in Flint after the city changed its water source in April 2014 was inexcusable. But it's important to understand the larger context of lead poisoning in Michigan's children. In 2014, slightly more than 5,000 Michigan children had blood-lead levels exceeding the level established for public health concern. And 36 Michigan zip codes – half of them in Detroit – had higher percentages of young children with elevated blood-lead levels than in the two Flint zip codes where the study by Dr. Mona Hanna-Attisha and the Hurley Medical Center found the highest percentage of lead-poisoned children in Flint after the water switch. The state data was provided by the Michigan Department of Health and Human Services.

While the lead poisoning in Flint was linked to public water supplies, flaking paint and the dust from paint in and around older homes is considered the primary source of elevated blood levels in children today. A number of schools across the state have begun checking their water in the wake of the Flint disaster.

CHAPTER 18

DEC. 10, 2015

LEAD POISONS KIDS ACROSS MICHIGAN

RESOURCES DON'T MATCH THE NEEDS

Editor's summary: This is one of the most important, and perhaps unexpected, stories Bridge Magazine reported during the water crisis. While not minimizing what happened in Flint, it gives a broader historical and contemporary context to the elusive issue of eradicating lead poisoning in Michigan and the nation. In neighborhoods across Michigan, several thousand children – mostly in urban areas – have been exposed to levels of lead poisoning higher than those in Flint. Old houses with flaking lead-based paints are the biggest culprits.

By Mike Wilkinson
Bridge Magazine

Beyond Flint in cities large and small, Michigan children are suffering from lead poisoning, limiting their school and playground abilities and their futures.

While the focus has rightly been on Flint's lead-poisoned water, thousands of children across the state have had higher levels of lead exposure – as measured in annual blood testing – than those in Flint. They live in Detroit, Grand Rapids, Jackson, Saginaw, Holland, Muskegon and other neighborhoods around Michigan.

The high blood-lead levels are proof that the lead scourge has not been eradicated despite decades of public health campaigns and hundreds of millions of dollars spent to find and eliminate exposure.

"This is still an issue. It's not going away," said Dr. Eden Wells, chief medical executive of the Michigan Department of Health and Human Services.

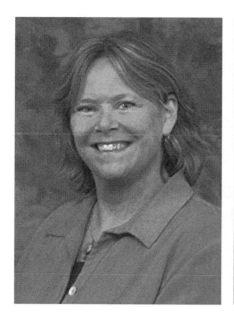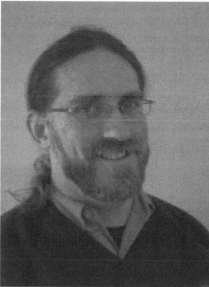

Left, Dr. Eden Wells, chief medical executive with the Michigan Department of Health and Human Services.

Photo courtesy of State of Michigan

Right, Paul Haan of the Healthy Homes Coalition of West Michigan, which works to eliminate household dangers.

Photo courtesy of Healthy Homes Coalition of West Michigan

In most areas with serious lead problems today, the source has been the traditional culprits: flaking lead paint on older homes and lead residue in dust and soil. In the United States, lead was banned in paint beginning in 1978 and phased out in gasoline from 1975 through 1996.

Young children are particularly susceptible to lead exposure because of their proximity to the most common sources of lead – on the ground. They crawl, pick up dust and dirt and put their hands in their mouths.

The findings in Flint were shocking: After a steady decline in lead levels measured in the blood of the city's young children, levels began to rise in 2014 after the city switched its water source from Lake Huron to the Flint River. That change in water supply, experts say, triggered the increase in lead poisoning because more corrosive river water stripped lead from older pipes, allowing it to leach into tap water.

The higher levels of lead in the blood of Flint's children, as proven in a groundbreaking study by Hurley Hospital pediatrician Dr. Mona Hanna-Attisha, finally forced state officials to confront the threat in the city's water. About 5 percent of Flint children tested had elevated levels of lead. The percentage of children with elevated levels was much higher in zip codes with the most residents in poverty.

Consider lead exposure rates in some other parts of Michigan:

In Detroit, five zip codes had over 700 children test positive in 2013, or nearly 15 percent of the 4,910 children tested.

In Grand Rapids, nearly one in 10 children of those tested in five zip codes tested positive.

And in Ludington, nearly 13 percent of the 229 children tested in 2013 registered elevated lead levels.

"We do have areas in our state and areas in our country where children are at risk," Wells said. "We've got to do as much as we can."

Flint's water crisis once again brought front and center a danger long known to rob children of cognitive and physiological function and impulse control. High levels of lead found in students in the Detroit Public School system have been linked to the city's extremely low school test scores.

In the 48206 zip code on Detroit's west side, 20.8 percent of the 701 kids tested had elevated levels in 2013.

Because of the well-documented dangers of lead, pediatricians regularly test children. "And every week there are more kids on" a weekly statewide report of elevated lead levels, said Paul Haan of the Healthy Homes Coalition of West Michigan, which works to eliminate household dangers to make children safer and healthier. Parts of Grand Rapids have some of the highest concentrations of children with lead, he said.

From a historical perspective, far fewer Michigan children are testing positive for lead poisoning in recent decades. In 2012, 4.5 percent of those tested in Michigan showed elevated lead levels. A decade earlier, 25.6 percent breached the same poison level.

In 2013, the percentage sank to 3.9 percent. But that percentage still represents nearly 5,700 children under age 6 who were tested. Each had lead levels above 5 micrograms per deciliter. (Although no amount is considered safe, experts use a reference level of 5 micrograms per deciliter to identify children with blood lead levels that are much higher than most children's levels.)

The impact on a child's nervous system and brain is obvious to parents and teachers: They see children easily distracted or challenged to retain information or progress academically and socially. Even lower levels of lead exposure can steal points from a child's intelligence – cognition they cannot get back.

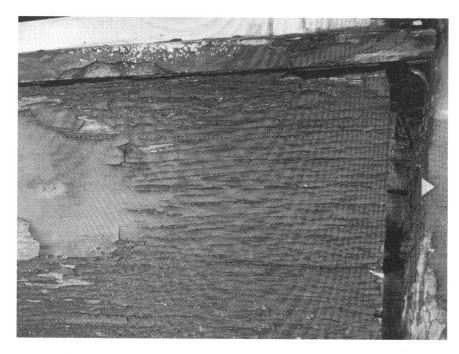

Flaking lead paint from window sills and other wood framework of homes is today considered the biggest cause of lead poisoning in young children.

Photo courtesy of Lester Graham/ Michigan Radio

Some researchers have suggested the sharp reduction in lead levels in recent decades, mainly from the elimination of lead in gasoline, explains the decline in violent crime in the United States and elsewhere. But in children suffering lead poisoning, the historical trend is meaningless and the implications are profound.

Kieya Morrison is a preschool teacher in Detroit, and formerly a longtime kindergarten teacher. Recently, she had a girl in her class with elevated blood lead levels (teachers are informed of health issues their students have).

Learning was difficult for the girl, and Morrison often would go over and over simple shapes: This is a triangle, this is a square. For the girl, the struggle was constant.

"She had cognitive problems. She had trouble processing things," Morrison said. "She could not retain any of the information."

At her pre-school in Detroit, where the teacher-student ratio was one to eight, Morrison gave the girl more attention and could "catch her" when she fell behind.

Morrison said she worried about what happened to the girl – her family moved out of the area after preschool – once she got to kindergarten and first grade, where there could be just one teacher for every 30 students.

"You really get lost," Morrison said of the older grades. "There's nothing to catch you."

Besides the federal and state money, foundations are supporting programs across Michigan that help pay for eliminating lead sources in older homes when a family cannot afford to pay for it. In the last decade, those programs have paid for lead abatements in 1,500 homes in western Michigan. Yet an estimated 60,000 homes need lead abatement in just that part of the state, said Haan of the Healthy Homes Coalition of West Michigan.

Even quantifying the extent of the problem is difficult. A 1998-2000 study estimated that 38 million U.S. homes had lead-based paint and 24 million had "significant lead-based hazards." In many cases, homeowners eliminate the danger themselves when they repaint a home or replace older plumbing.

But in many places where the housing stock is the oldest and incomes the lowest, places such as Detroit and Muskegon, problems persist, especially when paint is flaking from windowsills and frames and into the ground outside homes. Foundations and HUD have spent heavily to tackle the lead paint problem.

Although the state has its own program to help people pay for abatement, its funding only covered remediation in 180 homes in the last year.

Besides the ban on lead in gas, much of the decline in child blood lead levels in recent decades is attributed to changes in construction materials and public health awareness campaigns. The state gives parents and health care providers information on where to turn for help.

Pediatricians are encouraged to test all children ages 1 and 2 for blood lead and it is required for children of low-income parents who qualify for Medicaid. A positive test requires a second confirmation test. Family and home histories are then taken to determine the source of lead – possibly the home or a parent's workplace.

Haan said lead is treated as a medical problem, but it's a societal challenge, too. Beyond cognitive and physiological scars, lead exposure has been correlated to lower wages, higher incarceration rates and a greater likelihood of need for public assistance of all kinds.

"The problem is," Haan said, "we're still using kids as lead detectors."

CHAPTER 19

JANUARY 2016

SNYDER TO FLINT: 'I'M SORRY AND I WILL FIX IT'

DEMOCRATS TO SNYDER: YOU POISONED FLINT

Editor's summary: For even those who've paid casual attention, the Flint water crisis story has exploded beyond Michigan to the rest of the county and beyond. Gov. Snyder activates the National Guard to distribute water and seeks federal disaster aid, leading up to his apology in his annual State of the State address; Democrats and activists say the governor poisoned Flint's children with an agenda emphasizing cost-cutting over public health stewardship. Two MDEQ employees are suspended, and the blame game rages. State Attorney General Bill Schuette names a special prosecutor to investigate possible criminal wrongdoing.

"THE U.S. ENVIRONMENTAL PROTECTION AGENCY IS DEEPLY CONCERNED BY CONTINUING DELAYS AND LACK OF TRANSPARENCY AND HAS DETERMINED THAT THE ACTIONS REQUIRED BY THE ORDER ... ARE ESSENTIAL TO ENSURING THE SAFE OPERATION OF FLINT'S DRINKING WATER SYSTEM AND THE PROTECTION OF PUBLIC HEALTH."

— GINA MCCARTHY

TIMELINE: JANUARY 2016

By John Bebow
Bridge Magazine

2016

JAN. 4: Genesee County Commission declares a state of emergency.

JAN. 12: Gov. Snyder activates the National Guard to distribute bottled water to Flint residents and asks the Federal Emergency Management Authority to coordinate an inter-agency plan to provide resources to Flint. He says, "Flint residents can continue to pick up free bottled water, water filters, replacement cartridges, and home water testing kits at the water resource sites."

JAN. 13: Snyder announces 87 cases of Legionnaires' disease in Genesee County, including nine deaths, since spring 2014. It's not clear if the outbreak is linked to Flint River water. This is the first public notice, 10 months after the MDEQ notified Snyder's urban affairs advisor, Harvey Hollins, that the outbreak coincided with the switch to Flint River water. State officials didn't connect the outbreak to Flint water. Marc Edwards, the Virginia Tech professor, says there is a "very strong likelihood" the water is linked to the disease outbreak.

JAN. 15: Michigan Attorney General Bill Schuette announces his office will investigate possible criminal wrongdoing in the Flint water crisis.

JAN. 16: President Obama declares a federal emergency in Flint.

JAN. 16: Professor Edwards writes on his blog: "Even worse, many residents currently refuse to believe that Flint's water is acceptable for bathing and showering, which is a concern because the public health benefits from basic sanitation, outweigh the relatively low dangers from lead and legionella."

JAN. 19: Snyder's State of the State Address focuses on the Flint crisis. He tells Flint's citizens: "I'm sorry and I will fix it. … You did not create this crisis, and you do not deserve this. ... Government failed you at the federal, state and local level. … We need to make sure this never happens again in any Michigan city."

JAN. 19: Impassioned, bordering on outrageous, statements are made all around on WKAR's "Off the Record" show after Snyder's speech:

Longtime political analyst, founder of the Inside Michigan Politics newsletter, and former state Sen. Bill Ballenger: "I run water over my rice every weekend in Flint and we've got no problems ... and the situation in Flint is nowhere near as bad as you are depicting."

Former state Sen. Gretchen Whitmer: "I trust the doctors who have looked at the lead levels in those children that the governor has poisoned."

JAN. 20: Snyder appeals federal denial of major disaster declaration for Flint, which had it been granted would have made Flint eligible for more relief money than the earlier state of emergency. "This situation poses an imminent and long-term threat to the people of Flint.... The problems will contribute to years – and potentially decades – of health problems and economic loss as well as require repairs to the infrastructure that neither the city, county nor state has the capacity to carry out."

JAN. 20: Michigan House passes a $28 million supplemental spending bill to help Flint's recovery from the crisis. "My further commitment is the $28 million is just one more step toward a long-term solution. There is more to come," Snyder says in a press release. The bill is signed on Jan. 29.

JAN. 21: EPA Region 5 Administrator Susan Hedman resigns over the Flint water crisis. She was a 2010 appointee of President Barack Obama. On Jan. 12, the Detroit News published an interview with Hedman in which she defended her actions and deflected blame. "Let's be clear, the recommendation to DEQ (regarding the need for corrosion controls) occurred at higher and higher levels during this time period," Hedman told the News. "And the answer kept coming back from DEQ that 'no, we are not going to make a decision until after we see more testing results.'"

Professor Edwards refutes Hedman, saying state and federal agencies should have moved quickly to protect Flint citizens as soon as it was known that the Flint River water wasn't treated for corrosion. Edwards told the News: "At that point, you do not just have smoke, you have a three-alarm fire and respond immediately. There was no sense of urgency at any of the relevant agencies, with the obvious exception of Miguel Del Toral, and he was silenced and discredited."

JAN. 21: President Obama announces $80 million in aid to Michigan, some of it to help with Flint's water infrastructure repairs.

JAN. 21: EPA issues Emergency Order concerning Flint Water. The cover letter from EPA Administrator Gina McCarthy is addressed to Gov. Snyder:

"The U.S. Environmental Protection Agency is deeply concerned by continuing delays and lack of transparency and has determined that the actions required by the order ... are essential to ensuring the safe operation of Flint's drinking water system and the protection of public health."

And then the order itself:

"On or about April 24, 2015, MDEQ notified EPA that the City did not have corrosion control treatment in place at the Flint Water Treatment Plant.

"During May and June 2015, EPA Region 5 staff at all levels expressed concern to MDEQ and the City about increasing concentrations of lead in Flint drinking water and conveyed its concern about lack of corrosion control and recommended that the expertise of EPA's Office of Research and Development should be used to avoid further water quality problems moving forward.

"On September 27, 2015, EPA Region 5 Administrator Susan Hedman called MDEQ Director Dan Wyant to discuss the need for expedited implementation of corrosion control treatment, the importance of following appropriate testing protocols, urged MDEQ to enlist Michigan Department of Health and Human Services' involvement and discussed options to provide bottled water/premixed formula/filters until corrosion control is optimized.

"On November 25, 2015, the EPA Flint Task Force requested information that would allow EPA to determine the progress being made on corrosion control in the City. This information has not been received by EPA. This information includes water quality parameter measurements (pH, total alkalinity, orthophosphate, chloride, turbidity, iron, calcium, temperature, conductivity) in the distribution system.

"On or about December 9, 2015, the City began feeding additional orthophosphate at the Flint Water Treatment Plant to begin optimizing corrosion control treatment. Notwithstanding the orthophosphate additions, high levels of lead and other contaminants are presumed to persist in the City's water system until LCR optimization process, utilizing sampling and monitoring requirements, have confirmed lead levels have been reduced.

"The presence of lead in the City water supply is principally due to the lack of corrosion control treatment after the City's switch to the Flint River as a source in April 2014. The river's water was corrosive and removed protective coatings in the system. This allowed lead to leach into the drinking water, which can continue until the system's treatment is optimized.

"The City, MDEQ, and the State have failed to take adequate measures to protect public health.

"EPA remains concerned that the City lacks the professional expertise and resources needed to carry out the recommended actions and to safely manage the City's PWS.

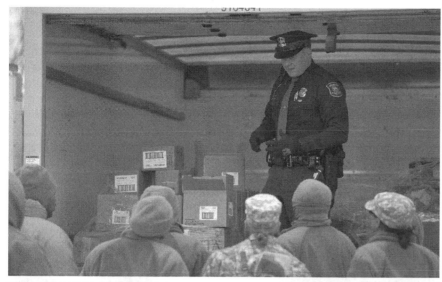

Michigan State Police coordinate the delivery of bottled water to Flint residents after Gov. Rick Snyder ordered the National Guard to Flint to help with water distribution.

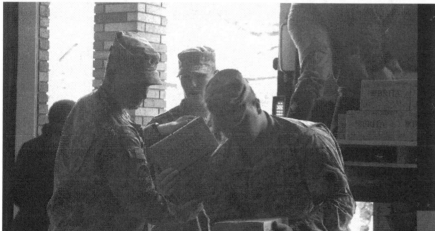

National Guard members unload water for Flint residents.

Photos courtesy of Michigan State Police

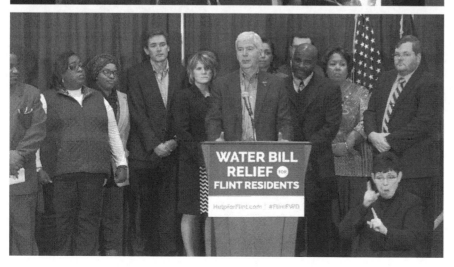

Gov. Rick Snyder signs a bill to provide millions of dollars in water- and sewer-bill reimbursement.

Photo courtesy of Livestream

"As a result of the emergency, EPA will promptly begin sampling and analysis of lead levels and other contaminants in the City to assure that all regulatory authorities and the public have accurate and reliable information. EPA will make its LCR sampling results available to the public on the Agency's website.

"The lead and other contaminants will remain present in the PWS and will continue to present an imminent and substantial endangerment to the health of persons until the underlying problems with the corrosion control treatment and fundamental deficiencies in the operation of the PWS are corrected and sampling results confirm the lead and other contaminant are adequately treated.

"The EPA finds that there is an imminent and substantial endangerment to the people drinking water from the public water system of the City of Flint and that the actions taken by the State and/or the City are inadequate to protect public health."

JAN. 22: Snyder goes on the "Morning Joe" show on MSNBC and takes state workers to task. "The heads were not being given the right information by quote-unquote experts.... I use that word with great trial and tribulation because they were considered experts in terms of their backgrounds."

JAN. 22: The Detroit Free Press reports: "The activist hacker group Anonymous has launched a Flint operation and is calling for Gov. Rick Snyder to be charged with 'voluntary or involuntary manslaughter. ... The crimes committed by Gov. Snyder as well as other city officials will not go unpunished.'"

JAN. 22: The Flint Water Advisory Task Force calls for Gov. Snyder to engage with USEPA staff experts "versed in Lead and Copper Rule requirements. ... These individuals should be empowered to guide implementation of a comprehensive LCR sampling program in Flint that will monitor lead levels now and throughout the conversion to raw water supply by the Karegnondi Water Authority and full-time use of the Flint Water Treatment Plant." The first among EPA experts the task force recommends is Miguel Del Toral, whose alarms about Flint were dismissed and hidden by the EPA and MDEQ in 2015.

JAN. 22: Snyder returns additional executive powers to the mayor of Flint. "Mayor Weaver will now have the authority to appoint the city administrator and all department heads. Today's action is the next step in transitioning to full, local control in Flint," Snyder says in a statement.

JAN. 22: Two MDEQ employees are "suspended pending an investigation, in accordance with Civil Service rules," says a press release from Snyder's office. The employees are not named. They soon are identified in media reports and state correspondence as Stephen Busch, a district supervisor, and Liane Shekter Smith, former chief of MDEQ's drinking water office.

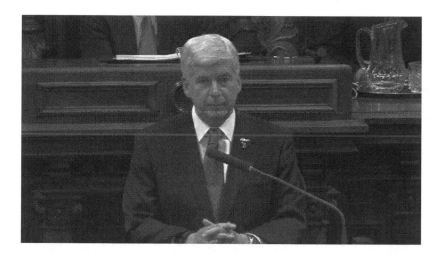

In his state of the state address on Jan. 19, Gov. Rick Snyder spent much of his speech on Flint; "I'm sorry and I will fix it... You did not create this crisis, and you do not deserve this."

Photo courtesy of Michigan Radio

JAN. 22: New MDEQ Director Keith Creagh responds to an EPA emergency order of the day before, says the state "looks forward to working cooperatively" with EPA and the City of Flint on the drinking water issue, and then takes a more combative stance: "The Order does not reference the tens of millions of dollars expended by or in the process of being expended by the State for water filters, drinking water, testing, and medical services."

"The Order demands that the State take certain actions, but fails to note that many of those actions, including those set forth above, have already been undertaken."

"From a legal perspective, we also question whether the USEPA has the legal authority to order a State and its agencies to take the actions outlined in the Order. We will fully outline our legal and factual concerns with the Order in writing or would be happy to host a meeting in Lansing or Flint. ... Subject to the above comments, we are committed to implementing the measures in the Order. ..."

JAN. 25: Michigan Attorney General Bill Schuette taps attorney Todd Flood (a defense attorney and former Wayne County assistant prosecutor) and former Detroit FBI bureau chief Andy Arena to lead a wide-ranging investigation into potential misconduct in office concerning the Flint water disaster. At the same time, state Rep. LaTanya Garrett, D-Detroit, files a petition with U.S. Attorney General Loretta Lynch to remove Schuette's office from the Flint water-crisis investigation claiming conflicts of interest.

JAN. 29: Progress Michigan, a liberal advocacy group, reveals state emails showing that state workers in Flint offices switched to purified water coolers as early as January 2015, even as state agencies were telling the Snyder administration and Flint residents that Flint water was safe.

Researchers working with professor Marc Edwards' Flintwaterstudy.org are shown testing tap water samples from Flint's for lead content in their Virginia Tech laboratory. Pictured are Anurag Mantha (striped shirt), Dr. Dongjuan Dai (green goggles), and Kristine Mapili (reaching for bottle) and Siddhartha Roy, partially blocked.

Photo courtesy of Logan Wallace/Virginia Tech

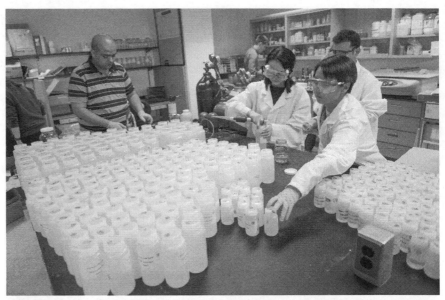

Gov. Rick Snyder and U.S. EPA administrator Gina McCarthy are sworn in at a March 17 hearing of the House Oversight Committee.

Screen capture courtesy of CSPAN

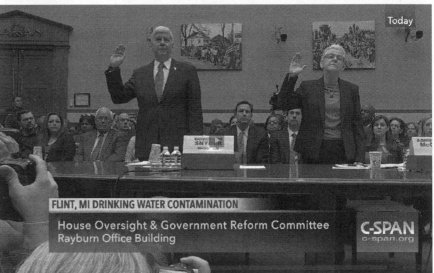

CHAPTER 20

FEBRUARY – MARCH 2016

IT ALL COMES TO LIGHT – THROUGH EMAIL

POLITICS TURNS THE FLINT CRISIS INTO A PARTISAN FOOD FIGHT

Editor's summary: Much of the ugly and incompetent government bungling of the Flint water crisis may not have come to light – at least not nearly so soon – if not for the extraordinary public release of Snyder Administration emails. Normally, governors' aides work behind a wall of secrecy – their email communications are protected from public release. Governor Snyder – facing immense pressure from the public, the media, and from advocacy groups steadily making various revelations from seemingly random state email records – waived his executive privilege and opened thousands upon thousands of email records to public view. The records provided a never-before-seen view of daily deliberations and management decisions at the highest levels of state government. Indeed, this book would not have been possible without all those emails. As media coverage focused on every intricacy of the email records, the Flint crisis took on a sharply partisan theme in presidential debates and Congressional hearings.

"PUTTING THE WELL-BEING OF MICHIGANDERS FIRST NEEDS TO BE THE TOP PRIORITY FOR ALL STATE EMPLOYEES."

— GOV. RICK SNYDER

TIMELINE: FEBRUARY – MARCH 2016

By John Bebow
Bridge Magazine

2016

FEB. 2: The U.S. Attorney's office in Detroit confirms that the Federal Bureau of Investigation and the EPA Criminal Investigation Division are conducting a criminal investigation of the Flint water crisis.

FEB. 3: The first of what will be three hearings of the U.S. House Oversight and Government Reform Committee is held in Washington. Witnesses include professor Marc Edwards, Flint mother Lee-Anne Walters, newly appointed Michigan Department of Environmental Quality director Keith Creagh and Joel Geauvais, acting director of water quality for the U.S. Environmental Protection Agency. But key committee members were more steamed about who wasn't there. Democrats wanted Gov. Rick Snyder, but committee chairman Jason Chaffetz, R-UT, didn't invite him. And Chaffetz was peeved that former Flint Emergency Manager Darnell Earley, whom he did invite, wasn't there. (Both Snyder and Earley would testify before the committee in March.)

FEB. 5: Gov. Rick Snyder announces that Liane Shekter Smith, head of the Office of Drinking Water and Municipal Assistance for the state DEQ, was fired. Four months prior, Shekter Smith had received a performance bonus of $2,652, according to the Detroit News. She is the first to be fired in connection with the Flint water crisis. Putting the well-being of Michiganders first needs to be the top priority for all state employees," Snyder says in a statement.

FEB. 12: At Snyder's direction, the state opens a new website containing thousands of pages of emails related to the Flint water crisis. The emails were those requested from state agencies. The details have been covered in earlier chapters based on the date they were sent.

FEB. 26: Snyder's office releases another email batch estimated at up to 8,000 sent to or from the governor's staff and the governor himself dating back to 2011. These emails were not subject to Michigan's Freedom of Information Law, which exempts the governor's office and Legislature from FOIA requests. Among many major revelations are emails between several of Snyder's top advisors urging a return to Detroit water as early as Oct. 2014, but apparently they didn't relate their concerns to the governor. As is the case with the content of previous releases, the details are covered in earlier chapters based on the date the email was sent.

FEB. 26: Snyder signs a $30 million supplemental budget bill for Flint. Among other things, it provides water bill credits to Flint residents for the portion of their water they could not safely use for drinking, bathing and cooking.

MARCH 5: Fitch Ratings declares that it could cost $275 billion nationwide to replace drinking water service lines containing lead.

MARCH 6: Democratic presidential candidates Hillary Clinton and Bernie Sanders debate in Flint and blame the water crisis on the Republican Party. Both call upon Rick Snyder to resign. Snyder responds and issues a press release documenting his administration's responses to provide bottled water, National Guard help, millions of dollars in funding, and other assistance to the city and repeats his declaration that he will fix the problems in Flint.

MARCH 11: Snyder calls for a full investigation of how the Michigan Department of Health and Human Services handled lead poisoning and Legionnaires' disease issues throughout the crisis. The governor tasks the state's Auditor General and MDHHS Inspector General with the probe.

MARCH 15: The second of three House Oversight Committee hearings are held on Flint with more partisan finger-pointing. Resigned EPA Region 5 Administrator Susan Hedman, who is among four witnesses, is the primary target of Republicans, while former Flint Emergency Manager Darnell Earley and Gov. Snyder (who will testify two days later) get most of the scorn from Democrats.

MARCH 17: It's barb-trading all around in Congress as Snyder and EPA Administrator Gina McCarthy testify. Republicans slam McCarthy. Democrats slam Snyder. And Snyder and McCarthy slam each other. Little new information arises about the Flint water crisis. The Snyder-McCarthy testimony highlights congressional hearings filled with finger-pointing but little in the way of future-oriented preventative strategy or new revelations.

MARCH 23: Flint is a case of "environmental injustice," the Snyder-appointed Flint Water Advisory Task Force declares in its final report, laying the blame squarely on the Snyder Administration and its state agencies. The report also is highly critical of the state's emergency manager law, saying the unilateral authority of emergency managers in Flint played a significant role in causing and prolonging the crisis and presented a lack of decision-making checks and balances. Emergency managers were too narrowly focused on financial issues in the water switch, the task force concludes. As in the task force's preliminary reports, it finds that the MDEQ and MDHHS both fundamentally failed in their missions to protect public health.

MARCH 29: Flint utilities manager Mike Glasgow says in a Michigan legislative hearing that it was a "bad decision" to switch to the Flint River. He explains that the city had 26 employees to handle water treatment at the time of the switch in 2014. By comparison, the city had 40 water treatment employees a decade earlier when the treatment plant only served as a backup to water supplied by the city of Detroit.

CHAPTER 21

FEB. 4, 2016

WHO'S TO BLAME FOR THE FLINT WATER CRISIS?

IT'S NOW CLEAR THERE WERE FAILURES AT ALL LEVELS

Editor's summary: As debate about Flint's water crisis intensifies after Gov. Snyder released thousands of pages of email records, John Bebow, president and CEO of the Center for Michigan and a former investigative reporter for major newspapers, plows through the evidence to produce a massive timeline and Michigan Truth Squad analysis of how the crisis unfolded. (The Michigan Truth Squad is a Bridge Magazine project that separates fact from fiction in political speech and campaign advertising.) What follows is Bebow's shorthand version of the Truth Squad findings.

By John Bebow
Bridge Magazine

The litany of mistakes that caused lead poisoning in Flint's drinking water – and responsibility for those gross errors – will be debated for years by investigators, lawyers, politicians, the media, and Michigan citizens.

As more news and finger-pointing arrives daily, questions abound.

No one is exactly sure how many Flint residents – especially young children – had elevated blood lead levels after Flint switched its drinking water source to the Flint River in April 2014. The full extent of the damage may be impossible to determine, especially among Flint's vulnerable, low-income residents who already face so many challenges.

Resolution of the ongoing water crisis remains distant. The U.S. Environmental Protection Agency recently announced that new filters given to Flint residents to screen lead from their tainted water likely did not fully protect those with extreme lead levels coming from their taps. Long term, the EPA has said it has serious concerns that the City of Flint "lacks the professional expertise and resources" to "safely manage" its drinking water.

Today, Bridge Magazine's Michigan Truth Squad publishes the most comprehensive timeline to date in one place. It is intended as an informal public repository of all major public records relating to Flint's water crisis. It is presented for local residents and a wider audience to help separate fact from fiction and understand the dimensions of this man-made tragedy. A complete portrait of the Flint disaster likely will take many months of official investigation and years of litigation.

When it comes to identifying who's at fault, reams of currently available information point in five directions. Readers can draw their own conclusions as to who or what agency is most to blame.

MICHIGAN DEPARTMENT OF ENVIRONMENTAL QUALITY

MDEQ is responsible for drinking water safety and regulation across our state. MDEQ failed the people of Flint and did so with arrogant disrespect.

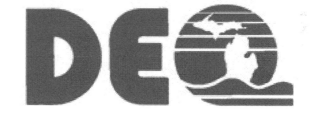

MDEQ's failure to anticipate and prevent the Flint water disaster is so drastic that it calls into question the agency's ability to regulate and safeguard public drinking water systems anywhere else. Indeed, the U.S. Environmental Protection Agency is now investigating MDEQ's competence to do just that.

MDEQ failed in these ways:

MDEQ drinking water regulators allowed the City of Flint to switch drinking water sources to the Flint River in April 2014 without requiring treatment to help neutralize the water and protect the water system's old pipes, many of them made from lead. Flint River water is highly corrosive. It rusts steel pipes and it destroyed a protective layer in the pipes in the lead pipes, mostly city-owned service lines from water mains to customer-owned plumbing. That allowed lead to flake into the drinking water. The chemical reaction is well known to professionals charged with protecting public water. MDEQ did not act to anticipate the problem after the switch to the Flint River, which resulted in disaster.

MDEQ drinking water regulators grossly misinterpreted federal regulations requiring chemical treatments to control corrosion.

MDEQ drinking water regulators ignored, and attempted to discredit, numerous serious warning signs of corrosion leading to lead poisoning in the Flint drinking water system. A General Motors engine plant declared within six months of the switch that the Flint River water was corroding its parts and switched back to using Detroit water purchased from a neighboring township.

MDEQ regulators said GM's issues were unrelated to the water's suitability for drinking, cooking and bathing. Within weeks of the water supply switch, Flint residents complained of discolored, smelly, bad-tasting water and related health problems with rashes and other impacts. MDEQ issued minor violations, but reacted with no urgency. In a February 2015 memo to Gov. Rick Snyder, MDEQ acknowledged "hiccups" in Flint's drinking water quality but concluded: "It's not like an eminent (sic) threat to public health."

MDEQ drinking water regulators disputed, ignored, and tried to discredit crucial alarms issued by EPA drinking water regulator Miguel Del Toral. Beginning in February 2015, he repeatedly warned MDEQ that the lack of corrosion control would lead to a serious health hazard, as lead would leach into drinking water supplies. In response, MDEQ staff denigrated Del Toral as a second-guesser and "rogue" employee; the state agency fought Del Toral's contention that corrosion control should have been done immediately when Flint switched to Flint River for drinking water. Not until mid-October 2015, when the crisis was full-blown, would MDEQ acknowledge the mistake.

As the Flint crisis became public starting in mid-2015, MDEQ responded with many incredible public statements that likely will become classroom case studies. The MDEQ public commentary in statements and comments to reporters was dismissive, insensitive, arrogant and – critically – inaccurate.

In summary, the overwhelming weight of the currently available public record points directly to MDEQ as the party in the best position to have prevented lead from poisoning Flint's drinking water supply.

In December, the Flint Water Advisory Task Force, an investigative body established by Gov. Rick Snyder, concluded: "We believe the primary responsibility for what happened in Flint rests with the Michigan Department of Environmental Quality (MDEQ). Although many individuals and entities at the state and local levels contributed to creating and prolonging the problem, MDEQ is the government agency that has responsibility to ensure safe drinking water in Michigan. It failed in that responsibility and must be held accountable for that failure."

In January, EPA's national administrator issued an emergency order, which concluded that lack of corrosion control caused lead to leach into Flint's drinking water. The EPA order said: "The City, MDEQ, and the State have failed to take adequate measures to protect public health… The EPA finds that there is an imminent and substantial endangerment to the people drinking water from the public water system of the City of Flint and that the actions taken by the State and/or the City are inadequate to protect public health."

MDEQ Director Dan Wyant and Director of Communications Brad Wurfel resigned in late December 2015 over the Flint scandal. Two key MDEQ drinking water regulators, Liane Shekter Smith and Stephen Busch, were suspended pending further investigation. Shekter Smith has since been fired.

Without the crucial and vigilant research of an independent drinking water expert, Virginia Tech professor Marc Edwards, the early, solitary drumbeat of concern from Del Toral of the EPA, and the courageous and spot-on medical proof from Flint pediatrician Dr. Mona Hanna-Attisha and her colleagues, high lead levels in the Flint water likely would have continued to escape public view.

In Truth Squad's view, MDEQ deserves every ounce of scrutiny, scorn and public mistrust heaped upon it.

U.S. ENVIRONMENTAL PROTECTION AGENCY

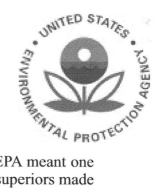

In its January 2016 emergency order, the EPA stated: "During May and June 2015, EPA Region 5 staff at all levels expressed concern to MDEQ and the City about increasing concentrations of lead in Flint drinking water and conveyed its concern about lack of corrosion control…"

The only way this statement is accurate is if "at all levels" the EPA meant one determined regulator, Miguel Del Toral, in its bureaucracy. His superiors made no serious moves for many months after Del Toral first raised serious misgivings about MDEQ and Flint water plant operators. In fact, in some ways, others at the federal agency undercut Miguel Del Toral's warnings.

For months, only Del Toral appears to have raised serious concerns about Flint's failure to use corrosion control on the river water. Public documents referenced in the Truth Squad timeline indicate that other EPA officials failed to act with any sense of urgency.

In a July 2015 email to Flint Mayor Dayne Walling, EPA Region 5 Administrator Susan Hedman said Del Toral's 8-page memo on June 24 to his boss raising grave concerns about Flint's water was just a "draft" and shouldn't have been released until it had been vetted and reworked. She even apologized "for the way in which this matter was handled" after Del Toral's concerns became public. Email records of one DEQ official claimed the federal agency "apologized profusely" after Del Toral's "unvetted draft" became public. EPA did not officially release Del Toral's memo about Flint to MDEQ until November 2015 – more than four months after it was drafted the memo and eight months after he sounded the first alarm to state regulators.

Also, in July 2015, another EPA water official, Jennifer Crooks, summarized ongoing MDEQ-EPA discussions about Flint, again with no sense of urgency. Crooks wrote: "Since Flint has lead service lines, we understand some citizen-requested lead sampling is exceeding the (federal) Action Level, and the source of drinking water will be changing again in 2016, so to start a Corrosion Control Study now doesn't make sense."

Moreover, in seeking to explain why the federal watchdog environmental agency didn't sound the public alarm earlier to Flint residents, the EPA said that was the role of the state agency. While technically true, EPA has the authority, the clout, and the moral obligation to set aside such protocols to address an emerging health crisis when a state is reluctant to do so. That's what the EPA did with its January 2016 emergency order.

To its credit, EPA has swung into action in Flint in numerous ways. But it was painfully slow to do so. For the agency to claim otherwise is disingenuous, based on the available public record. EPA Region 5 Administrator Susan Hedman resigned over the Flint crisis in January 2016.

The currently available public record suggests EPA bears considerable responsibility for delaying potential relief to Flint citizens until long after its own expert, Del Toral, made clear what was at stake.

MICHIGAN DEPARTMENT OF HEALTH AND HUMAN SERVICES (MDHHS)

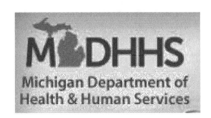

Just as the MDEQ is responsible for protecting drinking water supplies, MDHHS is responsible for monitoring blood lead levels in children – and taking action when they see a problem.

Just like MDEQ, the MDHHS failed the residents and children of Flint.

Flint pediatrician Dr. Mona Hanna-Attisha and the Hurley Medical Center, where she runs a pediatrics residency program, clearly linked a sharp increase in blood lead levels among young children to the switch to the Flint River for drinking water. In contrast, MDHHS whiffed and then disputed Hanna-Attisha's conclusions.

Two months before she released her results and broke the Flint scandal wide open, MDHHS experts looked for an elevated blood lead trend in Flint in response to concerns raised by Gov. Snyder's chief of staff. The MDHHS experts identified a spike in Flint blood lead levels shortly after the Flint River switch, but concluded it wasn't attributable to the drinking water.

On Sept. 24, 2015, the day Dr. Hanna-Attisha released her study, Wesley Priem, manager of the MDHHS Healthy Homes Section, wrote in an email to a colleague: "…This is definitely being driven by a little science and a lot of politics."

Days later, MDHHS Director Nick Lyons seemed to order his department to look for ways to dispute Dr. Hanna-Attisha's research. In an email, Lyons wrote: "I would like to make a strong statement with a demonstration of proof that the lead blood levels seen are not out of the ordinary and are attributable to seasonal fluctuations."

By Oct. 1, as MDHHS officials finally confirmed Dr. Hanna-Attisha's conclusions, Lyons prepared for a press conference by remarking in an email to a colleague, "I'd like to express my appreciation to the Hurley doctors for bringing this issue to our attention."

By year's end, the Snyder administration would conclude: "It wasn't until the Hurley report came out that our epidemiologists took a more in-depth look at the data by zip code, controlling for seasonal variation, and confirmed an increase outside of normal trends. As a result of this process, we have determined that the way we analyze data … needs to be thoroughly reviewed."

MDHHS experts' initial miscalculations helped delay confirmation of Flint's lead in water issue. If not for the work of Dr. Hanna-Attisha and other outside experts, Flint residents might still be drinking tainted water without warning from this state agency.

THE SNYDER ADMINISTRATION

The Flint disaster happened on Rick Snyder's watch. Emergency Managers whom Snyder appointed to reverse the city's fiscal calamity made critical decisions that led to choosing the Flint River as the city's drinking water source; those decisions were signed off on by state Department of Treasury officials. Flint's local elected officials also largely supported the switch.

Amid some calls for him to resign, Snyder has apologized to Flint's citizens and pledged to fix the problems. Since October 2015, he has provided considerable help with money, technical assistance and, though not until January 2016, boots

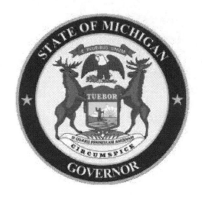

on the ground in the form of National Guard troops passing out bottled water and tap filters.

For the people of Flint, this was too little, too late.

To be fair, the governor could not be expected to know early on that water and health experts at two state agencies were wrong in dismissing warnings about an emerging crisis.

To Snyder's credit, in late July, his Chief of Staff Dennis Muchmore expressed worry to the agencies that Flint residents' complaints of brown water and skin rashes were being "blown off" by the state. That inquiry sparked a fresh round of denials of any serious problem by both MDEQ and MDHHS.

But, time and again, the Snyder administration followed the flawed guidance of the state agencies for many weeks as the crisis mushroomed.

Worse, in late-September 2015, after independent experts had clearly outlined serious concerns and provided evidence of a public health threat from lead in the Flint water, Muchmore's emails showed a more callous political calculation than a sense of urgency.

After the revelations of Virginia Tech's Edwards and Hurley's Dr. Hanna-Attisha were made public, Muchmore described Flint drinking water as "less than savory" and deflected that "it's really the city's water system that needs to deal with it." In these communications to the governor and other aides, he seemed to adopt the don't-worry conclusions of MDEQ and MDHHS, rather than considering an independent probe.

The question remains: Why did the governor and key aides keep relying on flawed briefings from the two state agencies as the crisis magnified?

We expect investigations will probe any culpability of officials in the Snyder Administration, including the governor.

To date, Gov. Snyder has released what he characterized as two years of his own email records relating to Flint (a release not required under the state's Freedom of Information laws). That's not good enough. Snyder has not released full email records of all in his administration concerning the Flint crisis. He must. Truth Squad encourages investigators to pursue public release of every word ever written by any government official at any level about the Flint crisis.

PUBLIC OFFICIALS IN FLINT

Had Flint not switched from the Detroit Water and Sewerage Department, the Flint crisis in all likelihood would not have happened.

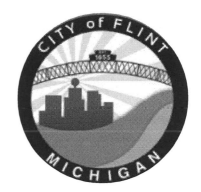

In a recent analysis, Truth Squad took Gov. Snyder and his appointed emergency managers to task for implying that the decision to switch from DWSD to the Karegnondi Water Authority and, ultimately, to the Flint River was made by Flint city officials. As Truth Squad noted, Flint's state-appointed emergency managers ran the city when every key decision was made. They signed the relevant orders and the state treasurer signed off.

Truth Squad would note, however, that lost in that narrative is ample public record that Flint leaders wanted to move from Detroit water service amid concerns about cost and local control. Flint leaders enthusiastically endorsed joining the new regional KWA scheduled to come online later in 2016. Although they did not make the decision to use the Flint River until KWA was ready, Flint leaders enthusiastically endorsed the Flint River decision – and toasted it the day of the water switch.

Neighboring Genesee County communities that were also getting Detroit water and had joined KWA stuck with the pricey Detroit water during the interim.

Two months after Flint made the source water switch, Mayor Dayne Walling declared to MLive.com that "It's a quality, safe product … I think people are wasting their precious money buying bottled water."

The actions of Flint officials going forward require ongoing scrutiny, especially since the EPA has declared it is worried the city "lacks the professional expertise and resources" necessary to "safely manage" the city's drinking water supply.

LESS BLAMEWORTHY: STATE E.M. LAW, UNIONS, AND OTHER FACTORS

Many factors, decades in the making, created the economic conditions that preceded the Flint water disaster. Flint's general economic decline has ravaged the city and its people, leaving Flint with a decrepit infrastructure and inadequate revenues to recover or maintain what little it has left.

Some say hard-line trade unionism drove big employers out of Flint decades ago, while others rail against manufacturers like General Motors leaving Flint helpless by pulling and taking thousands of good-paying jobs elsewhere. Some blame white flight, and others blame mismanagement of city finances. Still others lambast state policies and budget priorities that have shrunk revenue sharing dollars for cities like Flint.

In all of this worthy public debate, at least two narratives have been cited as possible contributors to Flint's water crisis.

THE MICHIGAN EMERGENCY MANAGER LAW

The public record does not support the suggestion that the state's emergency management law itself led directly to the lead poisoning of Flint's children. This narrative is amplified by national political and media pundits. MSNBC's Rachel Maddow is a leading proponent of this theory, also amplified by Washington Post columnist Dana Milbank. In late January, Milbank wrote: "Snyder undertook an arrogant public-policy experiment, underpinned by the ideological assumption that the 'experience set' of corporate-style managers was superior to the checks and balances of democracy. This is why Flint happened."

For several years, the emergency manager law has resulted in nearly constant, worthy, and unfinished debate about local control, threats to local self-determination, municipal finance policy generally, and what to do about municipalities and school systems facing unsustainable levels of debt and deficits.

At least two Flint emergency managers are facing questions about the decision to switch to the Flint River. If they are found culpable, they should face repercussions. But no evidence exists on the current public record that the EM law itself produced the Flint water crisis.

Beyond that, it remains unclear whether city officials, had they been in charge, would have made different decisions to avoid the Flint drinking water crisis, though they might have backed away from it sooner.

The record shows these officials broadly supported dropping Detroit as a drinking water source. A state-appointed emergency manager made the decision to use the Flint River as a water source, but officials didn't protest that choice. Some, in fact, toasted Flint water on the day of the switch. It's more than plausible that Flint officials would have followed the misguided regulatory orders of the MDEQ and fallen into a lead crisis of their own, had an emergency manager not been running the city.

On the other hand, the record shows that the City Council voted 7-1 in March 2015 to return to Detroit water service. The Snyder-appointed emergency manager, Jerry Ambrose, called the vote "incomprehensible" because it would have cost about $1 million more monthly. He kept Flint citizens drinking water sourced from their river.

UNIONS

The conservative American Legislative Exchange Council — which supports "limited government, free markets and federalism"— issued a tweet in late January 2016 blaming the Flint crisis on Flint itself. ALEC said: "Gov't failure, brought on by public employee pensions, poisoned Flint water. Stop blaming everyone else."

That is one of the single-most blatantly wrong and incredibly insensitive examples of naked political opportunism in the Flint saga. There is zero support for it in the public record.

CHAPTER 22

FEB. 10, 2016

EPA AUDIT FLAGGED MDEQ'S DEFICIENCIES YEARS BEFORE FLINT'S LEAD POISONING CRISIS

Editor's summary: A 2010 federal audit of the Michigan Department of Environmental Quality expresses doubts about how thoroughly the agency is testing lead levels as part of its municipal water safety program. The audit foreshadows many of the same issues that will arise in the Flint water disaster.

By Ted Roelofs
Bridge Magazine Contributor

Years before a lead-poisoning crisis made Flint an unenviable center of national attention, there were warning signs about the Michigan Department of Environmental Quality, the state agency charged with keeping drinking water safe.

Among them: federal government concerns about MDEQ's ability to detect lead in the water supply.

In 2010, the U.S. Environmental Protection Agency audit portrayed MDEQ as beset by budget cuts, staff shifts and limited resources, and willing to take regulatory shortcuts to safeguard water.

The agency's Drinking Water Program had just seen its annual budget slashed to about $1.5 million, down $300,000 from the previous fiscal year, the audit said.

"Frequent hiring freezes have impacted Michigan for about ten years," the report noted. "This has made it difficult to replace positions." Bans on contract services and a "cumbersome" employee hiring process didn't help.

Funding cuts forced MDEQ's Drinking Water Program to fill vacancies "with staff from other programs that have been cut or eliminated," the audit said. "While this practice preserves jobs, it decreases the technical knowledge of staff and requires tremendous resources to train these staff."

Almost as an aside, the audit suggested, "training for new staff would also be appreciated on fundamental public health issues and compliance decisions."

It is not clear whether the financial and monitoring shortcomings identified in the report were factors in MDEQ's much-criticized performance during the Flint water crisis, or to what degree they were addressed in the interim.

Melanie Brown, MDEQ's communication director, did not respond to requests for comment about the report. (After publication of this article, Brown wrote in an email to Bridge that MDEQ's new leadership "cannot immediately speak" to issues raised in the audit. She said MDEQ is working hard to test water in homes and school buildings and to "ensure our water sampling and testing protocols are the most effective methods as possible now and into the future.")

The EPA audit documented technical shortcomings in everything from monitoring radioactive pollutants known as radionuclides and coliform bacteria in water to how effectively MDEQ followed federal rules for tracking lead levels.

Lead in water is measured in parts per billion (ppb). Federal regulations require water utilities to certify that 90 percent of homes in a community contain 15 parts per billion of lead or less in drinking water. It's a standard some critics say should be tougher, for two reasons: One, even at levels below 15 ppb, lead poses serious health concerns, especially for young children. Second, the 90th percentile standard theoretically could allow cities to proclaim their water safe even if 10 percent of homes had lead levels higher than the 15 ppb EPA "action" standard.

Critics of the rule say that can leave lead "hot spots" that often correlate with high-poverty neighborhoods – as was the case in Flint – even if a water system is judged in compliance with EPA's 1991 Lead and Copper rule. A 2016 study led by Flint pediatrician Mona Hanna-Attisha found that lead blood levels had doubled among Flint children after the water switch, but increased even more in "socioeconomically disadvantaged neighborhoods."

The EPA audit said MDEQ failed to meet this federal standard, noting that it "does not calculate 90th percentiles, unless one sample exceeds one-half of the [15 ppb] action level. In that case, a potential violation will be identified and staff will use (a state database) to calculate the 90th percentile."

MDEQ's "practice does not meet the requirements of Federal Regulations, since it is required that all 90th percentiles be calculated," the audit concluded.

The audit also found MDEQ failed to submit 90th-percentile results to a federal water information system "in a timely fashion."

In "several cases," MDEQ also failed to make a timely report of lead readings that exceeded the federal action standards.

EPA was likewise troubled that MDEQ did not conduct the required number of water samples for lead, including during the summer months to conserve limited agency resources.

In the case of radionuclides – radioactive substances that can be found in certain rocks and minerals and sometimes enter water supplies – the audit found there were "no labs in Michigan certified for radionuclide analysis, so samples are sent out of state. The labs tend to be very slow and yield widely varying results."

The EPA also noted that MDEQ did not monitor whether water quality tests were done in schools or childcare centers. The agency left that task to local health departments, but had "no formalized oversight or enforcement to ensure" those reports were turned in, nor "specific programs to address drinking water contamination in schools or childcare facilities."

A BROKEN SYSTEM

An expert from the Virginia Tech scientific team that helped bring the Flint water crisis to public attention said the audit results weren't surprising.

Yanna Lambrinidou, a medical ethnographer and adjunct assistant professor at Virginia Tech, said deficiencies are common with water supply regulators across the nation.

"These are programs that are understaffed, underfunded and lacking knowledge and experience," she said.

She noted that in 2013, the Association of State Drinking Water Administrators found that 17 states had cut budgets for agencies regulating drinking water safety by more than 20 percent.

In Michigan, the EPA audit was conducted during the administration of Gov. Jennifer Granholm. It referred to "dramatic budget cuts" at MDEQ that had a "significant impact" on its water program.

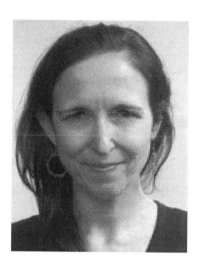
Yanna Lambrinidou, a water quality expert at Virginia Tech, said that MDEQ's budget-conscious approach to water monitoring is reflective of resource shortages in state environmental agencies across much of the country.

"Increased regulatory requirements coupled with a decrease in available funding, have required MDEQ to prioritize program activities" and sharpen its focus on "drinking water regulations that directly affect public health," the audit said.

Lambrinidou conducted research on lead contamination in drinking water in Washington D.C., exposed by the Washington Post in 2004. She also served on a working group for the National Drinking Water Advisory Council that issued recommendations for changing how lead and copper are regulated in drinking water.

Lambrinidou said the EPA audit's finding that MDEQ was not following the letter of the 90th-percentile reporting requirement was troubling. "It says to me that they are not following the law. It says to me the system is more broken than we think."

There's no indication the failings alleged in the audit led directly to the Flint water crisis. But the EPA's findings foreshadow much of what was to come when MDEQ regulators failed to quickly identify and mitigate the lead poisoning threat in Flint's drinking water after the city began drawing water in April 2014 from the highly corrosive Flint River.

On Dec. 29, the Flint Water Advisory Task Force, the team appointed by Gov. Rick Snyder to investigate what happened in Flint, concluded the MDEQ was primarily responsible for the failure. Some task force themes echoed the EPA audit findings – notably, it's description of MDEQ as an agency where "a culture exists in which 'technical compliance' is considered sufficient to ensure safe drinking water."

As a result of the Flint disaster, EPA is conducting a "full programmatic review" of MDEQ beyond its typical annual inspection to assure the agency "maintains reliable drinking water supplies that meet all of the requirements of the Safe Drinking Water Act."

The audit is expected to take several months.

Lambrinidou of Virginia Tech said the EPA audit in 2010 should have raised alarms at both EPA and MDEQ.

"What this says to me is that this report came out six years ago and six years later people in Flint have gotten poisoned water," Lambrinidou said. "What has happened in those six years? Who fixed what?"

CHAPTER 23

FEB. 16, 2016

WHAT FLINT LOST

'IT'S GOING TO BE HARD TO GET THE PEOPLE'S TRUST BACK.'

Editor's summary: This is a tough story to read. The comments of Flint residents interviewed in late January and early February 2016 about their total loss of faith in government agencies to do the right thing seems at first blush so paranoid, so irrational ... until you stop to try to put yourself in their shoes – being asked to trust the same people whose terrible decisions – or inaction – directly led to unsafe levels of lead in their drinking water.

By Chastity Pratt Dawsey
Bridge Magazine

About a year ago, Victoria Marx lost her balance while she stood on a ladder at Home Depot where she worked. It happened a few times. At about the same time, she noticed a tremor in her right hand.

Marx, 60, was diagnosed with Parkinson's disease, a chronic movement disorder that can result from a mix of genetic and environmental factors. A few months after her diagnosis, Gov. Rick Snyder was on television apologizing to the people of Flint, confirming they were exposed to high levels of lead after the city switched its drinking water source to the Flint River in April 2014.

A January 2016 test in Marx's bungalow showed her water was still unsafe to drink. She can't prove it, but she believes the lead in her water damaged her nervous system. As far as the governor goes, she doesn't believe anything he says.

"This is something I have to live with for the rest of my life," said Marx, who walks with a limp. "Things would've been fine if Snyder's emergency manager hadn't switched us over to the Flint River."

To be a resident in Flint now is to thrum with government mistrust. Coping for months with no fix, enduring a mix of bad information and too little communication, residents interviewed for this report say their faith in all levels of government is shattered. Instead they're beset by suspicion and, at times, paranoia as the government agencies implicated in the lead crisis are now in charge of the recovery effort.

Some residents say they don't trust that water filters distributed at fire stations can make their water safe. Others balk at accepting donated jugs of water for cooking and bathing because some containers have no labels. A few won't accept some brands of free bottled water, fearing E. coli contamination rumors that buzzed on Facebook. Still others reject the accuracy of blood and residential water tests conducted by government workers. Another blames lead for the deaths of her two German shepherds.

This visceral mistrust has only strengthened with the revelation that county, state and federal health officials dithered internally for most of 2015 before alerting the public that the water may have been linked to nine deaths from Legionnaires' disease in and around Flint.

Even months after lead contamination was confirmed, people say that they have yet to get answers as to why they're still getting rashes, or if their daily lives will return to normal by next year, the year after that, or ever.

At a recent NAACP meeting, one resident referenced police killings of unarmed African Americans nationwide and voiced fear of National Guard workers distributing water in Flint, saying, "If I open my door when they come, and take out my cell phone, they might shoot me because they think it's a gun."

ECHOES OF A DARK CHAPTER

The people of Flint speak of the cascading series of government failures in the language of betrayal. For many residents, a majority African American, the steady drip of disclosures echoes the most infamous chapter in the history of U.S. public health, prompting cries of, "Remember Tuskegee."

On Feb. 1, pastors from Flint and Detroit held a town hall meeting at which rap and business icon Russell Simmons and attorney Phaedra Parks, a cast member on the cable show, "The Real Housewives of Atlanta," both appeared.

Hundreds of people showed up. Ministers preached, local leaders spoke.

Several times speakers mentioned the Tuskegee experiment, the 40-year long, federally-funded experiment on 600 uneducated black men in Alabama. Government doctors told the men they were being treated for "bad blood." In fact,

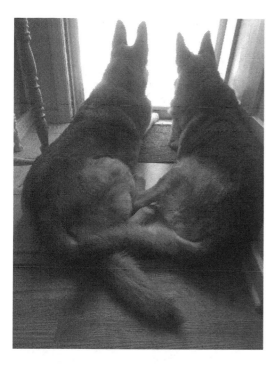

German shepherds Soldier and Kizzie died within a month of each other before the lead contamination was discovered in Flint. Their owner, Sonja Lee, suspects lead poisoning. The water in her home tested at a high lead level of 68 parts per billion, more than four times the action level of 15ppb.

Photo courtesy of Sonja Lee

most of them had syphilis and were unwittingly being studied to see how the disease would affect their bodies if left untreated, even after penicillin was available as a treatment. Dozens died.

As it happens, one objective of the Flint town hall was to introduce residents to doctors and lawyers they were told they could trust to address their health and legal problems, instead of having to rely on government agencies.

Benjamin Crump, a civil rights lawyer and president of the National Bar Association, a predominantly African-American group, told the crowd that while they should get water and blood tested for free with local and state agencies, they should share and compare those results with tests conducted by their own lawyers and family doctors.

"How can the person who caused me pain be trusted to test … the level of my pain?" Crump asked of government officials. "This begs the question of independent testing."

Frances Gilcreast, president of the Flint Branch NAACP, wrote an open letter to city officials and Gov. Rick Snyder in February 2015, chastising the government for putting cost savings above water safety. Her sentiments echo a year later.

"If this were Grand Blanc, or Oakland County," she wrote, "something would have been done immediately."

QUESTIONS AND DOUBTS

Two blood testing sites that screened children for lead exposure in early February offered a festive atmosphere. Someone dressed in a colorful monster costume danced the "Nae-Nae" with children. Face painters, snacks and balloon animals kept kids busy while parents poured over health questionnaires.

Parents asked about their children's reaction to Flint's water struggled to keep their emotions in check. Shavon Hamilton took deep breaths and looked off into the crowd, eyebrows furrowed. She had bottle-fed her infant daughter using tap water to mix the powder formula in 2014.

Kiara Settle let the tears well up. Her 2-year-old son was tested once during a hospital visit and showed a blood lead level of 5.4 micrograms per deciliter – just above the level of 5 ug/dl at which health intervention is triggered. Her family drank tap water for the first year after the city switched to Flint River water as its source.

"My baby was born in 2013," said, Settle, 24. "They didn't even give my baby a chance from the jump. I don't care what they say about anything anymore. I'm trying to move."

Residents said they want to trust results from the free water testing conducted by the Michigan Department of Environmental Quality, but said results can be confusing.

And, any way, they haven't forgotten that MDEQ is the agency that is blamed as the chief regulatory culprit in Flint's water disaster.

Kathleen Fridline was puzzled by the letter MDEQ sent to her elderly mother's house. It said that her mom's residential water test in January showed a lead contamination level of 78 parts per billion. The "action" level is 15 ppb, the document stated.

As she noted, the letter does not list actions to take, other than to call the local health department with questions.

"What do we do now? Who do we wait to hear from? The city? DEQ? How do we address this," Fridline wondered aloud while reading the results in her mother's living room.

"I'd like to say I'm angry, but I'm just not an angry person. I'm concerned."

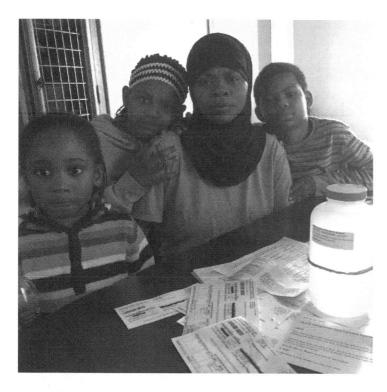

Mary Smith, 34, with two of her three children and her nephew. (L-R) Khamarri Key, 4, Kayla Dantzler, 9, and Kyrin Dantzler, 10. The city shut off their water service on Jan. 28.

Bridge photo by Chastity Pratt Dawsey

FILTERS, BOTTLED WATER QUESTIONED

Sometimes the information isn't so much vague as contradictory, residents say.

They note that local, state and federal officials have encouraged them to use water filters, saying they will remove lead. But then they heard that EPA experts worried that won't work if lead levels at their taps are too high for the filters to handle. Pregnant women and small children should continue to use bottled water, the EPA said.

That's the kind of direction that inspires distrust.

"I don't know what to believe," said JaMise Wash-Lang who took her son, JaCarie, to Carriage Town Ministries in Flint for a blood test.

His teachers say the 5-year-old has been more hyperactive. JaCarie has a mild rash that won't heal. The family has used bottled water for months, but bathed the boy in the tap water before a water emergency was declared in January.

Wash-Lang says she became anxious after a Facebook post went viral showing a woman, supposedly in Flint, testing several brands of bottled water and getting high lead content readings.

She knows how conspiracy theories about tainted bottled water and an uncaring government sound. Paranoid. Crazy, even.

Until it's your water. Your child.

"My main concern is the inconsistency of information, what to do, where to get help." She hadn't had her home's water tested, but was taken aback by the water test containers distributed along with free bottled water at the local fire stations. A questionnaire was attached to the plastic bottle with a rubber band.

"A rubber band?" she said. "What if the rubber band comes off? How is that saying that they value the accuracy of the test?"

Shavon Hamilton wants to avoid confusing information about filters and bottled water. She is considering buying a reverse osmosis system to filter impurities including lead from water where it enters her home. The system she wants could cost more than $3,000, or about $70 per month if she chooses a payment plan.

"It's going to be another bill I really don't need. But I'm doing it. I'm really scared," she said. "I don't feel like a good mother because I'm just now doing this."

Mary Smith lost her last shred of trust in city officials when she came home from dropping off her kids at school on a recent Thursday to find the water department shutting off her water. This was no ordinary shut off – workers drove up in a backhoe and dug several feet into the ground to reach the city service line.

At first, she thought, "They can keep their poison water." Then, she thought about her three children and nephew who live in the house. How would they flush the toilet?

The city said that it hasn't shut off any customer's water for nonpayment since August 2015. Officials said Smith's water was shut off because she didn't file documents to put the water bill in her name when she began the process to buy the house from the city in November.

She was infuriated, wondering why the city took time to shut off her water for what she considers a technicality, instead of focusing on making drinking water safe.

"This is the same government that told us for a year and half that we could drink the water. Nobody trusts the government anymore, especially not after all this," Smith said. "It's going to be hard to get the people's trust back."

Bridge computer-assisted reporting specialist Mike Wilkinson contributed to this report.

CHAPTER 24

FEB. 17, 2016

YEARS OF MISSED WARNINGS BEFORE FLINT RIVER SWITCH

WATER WAS 'VERY HIGHLY SUSCEPTIBLE' TO CONTAMINATION

Editor's summary: This report is based on the second big dump of Flint water crisis-related emails and documents from Gov. Rick Snyder's office. Many of the most telling documents are mentioned in Truth Squad analysis presented in previous chapters. In this story, John Bebow distills the most important findings.

By John Bebow
Bridge Magazine

I n the days, weeks, months and years leading to Flint's tragic switch to the Flint River as its drinking water source, experts repeatedly voiced misgivings. But with cost a driving factor, the Flint River plan would not be slowed down or stopped.

Missed warnings about the Flint River's suitability as a drinking water source are detailed in more than 20,000 pages of Flint-related emails and documents released last week by Gov. Rick Snyder's office.

Chief among them: Two days before former state Treasurer Andy Dillon formally recommended moving Flint off Detroit water, a Michigan Department of Environmental Quality drinking-water-safety regulator warned that using the Flint River would pose increased public health risk, including a higher risk of exposure to carcinogens.

In the days, weeks and months leading to Flint's tragic change of drinking water sources, experts expressed numerous misgivings about the switch. But with cost concerns among the driving factors, the Flint River plan flowed ahead – directly toward disaster.

This report recounts, in chronological order, missed warning signs about the Flint River as now detailed in the full Bridge Magazine Flint water-disaster timeline.

A FORGOTTEN REPORT FROM 2004?

For many years, the city of Flint bought treated water from Detroit. At the same time, the city's water treatment plant retained access to the Flint River for emergency service. But regulators have long concluded the river is a problematic drinking water source.

In 2004, a technical assessment declared that Flint's then-standby water intake from the river was "very highly susceptible" to contamination. The report – written by the U.S. Geological Survey, MDEQ and Flint water utilities department – noted that the treatment plant had effectively treated Flint River water to meet drinking water standards. But the report concluded that agricultural and urban runoff, as well as 96 potential contaminant sources upstream, made the river "very highly sensitive."

This report did not appear to get significant consideration among officials discussing the river option a decade later, state email records suggest. In fact, a veteran MDEQ engineer responsible for Flint drinking water oversight initially said he didn't know if such a report existed when he was asked about it in an email in early 2015, nearly a year after the Flint River switch.

2011-2012: WATER 'AESTHETICS'

Flint and Genesee County officials had long discussed how to move away from Detroit water, both to save money and gain local control over the region's water supply. The Karegnondi Water Authority was envisioned to supply Lake Huron water to Genesee County, Flint and other communities beyond Detroit's northern suburbs.

"The Karegnondi Water Authority has the potential to be a major factor in our region's economic development efforts," Flint Department of Public Works Director Howard Croft wrote to an MDEQ official in May 2012. "The City of Flint is pleased to be a partner in the process."

But the KWA is not scheduled to come online until late 2016. Long-running disputes with the Detroit system ultimately led Flint's state-appointed emergency managers and local elected officials to turn to the Flint River for a short-term solution. Water-safety officials raised concerns, but none reached red-flag

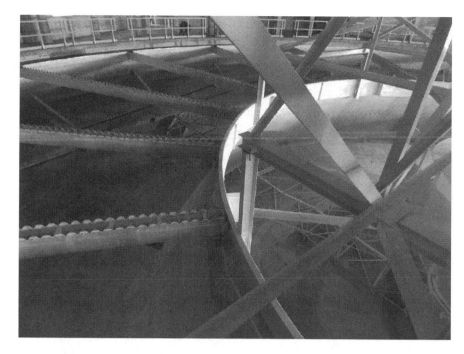

Inside the Flint Water Plant.

Photo courtesy of Michigan Radio

status. Instead, the same experts seemed to think the river's quality issues could be overcome through treatment.

In July 2011, a Rowe Engineering report analyzed the Flint River as a permanent water supply. It would require more treatment than Lake Huron water, and the river water "aesthetics" wouldn't be as good, but the river "can be treated to meet current regulations," Rowe concluded. The Rowe report did not predict the highly corrosive, discolored, smelly and ultimately contaminated water that would eventually flow through the taps of Flint homes.

2013: A NOD TO CARCINOGENS, THEN FULL SPEED AHEAD

As the talks leading to Flint's break with the Detroit system intensified in early 2013, concerns bubbled quietly in the depths of MDEQ. In January 2013, MDEQ District Engineer Mike Prysby emailed his colleagues about the prospect of switching to the Flint River. He raised concerns about the need to soften the river water and the possible need for "advanced treatment" to ward off potential contaminants. "I agree that the city should have concerns of fully utilizing the Flint River" for 100 percent of its drinking water supply, he wrote.

Two months later, Prysby's colleague, Stephen Busch, was more pointed.

"Continuous" use of the Flint River for the city's drinking water would "pose an increased microbial risk to public health" and "pose an increased risk of disinfection by-product (carcinogen) exposure to public health," Busch, a district manager in MDEQ's drinking water division, wrote to then-MDEQ Director Dan Wyant and other MDEQ officials on March 26. (Note: Busch's email had "carcinogen" in parentheses.)

The next day, MDEQ Deputy Director Jim Sygo emailed Busch: "As you might guess we are in a situation with Emergency Financial Managers so it's entirely possible that they will be making decisions relative to cost. The concern in either situation is that a compliant supply of source water and drinking water can be supplied."

The next day, March 28, Dillon wrote to Snyder: "I am recommending we support the City of Flint's decision to join (the Karegnondi Water Authority). The City's Emergency Manager, Mayor, and City Council all support this decision. Dan Wyant likewise concurs and will confirm via email."

Over the coming months, Flint, with state supervision, began the formal process of switching to Flint River drinking water as its interim water source, eventually flipping the switch on April 25, 2014. The change launched the crisis that has resulted in lead poisoning; water-safety violations for potentially carcinogenic trihalomethanes; a suspected link between the drinking water and a Legionnaires' disease outbreak that killed nine people; lawsuits; and numerous investigations, including criminal probes by the Michigan attorney general, the FBI and EPA's criminal division.

The regulator who raised those March 2013 concerns, Busch, was suspended over the Flint crisis. (Editor's note: Busch and Prysby of MDEQ and Michael Glasgow, operator of the Flint water plant, were also charged criminally in mid-April 2016). Wyant, who was copied on Busch's March 2013 concerns about the Flint River, resigned in late December over the Flint crisis.

SPRING 2014: LAST-MINUTE CONCERNS

On March 26, 2014, MDEQ's Busch told colleagues that the agency had a lot to talk about before the impending Flint River switch.

"… I would like to make sure everyone is on the same page on … what Flint will be required to do in order to start using their plant full time," Busch wrote in email. "Because the plant is set up for emergency use, they could start up at any time, but starting up for continuous operation will carry significant changes in regulatory requirements so there is a very gray area as to what we consider for startup."

A month before the switch, key MDEQ water safety officials were just getting their arms around that regulatory "gray area." Nearly two years later, after the Flint debacle unfolded, MDEQ Director Wyant would blame departmental "inexperience" for a failure of oversight.

MDEQ failed to require corrosion controls after the switch, and the agency held tightly to its regulatory misread for months as corrosive river water ate into old distribution lines, allowing lead to leach into the city's drinking water.

Despite their internal trepidations, MDEQ regulators thought the Flint River could work until the KWA water came online. It was a waiting game. Busch said as much on April 23, as he drafted departmental talking points by email before Flint made the switch.

"While the Department is satisfied with the City's ability to treat water from the Flint River, the Department looks forward to the long term solution of continued operation of the City of Flint Water Treatment Plant using water from the KWA as a more consistent and higher quality source water," he wrote.

Yet Busch's positive spin came a week after chilling disclosures from deep within the Flint Water Treatment Plant.

CONCERNS AT PLANT DON'T STOP THE SWITCH

On April 16-17, 2014, Michael Glasgow, the laboratory and water-quality supervisor at the city treatment plant, sounded alarms in emails to MDEQ.

Glasgow had expected big changes to water quality monitoring before the switch. But he said he hadn't received fresh direction from MDEQ beyond a months-old written comment that "things were subject to change."

"Any information would be appreciated, because it looks as if we will be starting the plant up tomorrow and are being pushed to start distributing water as soon as possible," Glasgow wrote on April 16. "I would like to make sure we are monitoring, reporting and meeting requirements before I give the OK to start distributing water."

A day later, Glasgow told MDEQ regulators the Flint water treatment plant would fire up against his best judgment.

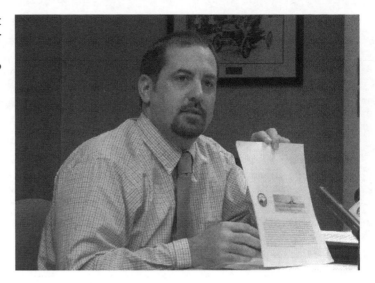

Michael Glasglow, Flint water plant supervisor

Photo courtesy Michigan Radio

"I have people above me making plans to distribute water ASAP," Glasgow emailed MDEQ. "I was reluctant before, but after looking at the monitoring schedule and our current staffing, I do not anticipate giving the OK to begin sending water out anytime soon. If water is distributed from this plant in the next couple of weeks, it will be against my direction. I need time to adequately train additional staff and to update our monitoring plans before I will feel we are ready. I will reiterate this to management above me, but they seem to have their own agenda."

A week later, on April 24, Daugherty Johnson, the Flint utilities administrator, was far more upbeat in his own email to MDEQ staff as he sought state approval to avoid working with Detroit for a backup water supply agreement.

"As you are aware, the City has undergone extensive upgrades to our Water Treatment Plant and its associated facilities," Johnson wrote. "Our intentions and efforts have been to operate our facility as the primary drinking water source for the City of Flint."

The next day, Flint River water officially became the city's drinking water source.

"It's regular, good, pure drinking water, and it's right in our backyard," Flint Mayor Dayne Walling said in toasting the Flint River switch. "This is the first step in the right direction for Flint, as we take this monumental step forward in controlling the future of our community's most precious resource."

CHAPTER 25

FEB. 17, 2016

WHY EVERY MICHIGAN RESIDENT SHOULD ASK ABOUT DRINKING WATER

PROBLEMS AND QUESTIONS EXTEND WELL BEYOND FLINT

Editor's summary: In this story, Bridge Magazine examines the larger implications of the Flint water crisis with consumer-focused, easy-to-understand reporting and writing that's not caught up in partisan finger-pointing.

By John Bebow
Bridge Magazine

The Flint water disaster is no longer just about Flint. It raises questions about drinking water safety for millions of citizens in Michigan and beyond.

Here are seven reasons why residents across Michigan and beyond should ask about the safety of their own drinking water.

NO. 1: MANY COMMUNITIES HAVE OLD LEAD WATER SUPPLY LINES

As the Flint lead problem exploded last fall, Michigan Department of Environmental Quality regulators traded emails about lead in drinking-water pipes across Michigan.

In September 2015, Liane Shekter Smith, chief of the MDEQ Office of Drinking Water and Municipal Assistance, emailed colleagues a list of dozens of communities with lead service lines. Some pipes may have been replaced, while others likely remain in use. Shekter Smith wrote: "We should be careful how we use this list at this time, but it is an indication of which communities may be facing similar issues to Flint."

The presence of lead service lines does not constitute an immediate problem. Many older communities nationwide have some lead service lines. Municipal water supplies are routinely protected with corrosion-control chemicals, which help keep old pipes from leaching lead. The lack of corrosion control when Flint switched to Flint River drinking water explains the Flint disaster.

Still, an August 2015 report to the National Drinking Water Advisory Council by a team of experts urges "proactive" replacement of lead lines, "strengthened" corrosion control treatments, and more intensive lead monitoring of tap water.

NO. 2: CHILDREN BEYOND FLINT HAVE HAD HIGHER LEAD EXPOSURE

In a December story, Bridge explained that in many zip codes, especially in older communities of Michigan, tests on young children show even higher blood lead levels than in Flint.

As government health agencies point out, there is no safe level of lead exposure for young children. Lead is a neurotoxin that damages the brain. It does its damage and is secreted from the body.

The sources of lead exposure are hard to track. The government's ban on lead in paint in the 1970s and phase out of leaded gasoline, which began in the late 1970s, correlate to a sharp decline in lead exposure for all citizens. Still, old homes with flaking paint on windowsills, walls and exteriors are a persistent source of exposure for children. Drinking water can be, but most often is not, a significant source of lead exposure.

If you are on a public water system, annual quality reports published by your local utility are the first place to look for lead levels in your drinking water – check your community's website. Still, such reports, and monitoring by the MDEQ and Michigan Department of Health and Human Services, didn't protect or warn Flint residents. It took independent, third-party water-safety and medical experts to uncover the problem.

One of those experts, Dr. Mona Hanna-Attisha, recently stated in a peer-reviewed medical journal study: "As our aging water infrastructures continue to decay, and as communities across the nation struggle with finances and water supply sources, the situation in Flint may be a harbinger for future safe drinking water challenges. Ironically, even when one is surrounded by the Great Lakes, safe drinking water is not a guarantee."

NO. 3: OTHER MICHIGAN COMMUNITIES FACE DRINKING WATER PROBLEMS

State email records released last week indicate that in 2013 and 2014, the MDEQ identified 1,100 drinking water regulation violations statewide, including what appeared to be 200 violations for exceeding maximum allowable contaminant levels. The violations came from 326 community water supplies.

State email records also show that between 2010 and 2014, 41 "non-community" drinking water supplies in Michigan exceeded the 15 parts per billion federal action level for lead.

Non-community drinking water supplies include schools, restaurants, motels, campgrounds and churches.

NO. 4: MDEQ'S WATER SAFETY PROGRAM HAS PROBLEMS

In October, Richard Benzie, MDEQ chief of field operations for the Office of Drinking Water and Municipal Assistance, described Flint in an email as the "biggest firestorm I have experienced in almost 40 years, and to think it is about a water system that has never exceeded an Action Level."

By "action level," Benzie appears to mean that MDEQ's official water testing in Flint in 2014-15 did not reveal a serious lead safety hazard. He's right. It's the rest of the story that's so troubling. In contrast to the MDEQ, independent technical researchers and a lone EPA regulator uncovered Flint's lead problem. And independent medical professionals discovered elevated blood-lead levels that the Michigan Department of Health and Human Service failed to find.

Also in October, MDEQ officials briefly discussed lead levels in Saginaw's drinking water in response to media inquiries. Lead in water is measured in parts per billion. Federal regulations require water utilities to certify that 90 percent of sampled locations known to have lead pipes in a community contain 15 parts per billion of lead or less in drinking water.

The MDEQ emails showed lead levels of 8 parts per billion in the last testing period in Saginaw. That's below the federal action level of 15 parts per billion. Flint's two most recent rounds of lead monitoring showed 6 parts per billion and 11 parts per billion. According to regulatory procedures, those results meant no further public safety action was required.

But independent researchers, led by Virginia Tech professor and drinking water expert Marc Edwards, found much higher lead levels in Flint drinking water last fall. Edwards alleged to federal investigators that lead testing in Flint homes was seriously flawed. A Michigan Auditor General investigation agreed.

Edwards said problems he and others found in Flint "without a doubt" call into question MDEQ-supervised lead sampling elsewhere in Michigan.

Last week, MDEQ Communications Director Melanie Brown said the agency is working to "ensure our water sampling and testing protocols are the most effective methods as possible now and into the future."

The U.S. Environmental Protection Agency has raised concerns before about MDEQ's drinking water regulation performance and is auditing Michigan's oversight.

NO. 5: NOT ALL COMMUNITIES WILL MEET ALL DRINKING WATER STANDARDS

In May 2015, Jon Allan, director of the MDEQ Office of the Great Lakes, asked MDEQ colleagues to react to a proposal calling for 98 percent of the community water systems in Michigan to have drinking water that meets all health-based standards by 2020.

MDEQ Water Resources Division Chief William Creal responded: "I think you are nuts if you go with a goal less than 100 percent for (drinking water) compliance in the strategy," Creal wrote. "How many Flints do you intend to allow???"

A day later, Liane Shekter Smith, then chief of the MDEQ Office of Drinking Water and Municipal Assistance, had a different reaction.

"The balance here is between what is realistic and what is ideal," she wrote. "Of course, everyone wants 100 percent compliance. The reality, however, is that it's impossible. It's not that we 'allow' a Flint to occur; circumstances happen. Water mains break, systems lose pressure, bacteria gets into the system, regulations change and systems that were in compliance no longer are, etc. Do we want to put a goal in black and white that cannot be met but sounds good? Or do we want to establish a goal that challenges us but can actually be accomplished? Perhaps there's a middle ground?"

Shekter Smith was fired in early February over the Flint water crisis.

In December, the staff of Rep. Adam Zemke, D-Ann Arbor, requested MDEQ feedback on a bill he planned to introduce to require that drinking water in schools be tested at least once every three years. Shekter Smith pushed back.

"Even if the proposal were to be for only lead and copper, this is a huge expense that would be placed on the supplier of water inappropriately," she wrote. "I understand the desire to have this kind of information, but if the legislature wants to require this monitoring, the burden for this should be on the schools or the board of education."

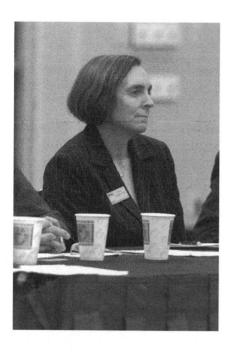

Liane Schekter Smith, former chief of the MDEQ Office of Drinking Water and Municipal Assistance. She was fired in February of 2015 over the Flint water crisis.

Photo courtesy of Michigan Radio

NO. 6: COULD WATER SAFETY BE 'MINIMALIST' IN YOUR COMMUNITY?

In December, the Flint Water Advisory Task Force, a bipartisan panel of policy makers and health professionals established by Gov. Snyder, laid much of the blame for the Flint crisis on the MDEQ's Office of Drinking Water and Municipal Assistance. The task force blamed MDEQ for a "minimalist approach to regulatory oversight responsibility" that is "unacceptable and simply insufficient to the task of public protection."

The task force characterized MDEQ's public response to the Flint crisis as "often one of aggressive dismissal, belittlement, and attempts to discredit" citizens and experts.

Exchanges between the EPA and MDEQ about lead worries in Flint, and blatant denials and deflections by MDEQ, are a central point in the narrative of the Flint disaster. The records recently released add greater context – with more intense worry from EPA officials, and more dismissive reaction from MDEQ officials.

"WOW!!!" EPA official Jennifer Crooks wrote to MDEQ regulators after lead readings in one Flint home topped 104 parts per billion. "Big worries here," she continued, and noted that the family living in the home had rashes and one child's hair was "falling out in clumps."

MDEQ staff reactions included this: "Not sure why region 5 [EPA] sees this one sample as such a big deal."

Two months later, as an EPA regulator pressed MDEQ about lead levels in Flint, MDEQ's Stephen Busch took offense. If the EPA official "continues to persist," Busch threatened to go to superiors "to help address his over-reaches."

In the end, Busch was suspended and later charged with criminal acts for his role in the Flint crisis. The aggressive EPA official, Miguel Del Toral, has been vindicated as a hero and the first government official to attack and identify the Flint crisis.

Finally, the story of state government workers in Flint receiving "alternative" drinking water supplies a year ago is well known. But a new part of the back-story revealed in records Friday provides more detail.

The logic for the special water supply, according to state email records: "… given that this state building has high public traffic (Flint citizens); it was felt prudent to offer an alternative supply of drinking water to citizens entering the building."

Richard Benzie, MDEQ's chief of field operations for the Office of Drinking Water and Municipal Assistance, took special offense.

"No doubt," he wrote in an email, the purified water in a state office building "will make it more difficult from a perception standpoint." Indeed, his MDEQ division continued to deny there was a serious problem with Flint drinking water for much of 2015.

But Benzie's first concern in his email was state employees' perceptions, not public perceptions. "Why does 'public traffic' deserve a higher consideration than concern for state workers?" he asked.

NO. 7: BECAUSE A FLINT CRISIS HERO STILL HAS QUESTIONS

Professor Marc Edwards' testing in Flint homes showed lead levels far higher than MDEQ had previously recognized. His tests of Flint River water showed it was highly corrosive, and the failure to properly treat it caused lead to leach into the city's drinking water. His research helped doctors pinpoint elevated blood levels in Flint children, especially in zip codes and wards with concentrations of poor residents.

Edwards, a Virginia Tech professor and 2007 MacArthur Fellow, is a nationally recognized drinking-water expert. He is a consultant to Flint as it seeks to recover.

In an email interview with Bridge, he wrote: "There is an attitude at some of these agencies … that by not meeting the health standards they will save money that would best be spent elsewhere. This has nothing to do with politics, but it is a self-serving argument by some, that is frankly an excuse to be lazy and sloppy and engage in illegal activities. I find this both arrogant and dangerous."

CHAPTER 26

MARCH 1, 2016

WHAT KEY SNYDER AIDES KNEW ABOUT FLINT AND WHEN

Editor's summary: A flurry of stories emerges when the Snyder administration releases its third dump of emails and memos – about 10,000 pages – on the last weekend in February. The most damaging are emails among Gov. Snyder's key aides – Valerie Brader, deputy legal counsel, Michael Gadola, chief legal counsel, and Dennis Muchmore, chief of staff. Brader and Gadola urge a quick return to Detroit water in October 2014, five months before lead issues emerged. They are told it would be expensive and that the water meets federal and state standards.

By John Bebow
Bridge Magazine

Among the most damaging government documents released on the Flint water crisis in recent months were emails showing that aides in Gov. Rick Snyder's office had serious concerns about Flint water long before the state took emergency action to protect residents.

In late February, the state released over 10,000 more pages of internal communications, including emails involving others in the governor's inner circle. Much of the conversation focused on the decision to switch the city's drinking supply to the Flint River in 2014 after decades of receiving water from Detroit.

Here are highlights from release, including the time period when the aides were given notice of problems with Flint's water:

VALERIE BRADER, SNYDER'S DEPUTY LEGAL COUNSEL (OCTOBER 2014)

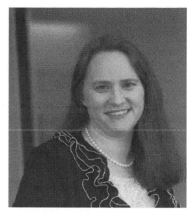

Brader sent an email to Chief of Staff Dennis Muchmore, Communications Director Jarrod Agen, Legal Counsel Michael Gadola, and Deputy Chief of Staff Beth Clement. She urges them to ask the Flint emergency manager to consider switching Flint off the Flint River and back to Detroit water from Lake Huron "as an interim solution to both the quality, and now the financial, problems that the current solution is causing."

Flint residents had been complaining about the water for months. A day earlier, General Motors said it would stop using Flint River water because it corroded parts at an engine plant in the city. Flint also had issued boil water advisories in late August and early September. Meanwhile, health concerns were increasing about chemicals Flint used to treat the river water.

"I see this as an urgent matter to fix," Brader wrote.

MICHAEL GADOLA, SNYDER'S CHIEF LEGAL COUNSEL (OCTOBER 2014)

Gadola responds 12 minutes later to everyone on Brader's email string.

"… (T)o anyone who grew up in Flint as I did, the notion that I would be getting my drinking water from the Flint River is downright scary. Too bad the (emergency manager) didn't ask me what I thought, though I'm sure he heard it from plenty of others. My Mom is a City resident. Nice to know she's drinking water with elevated chlorine levels and fecal coliform. I agree with Valerie. They should try to get back on the Detroit system as a stopgap ASAP before this thing gets too far out of control."

DENNIS MUCHMORE, CHIEF OF STAFF (OCTOBER 2014 - SUMMER 2015)

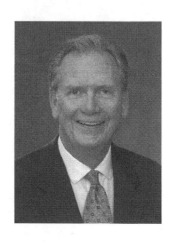

"Can you guys step into this?" Muchmore, Snyder's chief of staff, asks state Treasury Department officials the same day Brader and Gadola raise concerns.

This begins months of high-anxiety meetings and on-again, off-again brainstorming by Muchmore. But a wicked mix of financial, public perception, communication, policy and political problems vex Muchmore and those around him at every turn. For context, Brader's email is sent weeks before the 2014 election as Snyder is facing an unexpectedly difficult challenge.

In previously released emails, Muchmore expresses empathy for frustrated Flint residents and, at other times, shows bewilderment that activists and public officials would blame the state for the unfolding water crisis.

At one point in the newly released emails, Muchmore explores a reconnection to Detroit drinking water. Treasury officials and Flint's emergency manager's office warn it would be very expensive, and raise Flint's already extreme water rates by 30 percent. Bottom line: City residents keep drinking Flint River water.

Muchmore explores interim bottled water and water filter distribution ideas and makes limited progress. The city of Flint and Michigan Department of Environmental Quality insist the Flint drinking water meets safety standards.

Nine months later, Muchmore prods environmental and public health agency bosses saying, "I'm frustrated by the water issue in Flint. I really don't think people are getting the benefit of the doubt." Bureaucrats scurry but report back that the drinking water meets standards and find no evidence connecting Flint drinking water to elevated blood levels in children.

Not until independent water quality and health experts refute state agency deflections in October 2015 does Gov. Rick Snyder begin emergency action to remediate lead in Flint's drinking water and switch back to Detroit water.

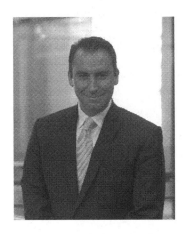

JARROD AGEN, SNYDER'S COMMUNICATIONS DIRECTOR (MARCH 2015)

Agen gets an email in March 2015 about a brewing Legionnaires' disease crisis that raises questions about whether the outbreak is linked to Flint's drinking water. After the email release, Agen told reporters that he never opened that email.

On March 16, 2015, MDEQ Communications Director Brad Wurfel copies Agen on a three-day old message that Wurfel first wrote to Snyder's urban affairs aide Harvey Hollins and MDEQ Director Dan Wyant.

"In December, our staff became peripherally aware that hospitals in Genesee were seeing an uptick in Legionnaires cases," Wurfel wrote.

Controversy ensues in coming months as local, state and federal agencies debate the cause and extent of the Legionnaires' outbreak and whether Flint drinking water is linked.

In January 2016, Snyder announces the Legionnaires' outbreak and says nine people have died from it. Later a 10th person dies. The governor says that he hadn't personally heard about the problem until days before. In the same month, Agen replace Muchmore as Snyder's chief of staff.

SARA WURFEL, SNYDER'S PRESS SECRETARY, AND DAVE MURRAY, DEPUTY PRESS SECRETARY (JANUARY-MARCH 2015)

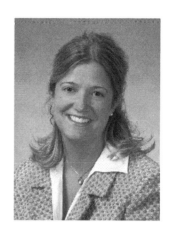

MDEQ spokesman Brad Wurfel began emailing colleagues on the governor's communications team about Legionnaires' in January 2015. On March 13, he clues in the governor's top two spokespeople on the Legionnaires' issue and urges action:

"Political flank cover out of the City of Flint today regarding the spike in Legionnaires cases. See enclosed. Also, area ministers put a shot over the bow last night … with a call for Snyder to declare state of emergency there and somehow 'fix' the water situation. It may be very advantageous to get Treasury, Gov's office, DCH, DEQ, and Flint EM around a table Monday to do the following:

- Update on what the city is doing.

- Update on what County Health Department is working on.

- Discussion of what we might all do next.

- Coordination of communication/messages.

"Did not want to reach out to Dennis without your approval/support. Please advise."

Ari Adler, special projects manager (January 2015):

"This is a public relations crisis – because of a real or perceived problem is irrelevant – waiting to explode nationally," Adler emails Agen.

"If Flint had been hit with a natural disaster that affected its water system, the state would be stepping in to provide bottled water or other assistance. What can we do given the current circumstances?"

Adler may very well spend most of the rest of his tenure with the Snyder administration answering that and related questions about the Flint water crisis. He became Snyder's communications director in late February 2016.

HOW SNYDER'S CHIEF OF STAFF WRESTLED WITH FLINT

Editor's summary: Dennis Muchmore was a generally well-liked veteran of Lansing's battles when he took the job as the governor's chief of staff. He could work both sides of the political aisle for solutions. But the Flint water crisis confounded him, despite his many overtures to key department heads responsible for protecting the safety of Michigan's drinking water and health of its children. His frustrations emerge in emails, and when he left his position at the end of 2015, it was clear that Flint had worn him down and left him with many regrets.

By John Bebow
Bridge Magazine

Deep in the Flint-related emails Gov. Rick Snyder released in late February is a fine-print, small-font spreadsheet of Dennis Muchmore's workload.

As the governor's chief of staff, Muchmore was responsible in 2015 for no fewer than 76 "priority projects," according to that document.

Possible 2016 ballot issues. An agricultural labor shortage. Speed limits in the Upper Peninsula. The Michigan Prescription Drug Task Force. Issues involving the transport of crude oil by railroad. Charity gambling. Regional transit issues. A Belle Isle Conservancy project. Medicaid. Regional projects ranging from Wayne County to Battle Creek to Benton Harbor. Something called "liquor stores and gas pumps." Another item called "Jobs for Scott and Nancy."

And … "Flint water issues."

A dominant question in the Flint water crisis is how key aides in the Snyder administration could raise early red flags about the city's water yet not coax answers or solutions from state agencies before lead poisoning became a full-blown public health crisis.

One lens through which to view that question is the emails and decision-making of the governor's long-time chief of staff. The records offer a view into a leadership culture where aides constantly juggled dozens of policy balls. And yet in

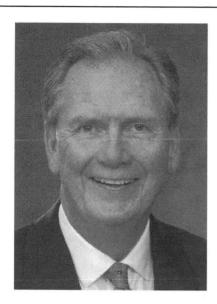
Dennis Muchmore

the crucible and complexity of the emerging Flint crisis, none among the many vastly experienced Snyder aides found the capacity to arrest the nightmare that gripped Flint, and now critically wounds a governorship.

In the high-minded times of early 2011, as Rick Snyder completed an unlikely climb to the governor's chair, he urged his appointees to work in "dog years," thereby implying he wanted to spur change in Michigan at roughly seven times normal human speed. As chief of staff, Muchmore was one of the key people in charge of the day-to-day work.

The team got off to a fast and sometimes controversial pace. Snyder et al ripped up the state's much-hated business tax. They led the nation in expansion of early childhood learning programs. They wrote special messages and launched task forces on dozens of policy issues. They signed Right to Work and various forms of controversial hot-button social issue legislation not originally on their agenda. They passed state budgets on time, grew the state's rainy day reserves, and addressed long-term pension and health care headaches. They helped negotiate Detroit in and out of municipal bankruptcy in a finance-minded motivation to get the city back on its feet. They won re-election just as the Flint crisis began to grow. And, while riding a fortuitous economic recovery from the Great Recession, they sent state-appointed emergency managers into Michigan's most financially troubled cities.

Like Flint.

By his final days in Snyder's office, after a year of Flint frustration, Muchmore, whose emails concerning the crisis have been among the most scrutinized, seemed to have had enough of the dog years.

"Welcome to the job," Muchmore wrote to his replacement, Jarrod Agen, as he cleaned out his office at the end of 2015. "It's one of those where tomorrow you'll have another set of even more ugly decisions."

Ugly decisions and dilemmas about Flint plagued Muchmore throughout 2015. In the end, emails indicate, the battle left him questioning himself.

"Of course, I have a lot of complaints about myself and this Flint thing," Muchmore wrote to a state Treasury Department colleague in October. "If I had acted more quickly on some of (Flint ministers') complaints we at least could have had a more robust discussion."

FEBRUARY 2015: 'WE CAN HARDLY IGNORE THE PEOPLE OF FLINT'

In the thousands of pages of email records released, Snyder himself says very little. To this day, Rick Snyder's day-to-day thoughts as the crisis unfolded remain largely a mystery. But Muchmore said a lot. And he attempted to lead numerous stopgap measures to deal with Flint. But he wasn't able to lead state government to solutions before the Flint water crisis mushroomed into a public health and public confidence crisis of epic proportion.

To what degree Muchmore (or other aides) broached possible solutions directly with the governor before fall 2015 remains unclear, at least from the emails released to date.

In February 2015, after Flint residents held up jugs of smelly brown drinking water in public meetings and Flint's mayor and ministers begged the Snyder administration for help, Muchmore pursued a switch from the Flint River back to Detroit drinking water.

"Since we're in charge we can hardly ignore the people of Flint," Muchmore wrote to state Treasury and public relations officials (the governor was not copied). "After all, if GM refuses to use the water in their plant and our own agencies are warning people not to drink it … we look pretty stupid hiding behind some financial statement."

But answers came back from Treasury and the Flint emergency manager that the switch would be costly and probably require a 30 percent increase in Flint water rates, which were already sky high.

MARCH 2015: 'WE'VE GOT TO DO SOMETHING'

Money and financial pressures in Flint were at the root of the city's brewing water problems for years as city officials waged battle with the Detroit Water and Sewerage Department over rates and control.

The Snyder administration, and its emergency manager (with the support of local officials in Flint) chose in 2013 to leave Detroit for a still-unbuilt Karegnondi Water Authority pipeline to Lake Huron. DWSD responded in kind, cancelling Flint's water contract with a one-year notice. With state approval, Flint, under its emergency manager, chose the problematic Flint River for its temporary drinking water source.

Not until October 2015, with Flint finally in full public health emergency, did the state, City of Flint, and the Mott Foundation find the money to re-connect to Detroit drinking water. And only then did Detroit find a way to reduce its past prices to make it possible. The switch came eight months after Muchmore first explored the idea in emails.

Stymied in February 2015, Muchmore pursued another Flint fix the following month, emails show.

As a former president of the Flint NAACP called the Flint water crisis "environmental racism at its worst," Kelly Rossman-McKinney, a prominent Lansing public relations executive, emailed Muchmore and warned "… this issue is out of hand. I'm concerned about the implications that this may have racial overtones. Ugh."

Muchmore responded: "It's an on-going issue that has to do with the long term viability of the city's finances." Yet, Muchmore reasoned, "We've got to do something for people in Flint because it's right to do more than it works financially. We've got to work on getting them water they can trust but there is no easy solution. This is a tough one, as everyone's position is correct just not easy."

That day, Muchmore emailed Treasury officials and Snyder aides looking for fresh solutions: "You can't expect (Flint) ministers to hold the tide on this problem.… If we procrastinate much longer in doing something direct we'll have real trouble."

In response, state officials explored providing bottled water, but Deputy State Treasurer Wayne Workman stated, "If this does happen, we need to figure out who would hand out the water. It should not be the City. It would undercut every point they are making." Flint officials and the Michigan Department of Environmental Quality were still insisting Flint drinking water was safe.

So Muchmore worked on a plan resulting in private companies donating 1,500 water filters that Flint ministers passed out over the coming months. But, again, Snyder's staff wrestled with a contradiction, according to emails: Flint city officials didn't want them to distribute filters because it countered their contention the water was safe.

JULY 2015: 'THEY ARE BASICALLY GETTING BLOWN OFF BY US'

In July, Flint haunted Muchmore again. As media reports began pointing to lead in Flint drinking water, Muchmore emailed then-MDEQ Director Dan Wyant and Michigan Department of Health and Human Services Director Nick Lyon. Again, the governor was not copied.

"I'm frustrated by the water issue in Flint. I really don't think people are getting the benefit of the doubt. Now they are concerned and rightfully so about the lead level studies they are receiving from DEQ samples. Can you take a moment out of your impossible schedule to personally take a look at this? These folks are scared and worried about the health impacts and they are basically getting blown off by us (as a state we're just not sympathizing with their plight.)"

MDEQ staffers reported back that the drinking water still met safety standards and there was no evidence connecting Flint drinking water to elevated blood levels in children.

"Frankly, the only way the issues will be totally resolved is when the (Karegnondi pipeline) comes online and the water is perceived to be cleaner and healthier," Muchmore told colleagues in three state departments at the end of July.

Not until independent water quality and health experts refuted state-agency deflections in fall 2015 did the Snyder administration take action.

SEPTEMBER 2015: MUCHMORE'S POLITICAL ANALYSIS

One of the key occasions in which Muchmore included the governor himself in Flint-related emails occurred as the crisis was breaking wide open in late September. A September 25 email made public earlier this year focused much on political analysis. Muchmore said "some in Flint are taking the very sensitive issue of children's exposure to lead and trying to turn it into a political football claiming the departments are underestimating the impacts on the populations and are particularly trying to shift responsibility to the state."

Indeed, independent experts were proving the connection between Flint water and elevated blood lead levels in children, and would soon force the state to acknowledge huge mistakes in drinking water and public health oversight. But, at that moment, in late September, Muchmore described "the incredible amount of time and effort" the administration had put into the Flint issue, criticized Democratic Flint-area Congressman Dan Kildee as a media hound, and said, "I can't figure out why the state is responsible," but for the state's involvement in the decision to switch Flint off Detroit water.

THE FRUSTRATIONS OF AUTUMN

Later in the autumn, Muchmore vacillated between working on complex Flint logistics and financial matters and occasionally losing his patience in emails.

On Oct. 1, after a whirlwind 24 hours in which he met with Senate Minority Leader Jim Ananich and State Rep. Sheldon Neeley (both Flint Democrats), Flint Mayor Dayne Walling, Flint ministers, and state Treasury officials, Muchmore emailed Snyder's legislative director and former Lieutenant Governor Dick Posthumus.

"Help," Muchmore said. "Get me out of this mess."

A few days later, Muchmore's wife, a Lansing public relations executive, suggested the Snyder administration get "an outrage management expert."

"I think you guys need someone … to help provide some forest for the trees help, message help, etc.," Deb Muchmore wrote." I don't like the way the issue is being handled, reported, etc. You need some help."

Indeed, public outrage flowed into the Snyder administration's constituent services office throughout the fall and winter:

"I remain convinced that if this had happened in a white, affluent, politically powerful community, none of this current obfuscation would be accepted."

"Tell the governor to stick his survey data up his #&*@. Cash your paycheck like a good drone and don't bother me with your $%#@. I don't believe it anyway."

"Whatever in God's name has happened to human kindness and compassion and doing the right thing? My question to you is … how can YOU sleep at night. Shame on all of you. I feel sick over this."

It's unclear if those public sentiments ever reached the desks of Muchmore and other top Snyder aides. But, along the way, Flint riddles kept coming Muchmore's way.

In October, the governor announced a bipartisan task force to investigate the mess and make recommendations so it doesn't happen again. As the task force was being formed, Senate Minority Leader Ananich asked for longtime former Democratic U.S. Sen. Carl Levin to gain a seat. Negotiations ensued by email. "I made the request," Muchmore replied, and records show that his request went to the governor. But Levin wasn't appointed.

In the negotiations, Muchmore asked Ananich's office to denounce a constant thorn in the Snyder administration's side: the liberal advocacy group, Progress Michigan.

"I assume these jerks don't represent the Minority Leader, but it would be nice to see a public denunciation of them from him," Muchmore wrote. "I'm sure they didn't volunteer any help to the Flint people or put any effort into alleviating the difficulties the city finds itself in since they never do anything positive."

DECEMBER 2015: ONE MORE CASUALTY

A few weeks later, on his way out the door, Flint gripped Muchmore as the casualties of the crisis broadened from the people of Flint to include a member of Snyder's cabinet – MDEQ Director Dan Wyant, who had just resigned.

"Just between you and I," Muchmore wrote to his replacement Agen on December 29. "I would have argued privately against this very strongly…. Dan is one of the most exceptional directors in state government history over the last forty years…. I'm not sure why this decision was made but if it's only optics, keep in mind that finding a replacement who has the trust of the business community will be very difficult."

Muchmore's concerns came too late to save Wyant.

And the many early Snyder administration email conversations and partial measures they pursued throughout much of 2015 didn't save Flint from the crisis.

In response to questions for this story, Muchmore released a statement.

"With the benefit of hindsight, it's clear that there were a series of breakdowns locally, with the state and with the federal government," the statement said. "Those with direct oversight should have ensured that corrosion controls were properly implemented and, when that did not occur, officials throughout the chain of command in the state should have caught the error and corrected it.

The Governor has accepted responsibility for this terrible situation. As part of that, he has taken the unprecedented step of voluntarily releasing volumes of communications in the interest of full disclosure, to help to restore the public trust and to underscore his absolute commitment to the people of Flint now and into the future."

CHAPTER 27

MARCH 1, 2016

SNYDER'S EMAILS HINT AT KEY ISSUES SOON TO TAKE THE PUBLIC SPOTLIGHT

Editor's summary: The late February release of emails from Gov. Snyder's office inspires another story – how those emails talk about significant issues that will soon grab public attention. This story talks about three: how to repair Michigan's crumbling infrastructure; whether the governor's office and legislature should be exempted from Michigan's Freedom of Information Act; and, finally, lead testing in Michigan schools.

By John Bebow
Bridge Magazine

The release of thousands of past Snyder administration emails regarding the Flint water crisis hint at emerging statewide issues.

Here are three:

CRUMBLING WATER INFRASTRUCTURE

Pipes aren't sexy. Politicians don't sweep into office talking about sewers and drinking water. Budgets aren't sexy in campaign season, either, unless they involve open discussion of taxes. Politicians often try to win elections by promising tax cuts. Both political parties have tried that approach in recent statewide elections.

In the wake of Flint, voters may hear much more from candidates about pipes, budgets and taxes. One question: Will that talk come as platitudes or real policy discussion?

As aides crafted early drafts of Gov. Rick Snyder's State of the State address late last year, Snyder adviser Rich Baird offered a warning for Michigan's future.

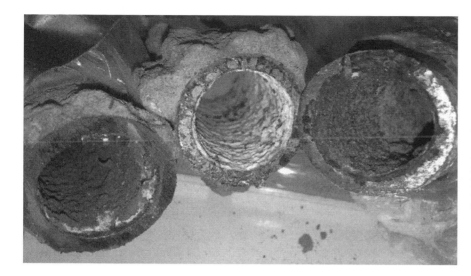

This photo dramatically shows the corrosion of three Flint water pipes removed after the city switched to Flint River-sourced water.

Photo courtesy of Min Tang and Kelsey Pieper/Flintwaterstudy.org

"Start framing the infrastructure problem," Baird wrote. "We have huge problems throughout the state with aged piping and plumbing. Ignoring it will be at the peril of future generations. We should put a number out there on what it is going to take to fix it or conclude it is safe for generations to come."

"If communities continue to use traditional methods to manage infrastructure, conservative estimates range in the billions to improve storm water, drinking water, and wastewater management systems over the next 20 years," according to Michigan's Draft Water Strategy published by the state's Office of the Great Lakes in 2015.

For drinking water systems alone, the cost would be $13.8 billion for improvements or upgrades over the next 20 years, according to Snyder Administration email documents released in late February.

For perspective, $13.8 billion is $3.8 billion more than the entire current annual state general fund budget. And it's $600 million more than the state will spend next year on public schools. In short, it's a huge number.

That price tag – plus billions more for sewer system upkeep – is the cost of preventing the next Flint drinking water crisis, preventing sewer failures resulting in pollution, and preventing industry from going outside Michigan for the water and sewer systems they need in the future.

That high-minded draft water strategy calls on Michigan to "establish sustainable funding mechanisms" for "water infrastructure management." But it's anybody's guess how all those needed water and sewer fixes will get funded in the next 20 years.

Some hope that a new Michigan legislative committee charged with investigating the Flint disaster will spread its inquiry into statewide infrastructure needs. But the current culture in Lansing is not to open the wallet willy-nilly for water infrastructure.

"I've heard some grumbling," Michigan Department of Health and Human Services Director Nick Lyon reported to colleagues in October as the Snyder administration sought stopgap funding to help Flint. "Some members feel it should be a loan, others worry that we are setting a precedent that the state will be asked to pay for similar upgrades in the future."

Yet some legislators, including Republicans, are now talking about framing an infrastructure ballot issue for 2016 or 2018.

STATE GOVERNMENT TRANSPARENCY

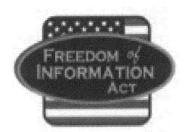

There's a rising call from government watchdogs and some members of both political parties to make publicly available the email and other records of the Michigan legislature and the governor's office, currently exempt from the Michigan Freedom of Information Act (FOIA). Michigan is one of two states that exempt the two bodies from giving the public access to those public records.

Snyder has turned that secretive custom upside down as he voluntarily – but under enormous pressure – released thousands of administration records.

"Michigan residents have a right to get answers to any questions they still have," Snyder said in a late February press release.

The records released provide an extraordinary window into decision-making, public and media relations, political calculation, financial analysis and policy making in the governor's office.

Don't expect to see it again, even if the law changes.

It's clear that writers of the many open, controversial, and often embarrassing Snyder administration emails never expected their thoughts to go public. In many cases, Snyder appointees and state bureaucrats stamped their emails with phrases like "privileged" and "not subject to FOIA."

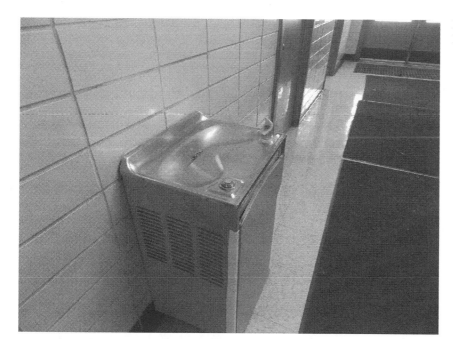

If future governors and legislators are subject to FOIA, reporters and residents can expect that policymakers may be less likely to put many of their communications in emails or text messages. They can avoid the prying eyes of journalists and the public by returning to face-to-face and telephone conversations to discuss sensitive negotiations, controversy, or the inevitable political intrigue.

Then again, how quickly we (and political figures) forget. Text messages were a major part of Detroit Mayor Kwame Kilpatrick's undoing a few years ago.

LEAD TESTING IN MICHIGAN SCHOOLS

In late February, Battle Creek-based W.K. Kellogg Foundation released a 75-page guidebook called "Managing Lead in Drinking Water at Schools and Early Childhood Facilities."

"School and early childhood facilities need to know if the drinking water they provide to children contains high levels of lead," the report declared. "Many parents, students, and communities across the country have found themselves in the position of discovering high levels of lead in their school's drinking water either through a media news story or through the school's sampling efforts."

The report called on schools to develop profiles of their plumbing systems and work with state drinking water safety agencies like the Michigan Department of Environmental Quality. The report further referred readers to a 12-year-old Environmental Protection Agency report to better understand lead monitoring in school drinking water. The EPA report stated that Michigan had no program for such monitoring.

Last fall, as the Flint crisis mushroomed, the MDEQ urged Michigan school districts with older plumbing to test their drinking water for lead. MDEQ's tests identified three elementary schools in Flint with elevated lead levels.

But there are no state requirements for schools to do so. Snyder administration email records show aides scrambling to get a handle on the situation last fall.

As of late October (2015), MDEQ staff charged with testing Flint schools "know, as we do, that this is likely a statewide issue," Anne Armstrong Cusack, the governor's associate director for the Office of Urban Initiatives, reported in email.

Another Snyder aide, Stacie Clayton, related an October conversation with John Felske, superintendent of the Muskegon Public Schools: "Felske has followed the developments in Flint during the past two months with concern, particularly since 'every building in our district' is more than 25 or 30 years old. Lead connections and plumbing fixtures with lead solder are likely in many buildings built before the mid-1980s. 'We produce 1,080,000 meals in our public schools each year,' Felske said. 'Obviously, we're using tap water to feed our children, let alone having them drink out of the water fountains.' "

Snyder aides called a number of school districts, according to email records, and found some testing for lead and some not.

In February, Howell found elevated lead levels in one elementary school.

In December, Rep. Adam Zemke, D-Ann Arbor, sought MDEQ feedback on a bill he planned to introduce to require that schools test for lead in drinking water at least once every three years. MDEQ water regulator Liane Shekter Smith pushed back on the idea, noting the huge potential cost for water suppliers.

"If the legislature wants to require this monitoring, the burden for this should be on the schools or the board of education," she wrote.

Shekter Smith was fired in early February for her role in Flint's water crisis.

CONGRESSIONAL HEARINGS

PARTISAN VENOM FLOWS FREELY AT HEARINGS BUT INSIGHTS ARE FEW AND FAR BETWEEN

By Bob Campbell

Three hearings of the U.S. House Oversight and Government Reform Committee in February and March 2016 produced few revelations, but lots of political heat from members of the committee and the final two witnesses – Gov. Rick Snyder and EPA administrator Gina McCarthy.

Republican committee members generally attacked the U.S. Environmental Protection Agency and its leadership. Democrats saved their harshest words for Gov. Rick Snyder and his administration.

Here are highlights or what was said or introduced into evidence, at the hearings.

HEARING 1 – FEB. 3: The witnesses were Joel Beauvais, an EPA water official, Keith Creagh, director of the Michigan Department of Environmental Quality, Marc Edwards, a Virginia Tech professor, and Lee-Anne Walters, the Flint mom whose home tap water lead test results began a process that ultimately led to exposing the lead problem.

Committee Chairman Jason Chaffetz, R-Utah, began the hearing angered that three witnesses didn't respond. He excused one, EPA's Miguel Del Toral, who was in Flint working on the water crisis. But Darnell Earley, one of Flint's former appointed Emergency Managers, and Susan Hedman, who was then the recently-resigned administrator of EPA's Region 5, both refused to testify, prompting Chaffetz to issue subpoenas and pronounce: "Participation....before this committee is not optional. When you get invited to come to the Oversight and Government Reform Committee, you are going to show up."

For Earley, he added: "We're calling on the U.S. Marshals to hunt him down and give him that -- give him that subpoena."

U.S. Rep. Matt Cartwright, D-Pa., one-upped Chaffetz when he asked (and then answered) his own question about a potential witness's whereabouts: "Can anybody tell me why Gov. Snyder is not here today? Because he's hiding, that's why."

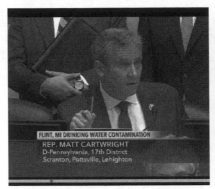

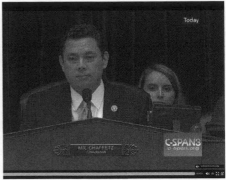

The ranking Democrat on the committee, Rep. Elijah Cummings of Maryland, who was also angry that Chaffetz hadn't invited Snyder, recalled the lyrics of songwriter Cat Stevens to describe what the lead-poisoned children of Flint face. Then, he said: "I've often said that our children are the living messages we send to a future we will never see. The question is, what will they leave us and how will we send them into that future? Will we send them strong? Will we send them hopeful? Will we rob them of their destiny? Will we rob them of their dreams? No, we will not do that!"

The Washington Post reported the crowd was silent until Chaffetz told them: "You should have applauded to that." So they did.

HEARING 2 – MARCH 15:

The witnesses were Susan Hedman, former EPA Region 5 administrator; Darnell Earley, former Flint emergency manager, Dayne Walling, former mayor of Flint, and Marc Edwards, professor at Virgina Tech and drinking water expert.

One of the more interesting details of this hearing came from an email put on the record from the EPA's Miguel Del Toral expressing his frustration that his bosses weren't moving quickly to stop the poisoning of Flint's children in late September 2015.

"At every stage of this process, it seems that we spend more time trying to maintain State/local relationships than we do trying to protect the children. I said this from the very beginning and I will say this again…you don't have to drop a bowling ball off of every building in every city to prove that gravity (and science) will work the same way everywhere. It's basic chemistry….

"Sorry for the rant, but I am very upset about this because I told people this was going to be the outcome. I watched this movie before in Washington, DC. And we are heading down the exact same path of denial and delay and meanwhile, the children are being irreparably damaged."

Del Toral's email was not the only criticism of the EPA at the second hearing.

Witness Marc Edwards, the Virginia Tech professor, said of the EPA: "….to this day, they have not apologized for what they did in Flint, Michigan. No apology from EPA. Completely unrepentant and unable to learn from their mistakes. I guess being a government agency means you never have to say you're sorry."

Hedman, more than any witness, seemed to annoy members of both parties. At one point she said: "I don't think anyone at EPA did anything wrong, but I do believe we could have done more."

Responding to Hedman's comments, Rep. Ted Lieu, D-Cal., said: "Why, in July or August, didn't you just stand up and scream, stop this? To me, this is negligence bordering on deliberate indifference."

HEARING 3 – MARCH 17:

The witnesses were Gov. Rick Snyder and EPA Administrator Gina McCarthy.

Democrats on the committee finally got their face-to-face opportunity to question and lecture Gov. Snyder.

Snyder didn't help himself in his opening statement when he – as he had done before – accepted blame, but also spread it.

"Let me be blunt. This was a failure of government at all levels. Local, state, and federal officials – we all failed the families of Flint. This is not about politics or partisanship. I am not going to point fingers or shift blame; there is plenty of that to share, and neither will help the people of Flint. Not a day or night goes by that this tragedy doesn't weigh on my mind…the questions I should have asked… the answers I should have demanded… how I could have prevented this. That's why I am so committed to delivering permanent, long-term solutions and the clean, safe drinking water that every Michigan citizen deserves."

Maryland Rep. Elijah Cummings, the committee's ranking Democrat, wasn't impressed. He said: "Gov. Snyder's administration chose to switch to the Flint River for a source of water, not the EPA. Gov. Snyder's administration ignored warnings from the Flint water treatment plant supervisors not to go forward with the switch, not the EPA….Gov. Snyder's administration caused this horrific disaster and poisoned the children of Flint."

But Cummings barbs were pale compared to what Rep. Matt Cartwright, D-Pa., had to say, using his skills as a former trial attorney and to ask a series of questions, often cutting off Snyder before he finished.

Then, Cartwright was set up for his knockout punch.

"Governor, plausible deniability only works when it's plausible and I'm not buying that you didn't know any of this until October 2015. You were not in a medically-induced coma for a year. And I've had about enough of your false contrition and your phony apologies. Susan Hedman from the EPA bears not one-tenth of the responsibility of the state of Michigan and your administration."

McCarthy also took plenty of heat. She put all the blame on Michigan officials for the Flint crisis, saying: "We were strong-armed. We were misled. We were kept at arms-length. We couldn't do our jobs effectively."

When Chaffetz repeatedly asked her whether EPA did anything wrong, she responded: "I don't know whether we did everything right, that's the problem. I would have hoped we would have been more aggressive."

Snyder was enraged because McCarthy accepted no blame. He pointed to emails that supported the contention that EPA officials were not pushing hard after they had evidence of a public health threat in Flint.

"When I read these things, I'm ready to get sick. We needed urgency, we needed action and they kept on talking," Snyder said.

Chaffetz, referring to McCarthy's statement that Hedman's resignation was courageous, told her: "If you want to do the courageous thing, then you, too, should resign."

CHAPTER 28

MARCH 22, 2016

OLD WATER AND SEWER LINES: THE MULTI-BILLION DOLLAR COST OF NEGLECT

Editor's summary: Bridge Magazine presses hard to give readers some of the harsh lessons emerging from Flint about the cost of ignoring a crumbling infrastructure of water and sewer lines under Michigan's also crumbling roads. Some of the numbers in this piece are staggering: $17.5 billion needed over the next 20 years for water and sewer line repairs and upgrades in the state; 25 billion gallons of untreated or partially treated sewage dumped into state waters over two recent years; 20 million gallons of clean, treated water lost in one water main break in Bay City. Get out your checkbook.

By Ted Roelofs and Pat Shellenbarger
Bridge Magazine Contributors

ike Gutow had fond childhood memories of fishing, swimming and skiing on its clear waters when he bought a Lake St. Clair waterfront home in May 2011

"Paradise," he said. "It's the best way to describe it."

A heavy rain fell just a few days after he moved in. He recalled that two or three days later "this glob appeared at the seawall that was about three-feet thick. Mixed in was a lot of dead fish. At first it was like, 'what the heck is this?' I'd never seen anything like it before, but, bad as it was to look at, the smell was even worse."

He now knows he was seeing and smelling the result of a sanitary and storm sewer system that is outdated, under-maintained and unable to handle the stuff flowing through its pipes, especially during a moderate or heavy rainfall.

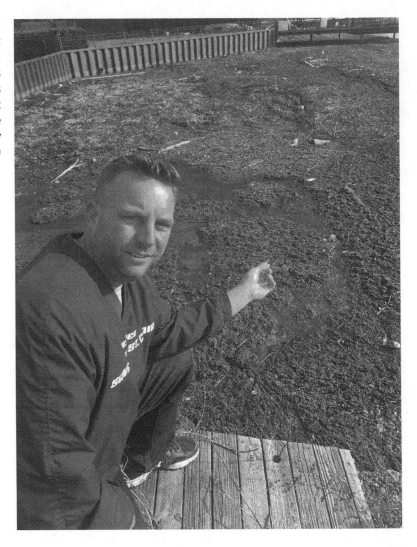

Mike Gutow learned hard truths about the deterioration of Michigan's underground pipes when he bought a home on Lake St. Clair. (Courtesy photo)

Drive along Michigan's streets and highways, and the poor condition of the roads is obvious. But buried beneath the roads are old pipes meant to deliver water for drinking and washing and carrying away waste that are in their own shoddy condition. Some have been in the ground for more than a century – well beyond their expected lifespans. In some cities, sewage still flows through hollowed out logs, although no one knows exactly where.

"Out of sight, out of mind, right?" said Ronald Brenke, executive director of the Michigan section of the American Society of Civil Engineers, or ASCE. "People don't think about it, because it's underground."

Much of Michigan's water and sewer infrastructure has been neglected for years and is in desperate need of repair, threatening public health. But experts say the undertaking could cost $17.5 billion over the next two decades.

That price tag doesn't even include replacing lead service pipes, a peril exposed by Flint's water crisis.

How shaky is Michigan's water infrastructure? Consider our faltering network of sewers. In 2013 and 2014, nearly 25 billion gallons of partially treated and untreated storm and sanitary sewage flowed into the state's waterways. One billion gallons is enough to fill more than 1,500 Olympic-sized swimming pools.

In its most recent report card, released in 2009, ASCE gave Michigan a D+ for its storm water sewers and a C for those that carry wastewater. Worse, ASCE graded the state's drinking water infrastructure a D.

"A significant portion of the state's primary (water) distribution system is nearing 100 years old," the report said, adding, "Much of the delivery system, including piping, valves and hydrants, are reaching the end of their anticipated design life, and routine replacement has been postponed for too long."

On March 10, Gov. Rick Snyder announced creation of a 21st Century Infrastructure Commission to recommend how to modernize the state's transportation, water, sewer, energy and communication infrastructures. He said he will ask the Legislature to approve $165 million in the state's 2017 fiscal year budget for the newly created Michigan Infrastructure Fund – a drop in the lake, by some estimates.

The ASCE report estimated that Michigan's municipalities would need to spend $13.8 billion to maintain and upgrade their water systems over the next 20 years. (The state ranked 27th in per capita spending for water improvement projects.)

The report estimated it would cost another $3.7 billion over the next 20 years to bring the state's wastewater systems up to standards.

"We haven't made any progress since the report card of 2009," Brenke said. "Our system is aging very fast, and we're going to need more repairs."

Buried in the ASCE's 2009 report, and largely ignored, was a dire warning that lead in the ancient pipes throughout the state could leach into the drinking water. That's what happened when Flint stopped buying water from Detroit in 2014 and began drawing its water from the highly corrosive Flint River.

"We have basically predicted a lot of things that happened in Flint," Brenke said.

While the Flint crisis has attracted national publicity and congressional hearings, Brenke contends that "Flint is just a symptom of a bigger problem."

On a recent visit to Flint, Tom Cochran, CEO of the U.S. Conference of Mayors, said he intends to cite Flint's water crisis to urge more federal investment in local systems.

"We're going to be meeting with the next president in December," he said at a Flint news conference. "This will be on the agenda – water infrastructure, and we will use Flint."

It's easy to find signs of Michigan's deteriorating water supply system:

- In December, a water main break along Detroit's Lodge Freeway shut down the road's northbound lanes on city's west side. Water covered all lanes for several hours, backing up traffic for two miles.

- In 2014, Bay City residents were told not to do laundry or water their lawns – and some large commercial water users were told not to use water at all – after a water main break drained 20 million gallons from the system and led to a big drop in water pressure.

- In 2012, Flint officials said a water main break leaked millions of gallons over the course of a year before they were able to find and fix it. The leak drained city residents of about $800,000 in lost water.

- In 2009, the mayor of Warren declared a state of emergency when more than 100 pipes failed in one winter month – three times the monthly average. A break near a shopping center spawned a sinkhole that swallowed a van and left the shopping center without water for several days.

Nationwide, the U.S. Geological Survey estimates water systems lose 1.7 trillion gallons of water a year to leaks, with 16 percent of water never reaching the tap.

LEAD LINES A FURTHER HEADACHE

The cost of fixing all those leaky pipes is in addition to what it would take to replace tens of thousands of lead service lines in cities and towns across the state – a measure gaining support from water safety advocates in the wake of Flint.

The American Water Works Association estimates there are 6.1 million lead service lines nationwide, down from an estimated 10 million in 1991. Most are in older homes in older cities, where lead was the material of choice for water service lines from the early 20th century into the 1950s.

In December, the National Drinking Water Advisory Council, which advises the U.S. Environmental Protection Agency on water issues, said, "removing the sources of lead in drinking water should be a national goal." In March, the board of the American Water Works Association, a nonprofit scientific and education group, voted unanimously to back those recommendations.

Still, with a few exceptions, there is no consensus among Michigan's drinking water systems to embark on removal of lead lines.

Lansing's Board of Water and Light spent $42 million over the last 12 years replacing 13,500 lead lines. Flint has just begun replacing lead lines, a project that is estimated to cost $55 million.

Grand Rapids estimates it has 17,000 lead service lines, although there seems to be little political impetus to spend the estimated $50 million to replace them despite the recommendations of the water advisory council.

Grand Rapids City Commissioner Ruth Kelly said she sees no immediate reason to replace the lead lines, since recent water testing found 90 percent of the homes had lead levels less than 2.2 parts per billion. The federal action threshold for lead contamination is 15 parts per billion.

Since 1994, when Grand Rapids introduced phosphate into the system, a remedy that puts a protective coating in lead pipes, lead levels in the city's drinking water have steadily dropped from 11 parts per billion in 1997. City Manager Greg Sundstrom has said he is satisfied the drinking water system is safe.

"I think it's working well. We've been testing it for years," Kelly said.

THE COST OF DOING NOTHING

While the price of replacing outdated water and sewer lines is high, doing nothing can be expensive, too. The American Society of Civil Engineers estimated that, without increased investment, waterborne illnesses would cost American households $413 million between 2011 and 2020. It calculated U.S. businesses would lose $734 billion in sales from 2011 to 2020 without added investment in water and sewer infrastructure.

Still, the question remains – where would the money to update Michigan's water and sewer infrastructure come from?

By and large, municipal sewer and water systems are funded by charges to their customers. So when a city loses lots of population – think Flint, Detroit and Saginaw – the system has few options but raising rates for those who remain.

In 2015, Flint's average $910 home water bill was the nation's highest – before a judge ordered it reduced by 35 percent.

"You still have the same infrastructure sitting in the ground. You end up with rates that go up substantially," said Anthony Minghine, chief operating officer for the Michigan Municipal League.

But Minghine said reduced revenues puts pressure on water or sewer system managers to defer long-term investments to avoid big rate increases. "Those (long-term investments) are the areas that are going to suffer," he said.

Ronald Brenke, the ASCE head for Michigan, said he's frustrated those warnings from groups like his have been ignored.

"Unfortunately, everything's got to be a crisis" before government officials will act, he said.

Sometimes that and a vocal citizenry is what it takes to spur elected officials into action.

State officials at first ignored Mike Gutow when he complained about the gunk clinging to the seawall of his Lake St. Clair home. That's why he formed the nonprofit group Save Lake St. Clair and began carrying his message to legislators, city councils and anyone else who'd listen.

State officials initially told him the gunk was algae, nothing to worry about. Eventually, a state test showed it contained human DNA. In other words, the stuff people flush down their toilets.

Part of the problem is that many Michigan municipal systems still have combined sanitary and storm sewer systems, which are prone to overflow in heavy rains. In the late 1980s, 46 Michigan communities had combined sewer systems, said Charlie Hill, an environmental engineer with the state Department of Environmental Quality. Since then, 16 cities have spent millions of dollars separating their systems, he said, and about 10 are in the process of separating.

The remaining 20 or so communities, including Detroit, have opted not to separate storm and sanitary sewers, but, instead, have built large retention basins to hold and partially treat the excess sewage during heavy rainfalls.

In 2013, combined sewer systems and retention basins in Michigan overflowed 423 times, spilling 11.4 billion gallons of untreated and partially treated sewage into the state's waterways – enough to fill more than 135 supertankers. That same year, another billion gallons of untreated sewage flowed out of the state's sanitary sewer systems, according to an annual report by the MDEQ.

In 2014, 11.6 billion gallons overflowed from the state's combined sewer systems and 750 million gallons from its sanitary sewers, the MDEQ's Hill said.

"I think there's a lot of work that needs to be done, but we've made a lot of progress from the raw sewage discharges we had 20 or 30 years ago," he said.

In recent years, when it rains hard, combined sewers and retention basins that serve the growing residential areas of Macomb and Oakland counties overflowed, sending untreated and partially treated sewage into the Clinton River and, eventually, into Lake St. Clair. Each year, Macomb County health officials often close beaches on Lake St. Clair when tests show high levels of E. coli, a bacterium that can cause illness and is an indicator of other pathogens.

In Harrison Township, a few miles north of his St. Clair Shores home, Gutow saw where the muck had built up four football fields long and well out into Lake St. Clair since 2001.

"When I saw that, my heart sank," he said. "I said, 'there's no way I can allow that to happen down by me.' "

When the DEQ said he'd need a permit to have machines remove the stuff, he donned waders, slogged through the muck and began heaving shovels full into the lake.

"It looked like poop," he said. "I'm even pulling up toilet paper. I could see what it was. I hated doing it. What was I doing? I was making my problem somebody else's."

Still, he's optimistic that he and other members of Save Lake St. Clair are being heard.

"The pressure is starting to come on," he said. "Yes, there are things being done. They're making vast improvements.

"What we're learning from Flint is that our infrastructure is well beyond the age that it should be allowed to exist anymore."

CHAPTER 29

MARCH 24, 2016

FLINT'S SWITCH TO RIVER WATER SAVED MONEY, BUT NOT FOR ITS CITIZENS

Editor's summary: Once again, a Bridge staffer finds an angle that brings fresh insight to the complicated Flint water crisis. Yes, Flint residents were paying the nation's highest water rates, and, yes, switching to the Flint River for its water source sharply dropped the city's costs for water. But Flint water rates continue to stay high because Flint's emergency manager decides the water and sewer fund, depleted to cover other costs in previous years, needs to be replenished. When power was returned to the city's elected mayor in April 2015, the terms of a $7 million state loan blocked Flint from leaving its new partner, the Karegnondi Water Authority, or cutting water rates.

By Mike Wilkinson
Bridge Magazine

Long before Flint's lead-tainted water brought national attention to the city, everyone in town knew the cost of its water was outrageous.

Huge price increases had brought Flint the nation's highest rates. When service and usage fees were combined, Flint's beleaguered residents paid an average annual bill of $864 in 2014. The next highest average in Michigan was $300 less. Predictably, in a city where 4 in 10 people live in poverty, thousands failed to pay their water bills.

"People in Flint cannot afford this," Randy Rauch, the Genesee County Child Welfare Director for the Michigan Department of Human Services, wrote in a February 2013 email to his supervisors in Lansing. Among his concerns: Rising water hook-up fees, ranging from $100 to $350. "Flint cannot live with these rates. I feel somehow the Governor needs to hear about this."

Within a day, Rauch's complaint had reached Gov. Rick Snyder's office, according to internal communications made public by Snyder's office.

Rauch was right – the people of Flint could not afford what they were being charged for water. But the back story is more complex than the easy narrative promoted by city leaders: that the Detroit Water and Sewerage Department was financially squeezing Flint, virtually forcing the city to look elsewhere for water, a decision that disastrously ended with the Flint River as an interim source.

Government emails and documents, and interviews by Bridge Magazine, show Flint's state-appointed emergency managers, with input from state treasury officials, continued to charge residents high rates after switching to the Flint River, even though the move had cut the city's water expenses to a fraction of what it had paid Detroit.

The reason: The cash-starved city needed every dollar it could collect from residents to replenish its water and sewer fund, money that had been reallocated over the years to close other gaps in Flint's budget, records show.

Residents, who may have anticipated the temporary switch to the Flint River would provide financial relief, saw no savings.

"That's when we really started getting angry," said Eric Mays, who was elected in 2013 to Flint's city council. "Why isn't that savings being passed along to the customers?"

Leaving aside the government failures that led most directly to lead from old city pipes leaching into the water supply, the tale of Flint's unyielding water rates shows the desperate choices cities like Flint must make between easing costs for impoverished residents and the imperatives of balancing the books.

A CITY ON THE EDGE

For years, Flint was shaped by the need for, and lack of, cash. Consider its attempts to stem a steady, decades-long decline in population and tax revenues and the decision in 2013, under the control of state-appointed emergency managers, to join the Karegnondi Water Authority and temporarily use the Flint River for drinking water.

How and why the city and state made those decisions raise questions about the sustainability of Michigan's model for municipal finance and its emergency manager law. In the end, the failures of government officials allowed a known neurotoxin to flow into the city's drinking water, sparking fear, medical crises, lawsuits and legislative and criminal investigations.

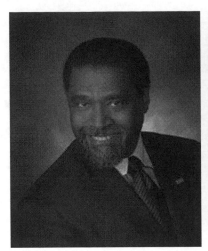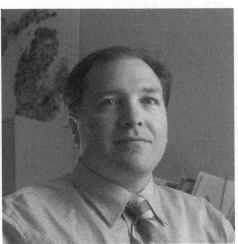

Flint Emergency
Manager Darnell
Earley

Photo courtesy State of
Michigan

Michigan State
University economist
Eric Scorsone

Two months after Rauch raised flags about the high cost of water in 2013, state Treasurer Andy Dillon agreed that Flint needed a cheaper water source. He gave the go-ahead for Flint's then-Emergency Manager Ed Kurtz to switch from the Detroit Water and Sewerage Department (DWSD) to the Karegnondi Water Authority (KWA), which was to build a new pipeline to Lake Huron by late 2016 to serve Flint and nearby communities and counties.

The city terminated its Detroit water service a year later and began getting water from the Flint River until the KWA pipeline was ready. Other communities within Genesee County, also members of the KWA, cut a short-term deal to stay with Detroit water. But Flint officials, contending their water treatment plant was safe, made the interim switch to the river.

Flint residents didn't see lower water rates and Darnell Earley, a subsequent emergency manager, told residents in 2014 that the savings would go towards upgrading a water system that was losing 20 to 40 percent of its water through leaking pipes.

By last April, when the state loaned the city $7 million, money that allowed the city to go back to local political control, the terms included provisions that blocked Flint from leaving the KWA – and said Flint could not lower rates to residents without the consent of the state treasurer.

BUDGETS BEFORE PEOPLE

Eric Scorsone, an economist and director of the Michigan State University Extension Center for State and Local Government Policy, has studied Flint's finances for several years. He contends the city's move to the Flint River was financially attractive to the state precisely because it would dramatically lower the city's water costs.

Keeping rates high, Scorsone says, allowed Flint to replenish water fund reserves to help pay its share of costs to build the KWA.

State officials also talked about needing money to pay for $8 million in upgrades to the city's water treatment plant. The money was necessary to treat water from first the river and later the KWA, and it would come from cost savings generated by using river water, according to a February 2015 letter from Tom Saxton, the state's chief deputy treasurer.

Emergency Manager Earley knew Detroit was willing to serve water until the KWA came online in part because Detroit was willing to (and still does) provide water to the Genesee County Drain Commission, a long-time DWSD customer like Flint that was also part of the KWA.

For Flint residents, "there was never a financial savings," said Valdemar Washington, a Flint resident and attorney challenging Flint's rates.

After residents' loud complaints about the odor, taste and color of the water and indications of health problems, calls to rejoin the Detroit system were rejected in early 2015 by Jerry Ambrose, who succeeded Earley as emergency manager. In March 2015, he mocked as "incomprehensible" a largely symbolic city council vote to make the switch back to Detroit water.

Again, Flint leaders' decision to stick with the Flint River was about money.

"That's what drove the emergency manager," said Mays, the city council member, "not health, safety and welfare."

AN EMERGENCY MANAGER'S PRIORITIES

Some who have studied Michigan's emergency manager law are troubled, too. Joshua Sapotichne, an MSU political scientist, has looked at Flint and other cities where Gov. Snyder has appointed emergency managers. He said emergency managers in Michigan have a limited tool box that relies heavily on cutting costs, at the expense of residents' health or other interests. Salaries, pensions and benefits for city employees were cut and services trimmed in the financially struggling city.

"All they can do is cut," Sapotichne said.

Peeling back the layers even more, another question emerges. Why did the city council and later the city's emergency managers borrow from Flint's water and sewer funds, which happened repeatedly from 2007 to 2013? Why did it have to dip a straw into the Flint River to save money?

The conventional wisdom has been the city of Detroit's high water rates pushed Flint to seek a cheaper long-term solution. It's true that costs had risen and the DWSD could not guarantee its rates. "It's an easy narrative to say Detroit raised the rates," Scorsone said.

But other places in Genesee County that paid the same base rate to Detroit had far lower bills. How Flint's became the highest in the nation is a mystery. "That's the tough part of all this is, we don't know that for sure."

What's clear, however, is those running Flint found it harder and harder to pay bills.

Flint, once home to nearly 200,000 people, now has fewer than 100,000. The city has lost tens of thousands of residents, jobs and the taxes they generated. Property values fell by half between 2001 and 2015 while personal income, over $2.5 billion in 2002, was just under $500 million in 2013.

Flint had been home to more than 80,000 well-paying GM jobs in the late 1970s, but by 2006, the company employed fewer than 8,000 in the city.

It was against that backdrop that city leaders struggled with finances. There were fewer people and businesses to spread the costs of an aging water and sewer system, and fewer taxpayers to fund the city's services. Income tax rates were capped by state law and the city's share of state revenue sharing fell by $63 million since 2003, including $7.7 million less in 2013 when compared with 2003, according to a March 2016 report by the Michigan Municipal League.

Like Flint, municipalities across Michigan face cuts in core services like police and fire – as well as infrastructure bills. Some communities ended up under state supervision or with emergency managers. Detroit, most famously, filed for bankruptcy.

In Flint, leaders before and after the first emergency manager chose to use its water and sewer money to balance other parts of the city's cash-strapped budget. In 2006, the city had "unreserved system equity" in water and sewer funds of more than $60 million.

"Flint used the water and sewer funds as a bank," MSU's Scorsone said. "In one sense, it made sense: That's where the cash is."

Mays, a colorful and controversial city official who recently was jailed for impaired driving, agreed. "The water and sewer funds always were the funds that had the money."

After settling a lawsuit over sewer overflows, the city dipped into the water and sewer reserves in 2007 for $15.7 million, a decision a judge later called illegal. Before the first emergency manager, the city council approved loans from the water and sewer funds and, later, emergency managers would do the same. By 2013, the funds were drained.

As a result, the city charged residents a rate increase of more than 20 percent in early 2011, and another 35 percent for water and sewer service later that year.

Washington, who is still fighting the rate hikes, said the increases didn't follow Flint's own ordinances requiring residents to be notified in advance. MSU's Scorsone said the hikes may have been "legal but not financially wise."

TOUGH DECISIONS STILL

Today, Flint's water budget still lacks money for basic maintenance. Faulty pipes need millions of dollars in repairs.

"Unfortunately, the city should have been using (water fund reserves)" for infrastructure, said Jerry Preston, a former president of the Flint Area Convention & Visitors Bureau. He has raised questions for years about the difference in water bills between those in Flint and surrounding communities, which also drew water from the Detroit system.

He said his suspicions have been confirmed.

"It's about a bunch of bad decisions," Preston said. "What's missing is the first decision: leaving the Detroit water system because the cost is too high."

More trouble looms, Scorsone fears. A $30 million state package to refund up to 65 percent of past water bills for Flint residents has lowered bills, but will run out next year. And no one suggests that the city's transition to the KWA will offer relief to residents on water bills.

"Within a year, this system's going to be in serious financial trouble," he predicts. "I don't see how water rates are going down."

By then, the water may be safer, but there's no guarantee it will be cheaper.

CHAPTER 30

MARCH 24, 2016

SNYDER'S TASK FORCE FINAL REPORT SLAMS DEQ, GOVERNOR AND STATE EMERGENCY MANAGER LAW

Editor's summary: Gov. Rick Snyder's critics who suspected a panel that he appointed to investigate the Flint crisis would go easy on state government and Snyder himself couldn't have been more wrong. The bipartisan panel, as seems obvious from the weight of evidence in emails and other data, laid heaviest blame on the Michigan Department of Environmental Quality. But it also slapped the governor for his ultimate failure when he appointed Flint emergency managers obsessed with cost savings over all else, including public health. The panel also expressed outrage at Snyder's appointment of department heads whose staffs failed them, and – in the aftermath – tried to lay equal blame on local and federal officials.

By Mike Wilkinson
Bridge Magazine

State government, especially the Michigan Department of Environmental Quality, is foremost to blame for failing to keep lead from poisoning Flint's water supply.

But decisions to switch the city's water supply to the Flint River, and stay there – despite mounting public outcry about the taste, odor, color and health effects of the city's tap water – were made by a succession of state-appointed emergency managers.

Those were among conclusions of the five-member Flint Water Advisory Task Force that Gov. Rick Snyder named to investigate the public health emergency in this poor, majority African-American city. Its report, released March 24, 2016, called for a review of the state's emergency manager system, which the

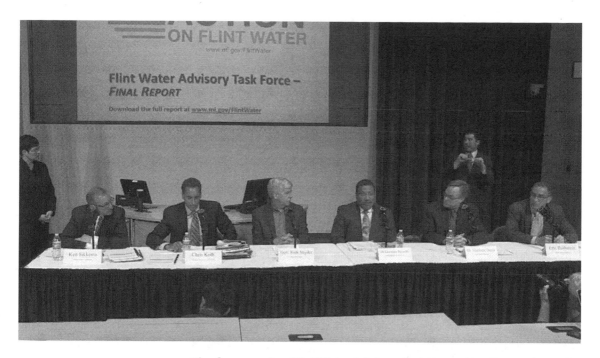

The five-member Flint Water Advisory Task Force that Gov. Rick Snyder appointed in October 2015 to investigate what went wrong in Flint and what needs to be done to fix it and make sure it doesn't happen again. The task force issued its final report on March 23, 2016, finding that the state government, especially the Michigan Department of Environmental Quality, was the primary cause of the water crisis. It also found state government, especially the Department of Environmental Quality, was the primary cause. It also criticized other state agencies, the governor himself, and the actions of emergency managers who Snyder appointed.

task force says played a major role in the government's sluggish response to the concerns and warnings of Flint residents.

"What was clearly evident was individual (emergency managers) made decisions and no one had checks and balances on those decisions," said task force member Chris Kolb, a former state representative and president of the Michigan Environmental Council. "Citizens had no ability to influence decision-making."

The 116-page report offered a rebuke to a signature tool of Gov. Rick Snyder and a legislature that has largely supported the emergency manager law. The law, resurrected by Republican lawmakers in 2012 weeks after state residents voted to drop it, was hailed after its implementation in Detroit led to that city's swift transition through bankruptcy. But the law has also been the subject of lawsuits as well as accusations that it disenfranchises minority residents, who argue that most of the financially troubled cities and school districts placed under emergency management have been majority black.

Snyder said he was open to adopting many of the task force recommendations. He said his office has already begun implementing some suggestions. "There are a lot of excellent recommendations here," Snyder told reporters at a news conference.

In Flint, the task force found, the Snyder-appointed emergency managers failed to consider, much less serve, the health interests of residents, a criticism the governor himself seemed to acknowledge in testimony March 17 before a congressional committee.

The task force report said Flint's emergency managers were too narrowly focused on saving money by switching from the Detroit Water and Sewerage Department to the Flint River as its drinking water source in 2014, and too reluctant to switch back to Detroit, also for financial reasons. As a result, local leaders and residents were marginalized. The report cited the citizens' economic and racial demographics.

"Flint residents, who are majority black or African-American and among the most impoverished of any metropolitan area in the United States, did not enjoy the same degree of protection from environmental and health hazards as that provided to other communities," the report noted, leading "to the inescapable conclusion that this is a case of environmental injustice."

The task force recommended review of the emergency manager law with focus on restoring "checks and balances" on emergency managers' decisions. Emergency managers also should have greater access to experts in public health and other areas, and should make sure local residents and officials have a voice in shaping policy, including the ability to appeal emergency manager decisions, the task force said.

If legislators adopt recommended changes, Kary Moss, executive director of the American Civil Liberties Union of Michigan, will welcome it. Last summer, Curt Guyette, an investigative reporter for the ACLU, broke stories about high lead levels in the water and the ACLU has called for changes in the emergency manager laws that had, at one point, been applied in cities and school districts in which more than half of the state's African-Americans lived.

"The task force is absolutely on the right track," Moss said. "None of this was possible a year ago. We're thrilled to see the dire consequences of this law are being taken seriously."

EM LAWS THAT WORK

Many of the task force's recommendations were outlined in a 2014 Bridge Magazine article examining why emergency manager laws are more popular in some states.

The article noted that while Michigan's law, which gives broad authority to emergency managers, was mired in controversy, states such as North Carolina and Rhode Island avoided acrimony by enacting laws that were more proactive and encouraged more input from local leaders. Experts told Bridge that Michigan should pay more attention to monitoring financially distressed cities before they are in crisis and, if intervention is needed, to give local leaders a more meaningful role in recovery.

"The reason why some (receiverships) succeed and others don't, I believe, is if you don't have buy-in, it'll never get through it," James Spiotto, a municipal bankruptcy expert and co-author of "Municipalities in Distress?: How States and Investors Deal with Local Government Financial Emergencies," told Bridge at the time.

"Nobody likes being told what to do from on high."

BROADER INDICTMENT OF STATE FAILURES

Much of the task-force report focused on other government failures, most notably by the much-maligned Michigan Department of Environmental Quality, which failed to enforce drinking water regulations, and the Michigan Department of Health and Human Services, which made mistakes interpreting data amid mounting of lead in Flint's water.

Both agencies, the task force wrote, "stubbornly worked to discredit and dismiss others' attempts to bring the issues of unsafe water, lead contamination and increased cases of... (Legionnaire's disease) to light."

The governor, meanwhile, had the "ultimate accountability" for the emergency managers he assigned to Flint, the report said. Likewise, it was Snyder who appointed the heads of the state environmental, health and treasury agencies, which bore "differing degrees of responsibility" for Flint's health crisis.

Without mentioning Snyder by name, the task force derided his insistence that the Flint debacle was a failure of local, state and federal levels of government. Such a statement "implies that blame is attributable equally to all three levels of government. Primary responsibility for the water contamination in Flint lies with MDEQ," the report concluded, while Flint was under the control of state-appointed emergency managers.

Anna Heaton, deputy press secretary to Snyder, supplied Bridge with a listing of all the task force recommendations via email that details how the governor's office is handling them. It is implementing some, considering others and referring the remainder.

THE CASE FOR EMERGENCY MANAGERS

Michigan has had an emergency manager law since 1988, though it was strengthened in 2011 before state voters dumped the law in 2012. The legislature enacted the current law weeks after the state referendum.

Dozens of states have emergency managers in response to an outgrowth of failing municipal and school district finance. "All constituents of cities are constituents of the state," said Mark Funkhouser, former mayor of Kansas City, Mo., and publisher of Governing magazine, who says such laws can be useful.

He estimates that of 1,000 cities in the country with more than 40,000 people, nearly one-third are in financial trouble. Emergency managers have helped cities like New York, the District of Columbia and Detroit, he said.

"While the jury may be out, the intervention in Detroit may have been successful," he said.

The Flint water task force would argue that, at least in Flint, it was not. The report found that emergency managers – Flint had four between 2011 and 2015 – made several questionable decisions, including the disastrous call to use the Flint River and then, amid mounting calls to return to water from Detroit, blocking the switch.

In the latter case, Emergency Manager Jerry Ambrose rejected a largely symbolic 7-1 vote in March 2015 by the Flint City Council, which urged a return to the Detroit system. Ambrose said the cash-strapped city could not afford it.

It was an example, said task force member Kolb, of how local residents and officials had lost their voice and the ability to influence local decisions.

Among the report's other findings:

- Emergency managers alone decided to use the Flint River for drinking water, and stay with that decision.

- State treasury officials, through the terms of a 2015 loan to Flint, told the city it could not return to the Detroit system without prior state approval.

- Emergency managers, often experts in financial matters, often don't have expertise in other aspects of effective government. "They don't know anything about public health," said Kolb.

- Without public input, residents and other local public officials didn't have the chance to raise meaningful questions about the move to the Flint River, Kolb said. Perhaps, he said, someone would have asked about corrosion control, the absence of which allowed lead to leach from the inside of city pipes and into the water entering residents' homes. The MDEQ should have required corrosion control, the report found.

"All those opportunities were missed because you had a few people making decisions," Kolb said.

Snyder created the task force in October 2015, the month he ordered the switch back to the Detroit water system.

Flint had been using the river's water since April 2014, a move which brought immediate outcries. But it wasn't until July 2015 that most residents learned about the potential lead problem. Still, it was three more months before state officials acknowledged lead was in the water and that a return to Detroit water was warranted.

"The causes of the crisis lie primarily at the feet of the state by virtue of its agencies' failures and its appointed emergency managers' misjudgments," the report concluded. "The significant consequences of these failures for Flint will be long-lasting. They have deeply affected Flint's public health, its economic future, and residents' trust in government."

Other members of the task force are:

- Ken Sikkema of Public Sector Consultants, and former member of the Michigan House and Senate.

- Dr. Matthew Davis of the University of Michigan Health System and an expert on public policy.

- Eric Rothstein, an infrastructure consultant with the Galardi Rothstein Group.

- Dr. Lawrence Reynolds, a pediatrician at Mott Children's Hospital.

CHAPTER 31

MARCH 31, 2016

THE UNHAPPY COUPLE

PERCEIVED SNUBS BETWEEN GOVERNOR, MAYOR STRAIN FLINT RECOVERY

By Ron French
Bridge Magazine

When Gov. Rick Snyder unveiled a 75-point plan in March to respond to the lead crisis in Flint, he forgot something:

Input from Flint's mayor.

Eight state agencies are listed in the governor's news release earlier this month as having formulated short, intermediate and long-term goals for the devastated city, but Flint Mayor Karen Weaver wasn't in meetings to help develop those goals. The mayor learned of the 75-point plan a week before Snyder held a press conference in her own city, after she believed the plan had been finalized. The state sent Weaver a quote written for her to be included in a news release. The mayor rejected it.

Two days later, Snyder was back in Flint for another press conference to unveil the final report of the Flint Water Task Force, an all-star commission appointed by the governor to investigate the causes for the crisis and recommend solutions. The task force, among other things, criticized the failure of state leaders to include local leaders in decision-making.

Mayor Weaver wasn't invited to that press conference, either.

She wasn't given an advance copy of the report – something even journalists received – and only learned of the time and location of the press conference through a call from someone at the Charles Stewart Mott Foundation.

To be sure, there's blame on both sides – the governor's office has at times not included Weaver in planning and press conferences, but Snyder's people counter that Weaver has at times either declined to participate or not attended meetings with state officials. "It's baffling," said Chris Kolb, co-chair of the Flint Water Advisory Task Force, who has navigated mistrust and bad communication between city and state. "I don't quite get what's going on right now."

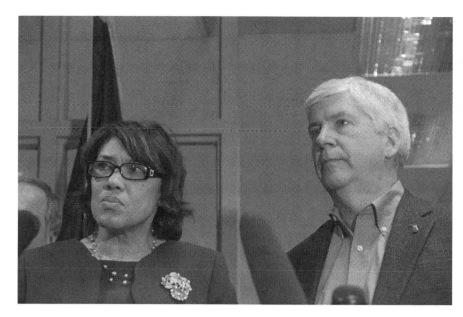

Gov. Rick Snyder and Flint Mayor Karen Weaver at a Jan. 27, 2016, press conference announcing help for Flint residents. Their body language made it clear even then that the relationship was strained.

Photo courtesy of State of Michigan

IRRECONCILABLE DIFFERENCES?

Call it a bad marriage. Say the governor is from Mars and the mayor is from Venus. There's no denying that there is a troubling communication breakdown that burdens efforts to restore clean drinking water and provide aid to Flint children who were harmed.

"Lack of communication is what got us into this problem," a frustrated Weaver told Bridge. "And it's still happening."

In July 2015, then-Snyder Chief of Staff Dennis Muchmore wrote in an email to Michigan Department of Environmental Quality officials: "I'm frustrated by the water issue in Flint. I really don't think people are getting the benefit of the doubt.… These folks are scared and worried about the health impacts and they are basically getting blown off by us (as a state we're just not sympathizing with their plight)."

The final report of the Flint Water Advisory Task Force drew the same conclusion – that the state was listening to its own expert staffers exclusively, rather than considering the views of outside experts or the people of Flint who were complaining of health problems.

"One of the biggest lessons we hope to impart in our report is the need for government leaders to listen to their constituents; in Flint that didn't happen," Kolb said at the press conference unveiling the task force report.

To Weaver, it appears that lesson hasn't been learned. She tore into Snyder and his team later that same day in a news release, scolding the governor for excluding Flint leaders from meetings about the future of their city.

"The continued failure to communicate with the elected officials here in Flint is simply astonishing," Mayor Weaver said in the news release. "I have avoided placing blame for the Flint water crisis, trying to focus the community's and my attention on moving forward. That can happen only if the state works cooperatively with local officials. But Gov. Snyder continues to ignore me, my administration, and the residents of Flint.

"He still doesn't seem to understand that the citizens of Flint no longer trust him or his administration. They don't want solutions imposed on them by the state, even if the efforts are intended to help."

POLITICAL FISSURE

Weaver was elected last year on a wave of voter anger about Flint's water crisis. On election night, she said she hoped her election would give residents upset about the crisis "a seat at the table."

A clinical psychologist by training and a small business owner in Flint, Weaver initially muted her criticism of Snyder, arguing that her role was to help assure Flint received the state funding it needed to emerge from the lead poisoning disaster. Weaver stood beside the governor at some press conferences last fall, saying it was important to work together on solution.

In early January, with his emergency managers under attack, the governor spoke of giving Weaver "more authority" over Flint's operations.

"I want to be partnering with the local official, which is the mayor," Snyder said. "I'm excited for the role she's playing there, and how we can work more closely together."

But relations have cooled. One reason may be that the city has cited far higher estimates than the state on the cost of replacing lead water lines. Snyder's 75-point plan doesn't commit to immediately replacing all lead pipes in the city, an action Weaver says should be a top priority. The city has begun digging up lead pipes on its own.

Partisan politics also may be playing a role in the relationship between the Democratic mayor and the Republican governor. In February, Weaver appeared in a Hillary Clinton campaign ad preceding Michigan's presidential primary that addressed the Flint crisis. "She's the one who brought it to another level of attention, and that's what we needed," Weaver says approvingly of Clinton in the ad.

Whatever the reason, Weaver wasn't given an advanced copy of the task force report or invited to attend the news conference in Flint where the report was released.

Neither was Dr. Mona Hanna-Attisha, the Flint doctor who helped expose high rates of lead in the blood of the city's children, and whose reporting was initially downplayed by state officials. Hanna-Attisha tried to attend the news conference, but was told the event was for media only, said Kolb and fellow task force co-chair Ken Sikkema.

Sikkema, former Republican Senate majority leader, and Kolb, a former Democratic legislator, told Bridge that the governor's office was in charge of logistics. Both men said they didn't know Flint leaders weren't invited.

Sikkema said he could understand why Weaver would be unhappy about the snub.

"It never even occurred to us that they wouldn't invite the mayor," Kolb said. "There have been several incidents like this. You would think there would be a hypersensitivity to making sure you're on the same page as the city, to build a really true partnership, because it's going to have to take a partnership."

Ari Adler, spokesman for Snyder, said he assumed his office was only handling logistics for the media, and that he thought "the task force was alerting the appropriate officials.... I don't know if the mayor was or was not invited but in hindsight, we should have closed that loop better."

STATE FRUSTRATIONS

State officials say they have had their own frustrations with Weaver. Snyder appointed the mayor to the 17-person Flint Water Interagency Coordinating Committee created early this year. The body is charged with making recommendations for upgrading the city's infrastructure and addressing health issues related to lead poisoning. But the mayor "has only been at one or two" of the six meetings held so far, Adler said.

In response to a question about Snyder scheduling events in Flint without informing the mayor, Adler pointed out that "the Mayor's Office has done a number of things without informing the Governor's Office. That's not a complaint but merely an observation over how both offices could be more proactive."

An illustration of the poor communications between state and city officials was the creation and unveiling of Snyder's 75-point plan. The Snyder administration sent Weaver a copy of the plan a week before the announcement. The plan was exhaustive, included short-term goals such as replacing plumbing in schools and daycares and long-term goals such as smoothing the eventual transition of water source to the Karegnondi Water Authority.

Weaver considered the plan to be a finished product, rather than something she and other city officials could still have input on. She didn't respond. Adler told Bridge that the governor's office was requesting feedback and didn't get it.

"Our office even offered to have the mayor participate by having a quote in the news release but she declined," Adler said. Weaver told Bridge that the governor's office wrote a quote for her and asked her to approve it, an action that, for the mayor of a city that had been run by the state by a series of emergency managers, felt patronizing.

"I would have preferred, if we were doing something, to be at the table," said Weaver, who had been working with Flint community leaders on a plan of their own. "When I found out, it had already been done; if there were people connected to Flint involved, I didn't know about it."

Weaver said Flint's plan, which has not been finalized, "is a very different plan" than the one released by Snyder, with different priorities. Weaver wants all lead pipes to be removed. Snyder's plan doesn't go that far, but does set a goal to "work with the city to plan and prioritize lead pipe service line removal."

"We have people who are trying to make decisions about you and for you, and they're not here," Weaver said of state officials. "We're the ones still using bottled water. We know what to do. We just need the resources to do it."

Having two plans is unsustainable, said task force co-chair Kolb, president of the Michigan Environmental Council. "The state can't just do this, the city can't just do this. This is somewhat bothersome that after all the lessons that should have been learned, this is still going on."

Meeting on a regular basis would be a start. For example, Lt. Gov. Brian Calley has worked in Flint three to five days a week since January, yet Weaver says she's only met with Calley twice, saying "he's doing his thing and I'm doing mine."

Adler told Bridge that "Gov. Snyder, Lt. Gov. Calley and many other members of the Snyder administration are regularly in Flint working on solving problems, meeting with elected officials, concerned pastors and other community leaders. Team members, including the governor and lieutenant governor, have met with the mayor and will continue to do so based on availability – which includes the availability of the mayor."

Meeting occasionally when everyone is available, and "doing his thing while I'm doing mine" is not good enough, Kolb said. "Someone high up with the state should be meeting with the mayor every week," Kolb said. "You can't just hand someone a 75-point plan. People buy in when they have true input."

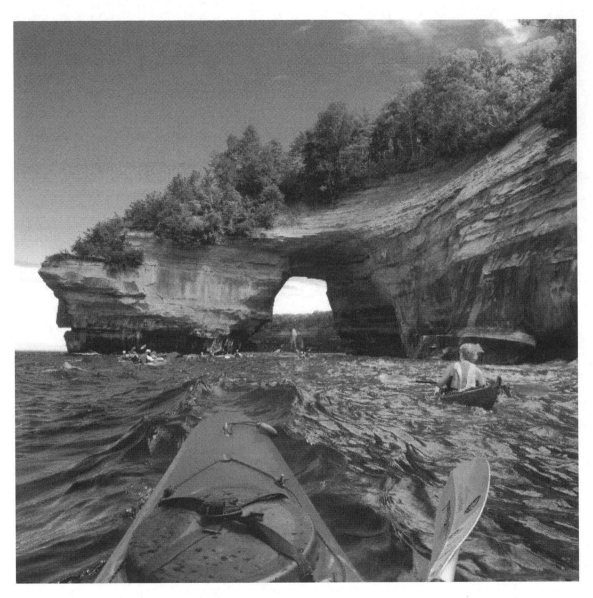

Pictured Rocks National Lakeshore near Munising on Lake Superior.

Photo courtesy State of Michigan

CHAPTER 32

MARCH 28, 2016

FLINT CRISIS IMPACTS PURE MICHIGAN CAMPAIGN

A RISK TO BUSINESS DEVELOPMENT, TOURISM

Editor's summary: It's probably inevitable that faraway businesses considering Michigan for expansion or relocation and travelers thinking about the state for visits or vacations would at least wonder about the state of the state, given the Flint mess. This story examines how the state and regional development and tourism officials are responding.

By Lindsay VanHulle
Bridge Magazine/Crain's Business Detroit

LANSING — The Pure Michigan campaign, in many ways, is about water.

The state's pristine lakes — the Great ones and the inland kind — are the frequent stars of television ads that portray Michigan as a recreation lover's paradise, a freshwater coastal dream.

Lately, the popular state tourism brand name is being linked, particularly on social media, to water of a different sort — the corrosive Flint River and the lead-tainted drinking water that poisoned the blood of Flint kids.

Bottom line: A company that relies heavily on water won't think about setting up in Flint right now, said Kate McEnroe, a Grosse Pointe native and president of Kate McEnroe Consulting, a corporate site selection firm with offices in Chicago and Atlanta.

"There are other choices of places to go almost 100 percent of the time," said McEnroe, who heard an NPR report about Flint while driving through rural Georgia. "Right now, people will wait until the dust settles, so to speak, and say, 'I'm not risking it right now.'

"The question right now is: How long does 'right now' last?"

The emergency in Flint has, for a time, been a knock against the award-winning brand that has shown up on TV, radio, print ads, billboards and even license plates since it launched in 2006 during Gov. Jennifer Granholm's administration.

Under Gov. Rick Snyder, the state adopted the Pure Michigan slogan for use in its business marketing. So if the brand is tarnished for the long term, it affects corporate recruitment and other efforts.

Economic development professionals say any damage done by the Flint crisis will be temporary. In the meantime, they added, the state and its regions must coalesce around a consistent message that Michigan remains open for business and tourists.

"It is too early to tell how much impact the Flint water crisis will have on the state's image. Certainly with our brand being Pure Michigan, it is more of an image problem," said Doug Rothwell, president and CEO of Business Leaders for Michigan. "We worked so hard to have Detroit not be a negative issue. Now, Flint puts a damper on it."

Corporate site selectors like McEnroe say they're increasingly having to offer out-of-state companies more nuance about Michigan when answering questions about Flint, similar to how they explained the state several years ago as Detroit headed closer to, and eventually through, bankruptcy.

BUSINESS DEVELOPMENT

The Michigan Economic Development Corp., which manages the $33-million Pure Michigan campaign, said the number of potential business deals in its pipeline has been down since the fall, which is when news of the Flint drinking water crisis began to break. But that's also the same time the MEDC cut its budget by 27 percent and laid off 65 employees due to a drop in tribal gaming revenue. As a result, fewer staff members are working on company outreach.

MEDC spokeswoman Emily Guerrant said deals now are generally smaller, more complicated and take longer to close; the state also has less money available for incentives. Taken together, she said, it's difficult to pinpoint the Flint crisis as the reason for a drop in business prospects.

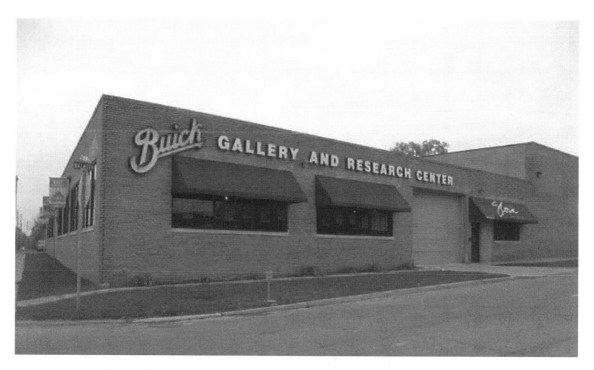

The Sloan Museum's Buick Automotive Gallery is one of the few attractions in Flint featured on the Pure Michigan website. The museum features more than 25 classic and concept Buicks, Chevrolets and other vehicles built in or near Flint.

On the tourism side, Guerrant said it's too early to have any tangible data to show whether the Flint emergency is keeping any vacationers away. The state won't receive estimates on the economic impact of this year's Pure Michigan campaign until next year. But winter tourism also suffered from lower-than-usual snowfall.

Steve Arwood, CEO of the MEDC and director of the new Michigan Department of Talent and Economic Development, said out of all the selling efforts put forth by the MEDC through the years, nothing tops Pure Michigan.

"It's iconic and award-winning," he said. "It has done more to market the state than anything we have done after that. It is the one thing that is continuing.

"When you do something for 10 years without interruption, it becomes very deep-seated and immediately recognizable. It's our brand in most of the U.S. and internationally."

Additionally, Arwood pointed to the success of the state with direct business marketing — the result of balanced budgets, improvements in workers' compensation administration and a flat corporate tax.

He said it is not hard to market Michigan as the automotive center of the country because few question that it is. But newer industries are showing strength in the state as well, such as aerospace, natural resources, agriculture and high-end food products.

He pointed to successes such as a Clemens Food Group pork processing facility in Coldwater that is under construction, a $325 million Arauco particle board manufacturing facility in Grayling Township and the American Center for Mobility at Willow Run. The latter project plans to transform the former Ford Motor Co. B-24 bomber plant at Willow Run in Ypsilanti Township into the nation's first autonomous vehicle testing site.

OTHER PRIORITIES

But how much money and effort for damage control and positive branding is appropriate and available as the state continues to reel from Flint stories? Last year, legislators in the state House proposed diverting money from the MEDC to pay for a $1.2 billion road-funding plan; MEDC administrators warned that could limit the Pure Michigan campaign. That proposal was dropped before the final package.

This year, Flint and a proposed $720 million debt restructuring of the Detroit Public Schools have dominated budget talks, though neither issue is expected to siphon money from Pure Michigan, said state Rep. Al Pscholka, chairman of the House Appropriations Committee.

Snyder's executive budget proposed leaving Pure Michigan funding at $33 million.

"I'm not advocating for any reduction to Pure Michigan," Pscholka, R-Stevensville, said. "Generally, I know in the House there's a lot of support for Pure Michigan."

Economic development agencies across Michigan say they have not noticed any loss of business interest because of Flint, though in some cases they are working harder to sell the state to prospective companies.

In Kalamazoo, where Ron Kitchens' team at Southwest Michigan First can talk with as many as 230 site consultants in a year, they now are making roughly three times as many phone calls to companies and site selectors telling them not to discount Michigan.

Deals are in the pipeline, he said, but he doesn't know how many will close.

"We're about selling the whole state. So when the water crisis broke, when the Detroit Public Schools hit the national news, there was a palpable gasp," said Kitchens, CEO of the regional economic development organization.

"I just think when people are in crisis, states are in crisis or regions are in crisis, the human reaction is not to run to the fire," he said.

MARKETING VS. SALES

Some economic development experts said they're concerned about the implications of using one brand to serve multiple types of marketing, especially in periods of negative attention, because the functions can't easily be distinguished.

Still others have suggested using recognized business leaders in Michigan to strengthen a corporate attraction campaign. Others say cuts to the MEDC, in dollars and staff, have had an impact.

"For Michigan to be the place that we need it to be, it's going to take a significant increase in the marketing and sales," Kitchens said. "Pure Michigan is a good marketing plan, but it's not a sales strategy. Sales strategies are people pounding the pavement, people who are at keyboards, looking at where companies are locating and how we can be more competitive than those locations."

Mark Winter, president and a founding partner of Identity, a public relations and marketing firm in Oakland County just north of Detroit, said the multi-pronged approach of Pure Michigan allows the MEDC to use its scant resources effectively.

He said an interconnected strategy, despite the single-brand risk, helps the state engage companies that employ millennials, for whom the live-work-play lines are blurred.

That could be important in the Flint recovery, said McEnroe, the site selector.

Positive messages

Several people said one of the main messages being shared in defense of Michigan is that Flint, much as Detroit was, is an isolated event not affecting other cities or regions.

While at a restaurant in Atlanta recently, "the waiter made a joke about the table water and referenced Flint," Winter said. "The first thing I did was stand up and support our state and all the things we're doing right."

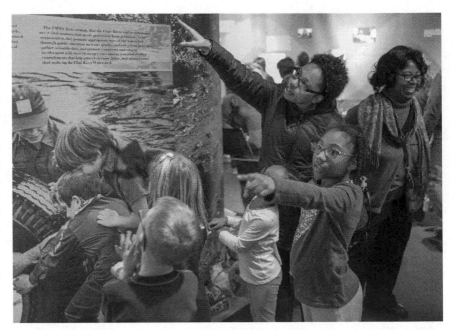

A family explores Water's Extreme Journey exhibit at Flint's Sloan Museum. Visitors learn about the history of Flint's water system, the science of filtration, examine current issues, and investigate the Flint River today. The museum is among Flint sites highlighted by Pure Michigan.

Photo courtesy of Sloan Longway Museum

The Pure Michigan campaign recently released a TV commercial focusing on Detroit's post-bankruptcy momentum. It is described as visually edgier than most Pure Michigan ads, including recent spots depicting Michigan's craft beer industry and farm-to-table restaurants.

State tourism promoters waited to tell Detroit's story until after the city's bankruptcy was resolved. They point to highlights such as improved city services, and construction of the M-1 Rail (now called QLine) and a new arena for the Detroit Red Wings.

Armed with the updated compelling messages, Dave Lorenz, vice president of state tourism agency Travel Michigan, said easing off the Pure Michigan throttle now would cause Michigan "to lose out on all that economic activity, and we would have then helped cause the problem that they're currently dealing with."

Tourism and economic development promoters should continue to tell Michigan's positive stories while rallying followers of official social media channels to spread the news, Winter said.

"Social media has provided an opportunity for people to vent and to share their thoughts, but unfortunately, more times than not, it's not balanced with the positive," he said. "Every bad message in a marketplace is just helping create distractions for the good things we're trying to say.

"If that positive information outweighs the negative, then we're going to be ahead of the game."

MARCH 28, 2016

MISSION IMPROBABLE: SELLING FLINT AFTER THE CRISIS

By Lindsay Vanhulle
Bridge Magazine/Crain's Detroit Business

In Flint, residents and businesses are trying to tell the world about their resilience in wake of the water crisis.

Jocelyn Hagerman, founder of a grassroots social media campaign called #FlintFwd, said she and others wanted to show the world beyond the city's limits that Flint is more than a bad headline.

"There's just this general consensus that, 'Why go to Flint? There's so little going on,'" said Hagerman, of Fenton. She and her husband, Phil, own several businesses in the region, including a real estate firm and Diplomat Pharmacy. "I don't want to make light of anything going on," she said of the water crisis, but "if we don't move away from the negative, we'll never move to anything positive."

The campaign began with T-shirts and bumper stickers. She said Ann Arbor-based marketing firm Phire Group agreed to help pro bono and teamed with Flint-based Digital Alchemy Films to make videos featuring residents and business owners talking about the city. "We see this as a long-term effort owned by the people of Flint – and we just helped create a platform for it to take place," said Jim Hume, principal of Phire.

The budget was small – maybe $10,000, Hagerman said – and she hasn't developed any metrics for success. She wants residents to share positive stories about the city on the #FlintFwd website and social media.

Since the water crisis became full-blown, traffic is down at businesses and restaurants and that has hurt what had been Flint's downtown development momentum, said George Wilkinson, a vice president of the Flint & Genesee Chamber of Commerce. Hotels are still busy, thanks in part to the many volunteers coming to help in Flint.

The chamber is working to get local, state and federal resources for business owners, including microloans, Wilkinson said, part of the effort to "let everyone know that Flint is open for business."

CHAPTER 33

APRIL – MAY 2016

TENSIONS, CRIMINAL CHARGES, LOWER LEAD LEVELS

PRESIDENT OBAMA VISITS AND DRINKS THE WATER

Editor's summary: The relationship between Flint Mayor Karen Weaver and Gov. Rick Snyder goes from lukewarm to icy. In order for the water system to function effectively, people have to use city water, but so many people aren't that officials, including the governor, urge greater use. Residents say Snyder should drink it first. He does and pledges to do so for 30 days. That draws derision from the mayor. Meanwhile, on April 20, the first criminal charges in the Flint water crisis are issued against two MDEQ officials and a Flint water-plant supervisor. Within weeks, the water-plant operator takes a plea bargain. On May 4, President Barack Obama visits Flint, drinking the filtered water and telling residents, "I've got your back." A week later, 10 foundations pledge up to $125 million in short and long-term relief to Flint.

"I'VE GOT YOUR BACK."

— PRESIDENT BARACK OBAMA

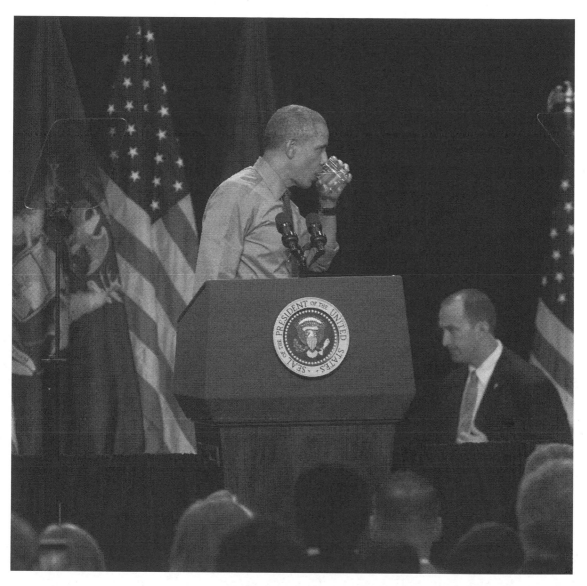

President Barack Obama came to Flint after getting a letter from Amariyanna (Mari) Copeny, known as Little Miss Flint. He told audiences "I've got your back." At two appearances, he drank filtered tap water: the first time to demonstrate that it's safe, and the second time because he needed it during a speech at Flint Northwestern High School.

Photo courtesy of Mark Brush/Michigan Radio

TIMELINE: APRIL – MAY 2016

By John Bebow
Bridge Magazine

2016

APRIL 1: Tensions rise between the Snyder administration and Flint Mayor Karen Weaver. The mayor claims she's being left out of the state's recovery planning for Flint. And the state warns Flint to withdraw threats of a lawsuit against the state over the water crisis.

APRIL 11: State health officials announce that the death toll from the Legionnaires' disease outbreak has grown to 12 in Genesee County. Five of the deaths occurred between June 2014 and March 2015, while seven were from May 2015 to October 2015. The switch to the Flint River as the source for Flint's water was in late April 2014. Epidemiologists have not confirmed a link to the city's water.

APRIL 13: The Michigan Legislature extends through the end of the summer a state of emergency in Flint because of the water crisis.

APRIL 15: As very high lead levels are found in nearly 20 Detroit schools' drinking water, the city's health chief urges citywide lead screening for children.

APRIL 15: Gov. Rick Snyder proposes that Michigan adopt some of the toughest anti-lead standards in the country – tougher than federal rules – including annual testing in all schools, day care centers, adult foster care, and substance abuse clinics.

APRIL 15: As the latest testing suggests, lead levels in Flint drinking water are dropping, but still potentially harmful, Snyder says he'd like to see Flint residents begin transitioning to filtered tap water instead of bottled water. Flint residents remain reticent. Some suggest that Snyder should come to their homes and drink the water first.

APRIL 18: Gov. Snyder accepts the residents' challenge to drink Flint water. He goes to Flint and starts 30 days of drinking filtered Flint water at a resident's home. But Snyder can't win. Mayor Karen Weaver would tell reporters two days later that she wasn't impressed. His spokesman also would later say the governor suspended the Flint water regimen while on a European trade mission the last week of April.

APRIL 20: Michigan Attorney General Bill Schuette announces criminal charges against two Michigan Department of Environmental Quality employees – Stephen Busch, a district supervisor, and Michael Prysby, a district engineer, and Michael Glasgow, a Flint water plant supervisor. Schuette promised that more charges would follow.

MAY 4: Michael Glasgow pleads no contest to a misdemeanor charge and prosecutors agree to drop a felony charge for tampering with evidence. In exchange, Glasgow agrees to work with prosecutors as they continue their investigation.

MAY 4: President Barack Obama visits Flint. He met briefly with Gov. Rick Snyder and then had community events. In the larger event, he spoke to about 1,000 people at Flint Northwestern High School, telling them not to despair that with health interventions the kids should be fine, telling the audience "I've got your back" and drinking filtered Flint water at two events. Obama said a letter from Amariyanna (Mari) Copeny, known as Little Miss Flint, convinced him to make the visit.

MAY 11: Foundations based in Michigan or with ties to the state commit up to $125 million, mostly to support recovery from the Flint water crisis. The hometown Charles Stewart Mott Foundation committed up to $100 million. "We envision a vibrant Flint with a robust economy, dynamic culture and healthy, thriving residents, and we're committed to achieving these goals," says Ridgway White, president of the Mott Foundation.

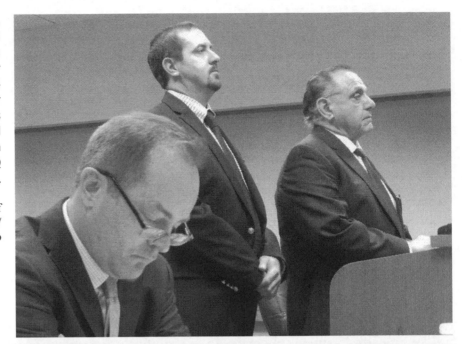

Michael Glasgow, center, pleaded no contest to a misdemeanor charge on May 4 two weeks after criminal charges were announced against him and two MDEQ employees.

Photo courtesy of Steve Carmody/ Michigan Radio

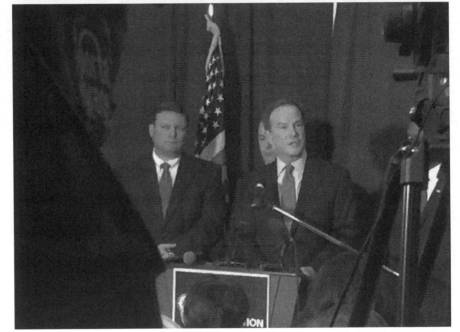

Attorney General Bill Schuette announces criminal charges in the Flint water crisis at a press conference in Flint.

Photo courtesy Steve Carmody/Michigan Radio

CHAPTER 34

APRIL 20, 2016

FELONY CHARGES FILED AGAINST THREE WITH A PROMISE OF MORE TO COME

Editor's summary: State and federal criminal investigations into the Flint water crisis began, respectively, in late January and early February, but it was still anyone's guess whether or when any charges would result. Then on April 20 the news broke: Attorney General Bill Schuette would be announcing felony charges against two Michigan Department of Environmental Quality employees who had been the key regulators working with Flint's water plant, and also the Flint plant's laboratory supervisor. At his press conference, Schuette all but promised that more criminal charges would follow. As of the publication of "Poison on Tap," the FBI and the criminal division of the U.S. Environmental Protection Agency had not announced charges.

By Nancy Derringer
Bridge Magazine

Promising they are only the first in a long investigation, Michigan Attorney General Bill Schuette announced felony charges against three government employees involved in the Flint water crisis.

Stephen Busch, a district water supervisor for the Michigan Department of Environmental Quality, and Michael Prysby, a district water engineer for the MDEQ, were both charged with multiple felonies and misdemeanors related to alleged misconduct in office and tampering with evidence.

Michael Glasgow, supervisor of the City of Flint water treatment plant, was charged with felony evidence tampering and misdemeanor willful neglect of duty. All the felony charges carry four- or five-year prison terms. (Editor's note: On May 4, Glasgow pleaded no contest to the misdemeanor count and the felony charge would be dismissed. In exchange, he is cooperating with prosecutors.)

The charges are "the beginning of the road back (to) restoring trust in Flint families in their government," Schuette said, adding they were likely to be only the first shot of legal consequences in the wake of the water crisis. "Each and every person who breaks the law will be held accountable," the Attorney General said.

The charges break down like this:

Busch and Prysby are accused of official misconduct for "willfully and knowingly misleading federal regulatory officials in the Environmental Protection Agency," as well as local officials, regarding the safety of Flint's drinking water, a felony carrying a potential five-year prison term and $10,000 fine.

Busch and Prysby are also charged with evidence tampering for allegedly mishandling water samples from the city and conspiracy to commit evidence tampering by concealing test results, a four-year/$10,000 felony.

Prysby faces an additional felony count of official misconduct for allegedly "authorizing a permit to the Flint Water Treatment Plant knowing (it) was deficient in its ability to provide clean and safe drinking water," Schuette charged.

Both men were also charged with two misdemeanor violations of the state's Safe Drinking Water Act, one for an alleged failure to add corrosion control to Flint's water treatment, and the other for manipulating water samples.

Busch and Prysby entered not-guilty pleas in Genesee County District Court and were released on personal recognizance bonds. Glasgow did not appear in court.

The charges generally reflect the findings of the independent Flint Water Advisory Task Force investigation. The report, released in late March, found the DEQ "failed in its fundamental responsibility to effectively enforce drinking water regulations."

"Given the magnitude of the crisis in Flint, it is important to know if laws were broken," task force co-chair Ken Sikkema told Bridge Magazine after the charges were announced. "It's also important to know that if they were, if they were broken intentionally or accidentally."

Busch and Prysby, both currently suspended without pay from the MDEQ, play parts in the narrative of the Flint crisis, as reflected in voluminous emails and other documents in Bridge Magazine's timeline. The timeline documents their key roles in the ill-fated decision to stop buying treated Lake Huron water from

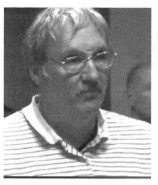 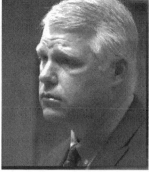 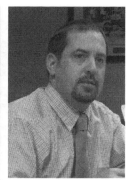

Left, Mike Prysby, MDEQ district engineer.

Center, Stephen Busch, MDEQ district supervisor.

Right, Mike Glasgow, Flint water plant supervisor.

Photos courtesy Steve Carmody/Michigan Radio

Detroit and begin using the city's treatment plant, which had been used only for emergency backup, and drawing water from the Flint River.

The decision was made while the city was under state-imposed emergency management, largely to save money, and had disastrous results: The failure to properly treat the corrosive river water led to the leaching of lead from the city water system's old lead service lines into residents' drinking water. Potentially thousands of residents were exposed to lead-tainted water, including many young children, who are most vulnerable to harm from ingesting lead.

The emails and other documents showed the MDEQ's apparent disregard of multiple warnings about the quality of Flint's water. After General Motors opted out of the Flint system, claiming the water was corroding its manufactured parts; and after residents complained of bad smell, taste and discoloration and after testing suggested potentially even more dire consequences – the MDEQ – with Busch, Prysby and others as key players – downplayed the complaints.

Reacting to Schuette's announcement, Gov. Rick Snyder repeated that "a handful of bureaucrats" who didn't use "common sense" bore most of the blame for the crisis. He said his office has been cooperative with the attorney general, as well as other agencies' ongoing investigations. He said he didn't believe he or anyone else in his office could be held criminally responsible for Flint's tainted water.

Task force co-chair Chris Kolb, president of the Michigan Environmental Council, said he "wasn't shocked that charges were filed," and that the actions "reflect what we saw in our investigation."

Left, Matthew Seeger, Wayne State University professor.

Right, Phillippe Grandjean, adjunct professor Harvard School of Public Health.

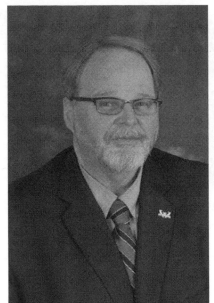 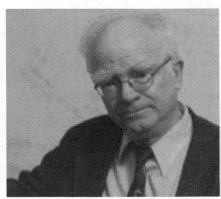

Left, Donald Conlon, interim chairman Eli Broad College of Business, Michigan State University.

Right, Lynn Wooten, associate dean Ross School of Business, University of Michigan.

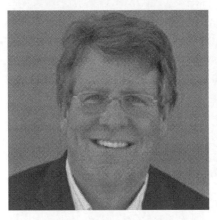 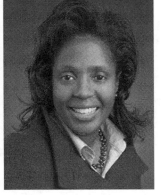

Marie McKendall, business professor Grand Valley State College.

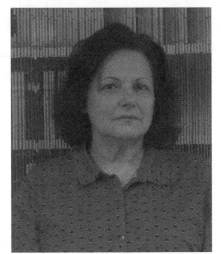

CHAPTER 35

APRIL 28, 2016

FLINT 101: IN BUSINESS SCHOOLS AND SEMINARS, A TOUGH GRADE FOR SNYDER

Editor's summary: Long before the Flint water crisis, Gov. Rick Snyder had said he'd like to teach after he leaves his job as governor. And then there was speculation that Snyder, again before Flint, might be on the short list as a cabinet member or even running mate for a Republican presidential candidate. Well, that was then and this is now. Snyder and his administration have made it into classrooms even before he's done as governor – but certainly not in the way he would have envisioned as "One Tough Nerd" who surprised Michigan's political establishment when he was elected in 2010.

By Ron French
Bridge Magazine

This is not how Gov. Rick Snyder wanted to make it into college classrooms.

Snyder's handling, or mishandling, of the water crisis that exposed thousands of Flint children to possible lead poisoning is being used in business school lectures as an example of epic organizational failure, along the lines of the BP Deepwater Horizon oil spill and the Catholic Church's response to the priest child molestation scandals.

"Crisis researchers will see this as one of the most important events in this time," said Matthew Seeger, dean of the School of Fine, Performing and Communication Arts at Wayne State University, and longtime expert on crisis communications. "We have other awful examples (of crisis management) such as the space shuttle Challenger explosion and Hurricane Katrina. Flint will be that big of a deal."

The state's mismanagement of the Flint water crisis will be the theme of a doctoral seminar at Wayne State this summer, and was the subject of a forum at Harvard University. It may be a case study in an upcoming issue of a national academic journal and will be incorporated into management classes at Grand Valley State University in the fall. It's already an area of study for several political science researchers at Michigan State University, as well as a senior capstone project for an MSU master's student.

The name of that master's project: "How Michigan Failed Flint."

Snyder has acknowledged the crisis will be an unfortunate part of his legacy, saying, as governor, he's ultimately responsible for the decisions and delays that led to lead leaching from pipes into the water system of Flint.

But the governor also has attempted to insulate his own office's decisions from the crisis, alternately blaming "career bureaucrats" or "civil service people" at various levels of government for giving his key advisers bad information. Snyder has been particularly biting in castigating the "culture" within the state Department of Environmental Quality and the Department of Health and Human Services, while denying similar problems in the governor's office.

The tone in college classrooms analyzing what happened in Flint is decidedly different.

"If he were a CEO, he'd be fired," said Marie McKendall, a business professor at Grand Valley State University. "There was a pronounced lack of problem-solving and communication. It almost seems in the end they forgot they were there to serve the people. That's an organization that is lost."

McKendall and colleague Nancy Levenburg are writing a case study for the North American Case Research Association journal, and say they will present findings at a national conference in October.

If their study is accepted for publication, business classes at colleges around the world may study for years the organizational missteps that led to the poisoning of Flint children.

McKendall says she plans to use Flint in her business ethics classes next fall. "There are lessons about structure, ethics, culture, decision-making," McKendall said. "It's a very rich case."

Harvard's Phillipe Grandjean, an expert on environmental pollution, called the state's handling of the water crisis "infuriating," where "decisions on water treatment were primarily made on the basis of cost and feasibility."

Staff members at Harvard's Global Health Education and Learning Incubator say they are building teaching tools for what the center calls "possibly the most egregious example of unsafe, lead-tainted water supplies in this country," ranging from multimedia video and simulation exercises, for secondary and university classes.

Wayne State's Seeger sees parallels to management decisions made by NASA before the space shuttle Challenger explosion, in which warnings of problems were ignored.

"Engineers had a good idea that the Challenger would not launch and tried to talk managers out of launching," Seeger said. "Almost every crisis has a failure of risk recognition, a sort of breakdown in decisional vigilance, not because of malicious intent, not because people are evil, but because of the way people process information."

Lead is a neurotoxin that hinders development of the brain and nervous system, particularly in young children. Thousands of Flint children were exposed to water with high levels of lead for more than a year, despite loud complaints from residents and outside experts.

Lead exposure among children in the United States has dropped sharply since the late 1970s when lead paint was banned and the phase-out of leaded gasoline began. But it's still a big issue: In more than 30 Michigan zip codes, most of them in Detroit, an even higher percentage of children had elevated levels of lead in their blood in 2014 than in two Flint zip codes with the most acute exposure. No level of lead exposure is considered safe in the rapidly developing bodies of for young children.

Emails released by the governor's office reveal that state officials stuck to (often faulty) data analysis generated by their own experts while ignoring, and at times trying to discredit, data analysis and recommendations of outside experts. Emails also reveal that Snyder's own inner circle of advisers discussed growing concerns about Flint water among themselves, but apparently failed to share concerns with the boss.

Seeger, who's authored several books on crisis management and communications, will lead a doctoral seminar on Flint this summer examining the failures of crisis communication in the ongoing man-made health disaster.

"It's hard to understate the capacity of humans to ignore risks," Seeger said. "You probably know some people who smoke. The surprising thing for people like me who study crises is that we don't have more cases like Flint, where people ignore the flashing red light."

Throughout the first three quarters of 2015, the governor and his then-chief of staff, Dennis Muchmore, said nothing publicly to contradict the official line of state agencies that the water coming from the taps in Flint met safe drinking water quality standards, even after residents and outside experts publicly contended otherwise – a trait Seeger said often happens as organizations create "tenacious justifications for what's going on. By trying to be on the same page, people lose track (of what's important)," he said.

For his part, Snyder disputes that the culture in his office is dysfunctional, or that aides were disinclined, or even afraid, to tell the governor of troubling information trickling in from Flint.

Snyder told Bridge in March that he has always made it clear that problems need to be addressed openly if they are to be solved.

"We need to create a culture where people can say, 'You know, we need to try things, be more open, be more inquisitive, and try different things.' And that's the culture we largely have," Snyder said.

But the released emails tell a more complicated story, including multiple instances in which staff members in his own office were trading concerns about Flint issues in the year before Snyder says he first learned there were high lead levels in the water system.

In one notable case, Harvey Hollins III, Snyder's director of Urban and Metropolitan Initiatives, was told in March 2015 about an increase in Legionnaires' disease in Genesee County that appeared to correspond with the switch to Flint River-sourced water. He didn't tell Snyder. Hollins said he didn't have enough information to take the concern to his boss.

That points to a culture problem in Snyder's inner circle, said McKendall, the Grand Valley business professor. "The culture is the culture the governor wants to create. And there were some very powerful norms these people were following."

Don Conlon, professor of management in the Eli Broad School of Business at Michigan State University, drew a parallel to another crisis - terrorist attacks in Paris and Brussels.

"People operate in silos and the data is so fragmented no one can draw conclusions," Conlon said. "In Europe, (police) have the same information-sharing problem. Perhaps there are some terrorists that all the countries know, and others that only one country may know of, and that information is not shared."

In the case of Flint, MDEQ officials were focused on lead levels in the water, while state health officials were independently examining lead levels in children.

Snyder has said he could "kick himself" for not asking more questions as Flint residents complained about the water coming from their faucets. But he also has said that, given the size of government, any governor must rely at least somewhat on experts.

"The challenge is, and I don't use it as an excuse but, when you've got 47,000 people (in state government), there's a lot of pockets that you need to get to and this is one that we didn't," Snyder said in New York.

"And it's tragic, it's just terrible, and ... I don't want to use that as an excuse, they work for me. And so, I'm trying to represent the values that you'd hope to see people do, to say that if it happens on your watch you need to take responsibility and you need to go fix it. And, if anything, people can see that I have a passion to fix it as much as anyone, given the fact that these people work for me."

Crises happen in all organizations, said Lynn Wooten, an associate dean at the Ross School of Business at the University of Michigan, and an expert on crisis leadership. But she said that how leaders respond to crisis can limit the damage, or worsen it.

"I don't know the inner workings of the governor's office, but it sounds as if you have a culture that isn't willing to face the brutal facts," Wooten said. "Everyone knows there is a problem, but they want to stay in denial."

Wooten compared Snyder's early response to Flint to the initial response of British Petroleum CEO Tony Hayward in 2010 to the Deepwater Horizon oil spill in the Gulf of Mexico.

In public statements, Hayward underplayed the amount of oil that was leaking from the well, and later said the Gulf of Mexico was so large the spill wouldn't do much damage. The spill ended up being the worst offshore, man-made environmental disaster in U.S. history. Hayward was ousted as CEO in the wake of his tone-deaf responses.

Wooten said Snyder and other state officials should have been more open to the data of outside researchers. For instance, pediatrician Dr. Mona Hanna-Attisha studied records that showed that a higher percentage of Flint children had worrisome blood lead levels after the switch to Flint River water. Similarly, Virginia Tech professor Marc Edwards found much higher lead levels in Flint's drinking water than city testing had shown. Both won accolades for exposing the lead threat, but both were initially dismissed by MDEQ and MDHHS experts. Wooten said it shows: "You need insiders and outsiders on a good team. They may drive you crazy in meetings, but you need people who are willing to tell you the truth."

Levenburg, the Grand Valley management professor, said: "There's a phenomenon called escalation of commitment to a bad decision. A group rationalizes its decisions (despite) increasingly negative outcomes. Under this phenomenon, once you start to see things go bad, you dig in."

Wayne State's Seeger said the state's mismanagement of Flint reveals the need to "build organization systems that are very sensitive to risks when (risks) come up. We need ombudspersons and anonymous tip lines so leaders can get these kinds of concerns."

Exploring how the state bungled the Flint crisis may be studied for years, but it is more than an academic exercise for Snyder and future governors. "I want the governor and the state to resolve this," Wooten said, before the next crisis.

CHAPTER 36

MAY 11, 2016

MOTT LEADS 10 FOUNDATIONS IN $125M COMMITMENT TO FLINT

Editor's summary: Flint residents have been the recipients of generous donations of water, food and other support from Michigan, other states and even internationally since the water crisis became widely known in early 2016. But with the Flint-based Charles Stewart Mott Foundation leading the charge, the giving announced in early May 2016 by 10 foundations based in or with ties to Michigan is a huge commitment to providing assistance to Flint residents well into the future.

By Nancy Derringer
Bridge Magazine

Flint's recovery received a welcome jolt on May 10, as 10 foundations based in Michigan or with roots in the state announced a charitable gift of up to nearly $125 million, with most support connected to Flint's ongoing water crisis.

Far from another bottled-water donation, the foundations vowed to support programs in such areas as early childhood education, health interventions for residents exposed to high lead levels, and economic development.

Up to $100 million of the gift will come from the hometown Charles Stewart Mott Foundation.

"Flint's water crisis is far from over," Ridgway White, Mott's president, said in the release. "While some funds and services have been provided, we're still waiting for the state and federal governments to step up, replace damaged infrastructure and make long-term commitments to the health and education of children. Today our foundations are stepping in to help. We envision a vibrant Flint with a robust economy, dynamic culture, and healthy, thriving residents, and we're committed to achieving these goals."

The foundations are among the biggest and most prominent in Michigan. Besides Mott, they include the W.K. Kellogg Foundation, The Kresge Foundation, the Ford Foundation and The Skillman Foundation (Disclosure: Kresge, Kellogg, Mott and Ford all provide financial support to The Center for Michigan or Bridge Magazine).

The Flint gift marks the second time in recent years that heavyweights in the nonprofit sector have made large contributions to correct, or try to correct, a crisis caused at least in part by government.

In 2014, the so-called "grand bargain" saved the Detroit Institute of Arts' collection from liquidation and was a major factor in the ultimate resolution of that city's bankruptcy proceedings. In that case, foundations led an effort that grew to include the state of Michigan and private donors in raising $800 million to protect both the art and the pensions of Detroit's retirees.

In Flint, a task force appointed by Gov. Rick Snyder concluded in March that government failure, mostly at the state level, was to blame for the disastrous decision to switch the city's water supply from treated water long supplied by Detroit's water system to the more corrosive Flint River in 2014, in part to save money. Failure to properly treat the river water resulted in lead leaching into residents' drinking water. Lead is a neurotoxin that can inflict irreversible brain damage, particularly in young children.

In an interview Wednesday with Bridge, White said the Flint grant is not intended to do government's work for it.

"We want to create a narrative of hope. We don't feel we're replacing government dollars. You can't prescribe a pill for lead poisoning, but you can prescribe good nutrition and good education. Some things, like fixing the water infrastructure, are clearly government's responsibility. There is opportunity to show how philanthropy can complement government and fill a void. But we're not going to replace pipes."

In broad strokes, the foundations said their gifts would focus on six areas:

1. Safe drinking water, including ongoing, independent water testing. Experts will develop modern, integrated management of drinking, storm and wastewater. The foundations did not mention in the statement which experts they were referencing, or whether they would seek water experts outside government. Water experts in Flint and state government absorbed much of the blame for the Flint crisis.

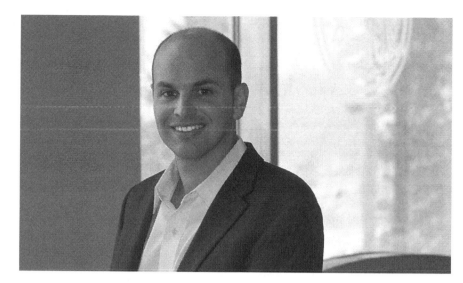

Ridgeway White, president of the Charles Stewart Mott Foundation.

Photo courtesy the Charles Stewart Mott Foundation

2. Family health, including a dollar-for-dollar match of up to $5 million in donations made to the Flint Child Health & Development Fund through the end of 2016. Dr. Mona Hanna-Attisha, the pediatrician who helped bring the seriousness of the water crisis to public attention, established the fund through the Community Foundation of Greater Flint. It will provide support over the next 20 years for interventions for Flint children exposed to lead.

3. Early childhood education, so that young children in Flint can be admitted to Early Start, Head Start and Great Start Readiness programs.

4. Improving the city's nonprofit sector, which the foundations said have been challenged by early response to the crisis.

5. Community engagement, through promotion of civic engagement and local decision making.

6. Economic development, to attempt to correct the damage done to the city's businesses by the water crisis. The foundations said this will include job training and entrepreneurship.

Rob Collier, president and CEO of the Council of Michigan Foundations, said the collaboration was intended to answer the question: "How can it be a strategic partner and leverage its resources to make sure the issues are addressed? Are we doing what government should be doing? I would argue we're not. But we're using our resources to enhance what government can do."

Philanthropy always responds to natural disasters, Collier said, and while Flint's was man-made, he said the foundations are playing a familiar role.

"What makes this one unique is the fact it has to have a long-term horizon because of the issue of lead," and its lingering effects on those who ingested it. Normally disaster relief is accomplished on a shorter timeline, but Flint's could have "a 20-year horizon," Collier said.

Mott's White said that beyond money and support the aid package offers intangible help. "I think it really shows that the citizens of Flint are not alone. The rest of the nation cares about Flint, and we will not be neglected."

Both Collier and White said the foundations were positioning themselves as an influential partner in both Flint's immediate recovery and its future, as indicated by the emphasis on economic development.

"There are short-term, intermediate and long-term needs," Collier said.

The foundations' statement said other partners will join their partnership. It did not go into detail about conditions for the various philanthropies to meet the full $125 million pledge.

The Mott Foundation has been heavily involved in helping to resolve the Flint crisis since the full extent of the problem was made public late last year. Mott picked up one-third of the $12 million cost of switching the city back to treated Detroit water last fall. As of mid-May 2016, Flint's tap water must still be filtered. In April, White wrote in Philanthropy News Digest: "Our decision to help pay for the switch was a no-brainer. ...We couldn't sit on the sidelines while the children of Flint were being harmed. Our role as a catalyst for the return to safer water speaks to one of philanthropy's most valuable attributes: the ability to respond swiftly when disaster strikes to help people meet their basic needs. But after taking swift action, the question then becomes 'What next?'

Later in the same piece, he wrote, "We firmly believe the state of Michigan and the federal government must provide the resources – financial and otherwise – needed to address the harm caused. There's little doubt that any government restitution Flint receives will fall far short of what will be needed to address long-term health, infrastructure, and economic concerns. That's all the more reason we must call on state and federal government to provide maximum resources to Flint. And it's partly why we haven't rushed to make subsequent commitments. We don't want government officials to think it's okay to send fewer dollars to Flint."

The 10 foundations, and their gifts to Flint, as they describe them:

CHARLES STEWART MOTT FOUNDATION, up to $50 million over the first year and up to $100 million total over five years, with grants across all six priority areas, as well as investments in K-12 education;

FLINTNOW FOUNDATION, committing continued support from a $10 million pledge to aid in a broad range of relief and revitalization efforts in Flint.

W.K. KELLOGG FOUNDATION, up to $5 million over the next year to support children's education, health and well-being, backed by significant investments in community engagement.

THE KRESGE FOUNDATION, up to $2.5 million for operations and recovery programs of select non-profit partners, to enhance civic capacity and community engagement.

CARNEGIE CORPORATION OF NEW YORK, committing $1 million to support the educational needs of children in Flint.

FORD FOUNDATION, committing $1 million to the health needs of the Flint community.

THE HAGERMAN FOUNDATION, $1 million over the first year to support the non-profit sector and efforts to revitalize Flint's economy, with plans to support education, health and wellness over the long term.

ROBERT WOOD JOHNSON FOUNDATION, $1 million to support children's health needs through the Flint Child Health & Development Fund of the Community Foundation of Greater Flint.

RUTH MOTT FOUNDATION, $1 million for the short- and long-term needs of Flint children and adults, in addition to investments already made.

SKILLMAN FOUNDATION, committing $500,000 immediately, with the potential for an additional $1.5 million over the next three years, to support civic capacity, as well as childhood health, nutrition and literacy.

CHAPTER 37

MAY 24, 2016

MANY IN FLINT'S LATINO COMMUNITY WERE LATE TO HEAR ABOUT LEAD IN WATER

Editor's summary: Once the state rolled out its plan to help Flint residents exposed to potentially harmful levels of lead in their tap water, members of one group – the community's Latinos, about 4,000 strong – did not all get the message. Language, fear of uniformed National Guard members distributing water and other factors were in play. The sad thing here is that some people drank and cooked with the water longer than others who got the word months earlier. There are lessons in the aftermath of all crises, and this report has suggestions for government and advocates alike.

By Jacob Wheeler
Bridge Magazine contributor

Embedded within Flint's nearly 100,000 residents are about 4,000 Latino immigrants, including an estimated 1,000 without legal documentation. Many among the community have lived in a netherworld where their greatest concern was not the foul taste, smell and color of the city's water the past few years.

Fear of deportation for themselves, their relatives or friends was paramount. Language complicated matters for many who spoke only Spanish, while others lived without online communications or even benefit of radio and television reports.

That helps explain why, according to Bridge interviews with advocates and officials involved in the aid efforts for the city, many Latinos were late to discover concerns and warnings about lead in the city's water.

Flint residents were told to stop drinking the city's water on Oct. 1, 2015, after the state confirmed water-service pipes and soldered joints were shedding flakes of lead into the water supply and home taps. News reports and government directives rolled out over the weeks and months that followed.

Many Latinos, for a variety of reasons, didn't get the message. In a city where delayed revelations about lead-poisoned water ignited international outrage, perhaps no corner of Flint learned of the threat later than its Spanish-speaking residents.

The reasons are complex, as are moral questions: Does government have a duty to take extra measures in an emergency to reach immigrant communities that may be wary of, or actively avoiding, government help? Activists say the missed connections with Latinos in Flint carry lessons for policymakers, first responders and community activists themselves.

January turned out to be a busy month for community outreach in Flint. On Jan. 5, Gov. Rick Snyder declared a state of emergency in Flint, as the city's story splashed across front pages worldwide. Six days later, the Michigan Department of Technology, Management and Budget printed 15,000 handbills in Spanish with relevant information about the water crisis.

National Guard members distributed the handbills door-to-door. But some wary residents, on edge from stepped up federal deportation raids, didn't read them or didn't trust the information. More alarming, community activists say, were inaccurate early announcements that Flint residents would need to show photo identification to get free water bottles. There also were confusing, inaccurate rumors about why the water tasted bad. The dearth of local Spanish-language media didn't help.

As community organizers, churches and other advocates worked to fill the communication gap in late January, they discovered that some local Latinos had learned of the water crisis from relatives in Mexico, who saw television reports broadcast from Flint.

Once the emergency was declared, the state quickly made free bottled water and filters available to residents. But two strategic decisions hindered outreach to some in the Latino immigrant community.

The state made the seemingly reasonable decision to deploy the National Guard, the State Police and Red Cross workers to canvass neighborhoods with bottled water for drinking and bathing. Advocates for Spanish-speaking residents said many were afraid of these uniformed visitors; afraid of being apprehended and deported for being in the United States illegally, or leery because of the legal status of someone in their household. Many didn't respond to knocks on their front door.

"The timing of the water distribution in Flint was unfortunate because it came at the same time as the Obama administration was stepping up raids for folks with recent removal orders," said Susan Reed, managing attorney at the Michigan Immigrant Rights Center. "We in the advocacy community were aggressively telling people – undocumented or not – not to open their doors to people without search warrants."

Meanwhile, some Flint fire stations, which were among the first water pickup locations, initially asked residents for government-issued photo ID in exchange for free water.

Eventually, fire stations stopped asking, but not before reports about photo IDs spread quickly among immigrant families.

David Kaiser, a spokesperson for the Michigan State Police, told Yahoo News the next day that photo ID "is not required, it's just requested" and that residents' addresses were only being tracked to ensure that free water, filters and supplies were actually going to residents of Flint and to get a better handle on where help was most needed.

Some didn't get the message. At Fire Station no. 1 – one of the fire stations turned into water distribution centers – a National Guardsman required a photo ID before handing over a case of bottled water to each car that lined up.

Ron Leix, a spokesman for the State Police, confirmed miscommunication prompted at least one fire station to ask for identification. The state issued a press release on Jan. 22 confirming that a photo ID was not required.

"During a disaster is not the time to think about someone's immigration status," Leix told Bridge.

As water donations picked up at local fire stations, members of the Michigan National Guard were going door-to-door to help residents.

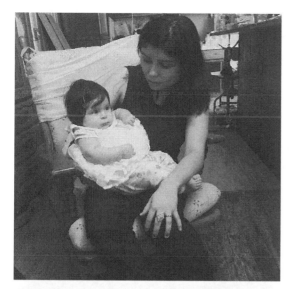

Like many in Flint's Latino immigrant community, Yaquelin Vargas said she didn't learn until late January that Flint's drinking water was lead poisoned. Vargas, a U.S. citizen, said she drank tap water while she was pregnant, and as she first began breastfeeding Lydia in September 2015. Tests showed Lydia with elevated lead levels in her blood.

Bridge photo by Jacob Wheeler

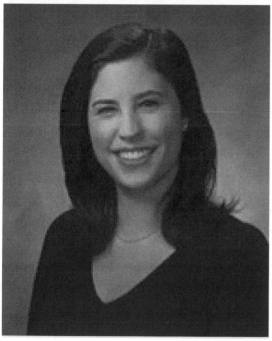

Natalie Zarowny of ABC12 WJRT in Flint.

Thomas Vega, staff sergeant and public information officer for the Michigan National Guard, arrived in Flint on Jan. 14 to begin overseeing the outreach effort. Within days, guard members began delivering palm cards printed in English and Spanish with information on nutrition, free water tests and instructions for using free filters. They left information sheets on doors when no one was home or attached them to the water bottles themselves.

"We heard rumors circulating through the community spread by activists that the National Guard was going to turn people's names over to immigration authorities and have them arrested," Vega said. "Those rumors were false and, as a Hispanic myself, I took them personally."

The difficulty in reaching Flint's Spanish-speaking community did not receive wide publicity until late January, with coverage by local television reporter Natalie Zarowny on ABC12 WJRT. A single mother, identified only as Lucia, told Zarowny: "I'm not here legally. And I'm always scared that they'll arrest me, and then deport me."

Community organizers met a family who learned of the danger after getting a call from relatives in Mexico City who had seen news of the Flint water crisis on Univision.

At Our Lady of Guadalupe in northern Flint, parish member and attorney Victoria Arteaga told Bridge she encountered "a few dozen families who came to us and said they didn't know" of the water crisis.

"When the crisis hit, I went to Guadalupe for help," said Maricela, an eastside resident, who asked to be identified by her first name only. "I trusted them. They were compassionate in those first days."

Juani Olivares, who chairs the Genesee County Hispanic/Latino Collaborative, an advocacy group, estimated that 95 percent of the people who volunteers encountered that weekend were unaware that lead had contaminated Flint's water supply and posed a health risk, particularly to children.

"We realized we needed to do something because the problem (of people not knowing) was bigger than we were told," Olivares said.

The impact was immediate. Deacon Paul Donnelly, of St. Mary's Catholic Church, was interviewed by reporter Zarowny and told viewers they could get water from the church without identification. Kathy Tomczyk, a church book-keeper and secretary, said she witnessed "an explosion" of people on Thursday morning who needed water to drink and bathe themselves.

"We've been taking care of them ever since," said Tomczyk, who adds that the need for more bottled water is even greater now than it was in January.

Yaquelin Vargas, 21, is a U.S. citizen, speaks English and was studying to become a nurse. But events conspired to leave her cut off from the larger world.

Vargas, a native of Nueva Rosita in Coahuila, Mexico, and her father, also a U.S. citizen, moved to Flint six years ago after successfully bidding on an affordable home. Three years ago, while enrolled at Genesee Early College, she won an American GI Forum beauty pageant. She was taking classes at University of Michigan-Flint and interning at the Hurley Medical Center to become a pediatric nurse.

Then her father became too ill to work, and Vargas quit her studies to care for him. They have no radio or television.

They knew E.coli bacteria had been found in their tap water, and they were told to boil it. She said they were then told they could drink the water if they used a filter. But during her pregnancy – and after Lydia's birth, on Sept. 12, 2015, as the infant breastfed – mother and grandfather said they were unaware of the lead problem.

During her pregnancy, Vargas said, her doctor insisted she stay hydrated with the foul-tasting water because "it will help the baby."

It was not until early January, when Lydia was not tracking the movements of her mother's finger, that Vargas suspected a problem. In late January a volunteer from nearby St. Mary's Catholic Church knocked on their door and said the Vargas family should stop using the tap water.

"I feel responsible for hurting my daughter," Vargas says now. "We had no idea."

Could the city and state have done a better job of reaching out to Flint's undocumented community at the height of the water crisis? Advocates say there are examples showing better ways to communicate.

Henry Fernandez, a senior fellow at the Center for American Progress, a progressive public policy research and advocacy organization, lauded then New York City Mayor Michael Bloomberg's effort to reach the city's undocumented immigrants when Hurricane Sandy hit in 2012.

Before the hurricane reached the city, the government released an online guide in Spanish and other languages answering questions about disaster assistance.

"They had the infrastructure in place, the people in place, and pathways for this to be done." Fernandez said. "…It's really important to lay that groundwork beforehand."

A law that guarantees government officials won't ask for photo ID during a crisis would help, said Ryan Bates, executive director of Michigan United, a nonprofit activist group.

Bates said he believes identification was initially required at Flint fire stations because officials were more concerned that residents would take commercial advantage of the handouts.

"There's an unfortunate gut reaction from public officials that folks in communities like Flint are suspect. We should treat people as victims who need help."

Fernandez said the outreach in Flint shows that governments need to take a broader approach to reaching immigrant or non-English-speaking communities. Schools could have been an important part of the outreach, he said.

When President Barack Obama introduced his 2012 Deferred Action for Childhood Arrivals (DACA) legislation commonly known as the "Dreamers Act," Los Angeles public schools sent home letters with each Latino immigrant student explaining how family members could apply.

Susan Reed, the immigration lawyer, said now that lead poisoning is being documented, it's imperative for Michigan to expand Medicaid eligibility to include children who are not U.S. citizens.

"We haven't seen clear communication from the state as to the health status for noncitizens," Reed said. "How do we ensure that folks who don't have status continue to have access to monitoring and intervention? They should have that after being poisoned by lead."

But Anna Heaton, the governor's press secretary, said federal law prevents undocumented immigrants from enrolling in Medicaid.

"This population most often seeks health care from free clinics and federally-qualified community health centers, of which there are several in Flint," she said.

"We are working with those locations as well as with charitable and religious organizations to encourage blood lead level testing and to ensure resources exist for follow-up health care. If more resources are needed in the future, we will work with these organizations."

By Bob Campbell
"Poison on Tap" Editor

Perplexed. That's how I felt five months ago when I started paying attention to Flint's water crisis. The decisions that led to the poisoning of Flint's water supply and, in turn, its residents (most acutely the city's vulnerable young children) were baffling. Surely, government regulators making critical public health decisions about risk would build margins of error into their calculations to avoid disastrous surprises. That's why we have a Michigan Department of Environmental Quality and a U.S. Environmental Protection Agency – to ensure and protect.

Our health risk is a complicated mix of things we can and can't control.

The citizens of Flint – among the nation's poorest, most abandoned, and most crime-plagued – certainly had risks they couldn't control, but they had every right to believe that getting clean water for drinking, making infant formula, cooking and bathing wouldn't be one of them. In "Poison on Tap," Bridge Magazine reporters tell us clearly that the regulators expected to protect their health did not.

Lee-Anne Walters, the Flint mom who battled so courageously when she knew the water was hurting her children, had a telling conversation she related to Michigan Radio reporter Lindsey Smith: "The state nurse told me, 'Oh, I understand your son has lead poisoning, but it's not as bad as it could be; he's only going to lose a few IQ points.'"

A few IQ points. What's the big deal?

Published, peer-reviewed studies have found that for every additional microgram per deciliter of blood-lead exposure in children five and younger, they lose up to one IQ point, though there are many variables. Dr. Mona Hanna-Attisha's study of Flint children found that the percentage of children with lead levels of at least five micrograms per deciliter of blood increased from 2.1 percent to 4.0 percent after the April 2014 switch to the Flint River as the city's water source.

In two southwest Flint zip codes, it increased from 2.5 percent to 6.3 percent. Gavin Walters, Lee-Anne Walter's son, had a blood-lead level of 6.5 micrograms per deciliter.

Put yourself in Walter's shoes. What would you think when a public health nurse dismisses your concerns over "a few IQ points." Maybe just enough to keep Gavin out of the elite college he'll want to attend someday. Or put him into a remedial classroom.

In John Bebow's exhaustive Timeline and Michigan Truth Squad analysis, "Poison on Tap" provides an insight into the perspective of regulators who made the worst calls.

In the Chapter 2 timeline, Stephen Busch, an MDEQ district supervisor, emailed several state colleagues in March 2013 to raise concerns about the prospect of the city using the Flint River as an interim water source after it disconnected from the Detroit water system. Jim Sygo of MDEQ responded: "As you might guess we are in a situation with Emergency Financial Managers so it's entirely possible that they will be making decisions relative to cost. The concern in either situation is that a compliant supply of source water and drinking water can be supplied."

In other words, our job is only to say whether "compliant" – not best or even clean or safe – water can be provided.

Just a few IQ points.

Beginning in February 2015, MDEQ regulators dismissed concerns about lead in the water when they were first raised by Miguel Del Toral, the EPA's lone voice of concern for Flint's children. The MDEQ also sanctioned water testing methods designed to pass tests, not protect children.

Still other emails between MDEQ and other EPA regulators reference rules that MDEQ employees argued would give Flint lots of time to determine compliance with federal rules before taking action to remediate the lead problem. So much time, they argued, that by then Flint would be switched back to Lake Huron-sourced water from the new Karegnondi Water Authority. Why bother worrying about lead?

And consider this email trail on May 10-11, 2015, among Jon Allan, director of Michigan's Office of the Great Lakes; William Creal, MDEQ's water resources division chief, and Liane Shekter Smith, the former head of MDEQ's drinking water program who was fired in February 2016 for her role in Flint's crisis. Their discussion is about proposed targets for health-based drinking water standards. Allan suggests a 98 percent compliance in community systems by 2020 and 90 percent in non-community systems. Creal responds: "I think you are nuts if you go with a goal less than 100 percent for (drinking water) compliance.... How many Flints do you intend to allow???"

Shekter Smith responds a day later: "Of course, everyone wants 100 percent compliance. The reality, however, is that it's impossible. It's not that we 'allow' a Flint to occur; circumstances happen. Water mains break, systems lose pressure, bacteria gets into the system, regulations change and systems that were in compliance no longer are, etc. Do we want to put a goal in black and white that cannot be met but sounds good? Or do we want to establish a goal that challenges us but can actually be accomplished? Perhaps there's a middle ground?"

A middle ground. A few IQ points. A little growth retardation. Some nerve damage. What's the big deal?

Why did the regulators accept this? Unlike the state-appointed emergency managers, their mission wasn't to save Flint $1 million a month. But they still decided the river was good enough and, since by the time the regulatory clock expired, they'd have Lake Huron water again, so there was no point fussing with corrosion control to keep the lead out.

Marc Edwards, the Virginia Tech professor and national expert on lead in water supplies, was pulled in to help with the Flint crisis on an incognito basis by the EPA's Del Toral in April 2015. Edwards, like Del Toral, has been widely hailed as a hero in Flint for the flintwaterstudy.org project he initiated that found much higher lead levels in tap water than city tests had shown.

In an interview for "Poison on Tap," he told me that Michigan isn't the only place he's seen bad decisions, obfuscations and outright lies by community, state and federal regulators. In Washington D.C., he said, tap water-borne lead poisoning that began in 2001 was "30 times worse than what happened in Flint," because it went undetected for six years.

"We have a culture of corruption at these agencies that destroys good people and promotes bad people," he said. "They become cynical and willfully blind. They distance themselves from the public. I saw it happen to my best friend. If you're in a corrupt culture, you learn to do things that you once would have abhorred. It's business as usual."

For all the hyperbole from commentators, Hollywood actors and politicians, the lead poisoning found in most of Flint's children wasn't extreme by historical or contemporary measures.

In 2014, the year of the Flint River water switch, at least 36 Michigan zip codes, half of them in Detroit, had a greater percentage of young children with blood-lead levels exceeding the U.S. "reference level" for health concern, than in the two Flint zip codes with the highest percentage of young kids exceeding the reference levels. These results are revealed in Chapter 18 of "Poison on Tap."

Other kids have it worse. Just a few IQ points.

Now consider, too, that the percentages of children with elevated levels of lead in their blood in Flint and everywhere in the United States has declined precipitously since lead was banned in paint in 1978 and leaded gasoline was phased out between the late 1970s and mid-1990s. The most extreme blood-lead measurements among Flint's kids were the median in many cities just a few decades ago.

In 2014, most of the Michigan kids with elevated lead levels were not victims of a 21st Century, regulatory miscalculation or, as some commentators would have us believe, political conspiracy. The biggest problem in today's hot spots of lead poisoning are old homes with flaking, peeling lead-based paint, typically found in poor neighborhoods. In a few of those zip codes, one in every five children still have lead levels of public health concern. Little kids pick up and eat paint flakes, they get paint dust on their hands and put their hands in their mouths. Poison.

By contrast, in Flint's two most affected zip codes, about one in every 16 children under five years old had elevated blood-lead levels after the April 2014 water source switch, Hanna-Attisha's study showed. But what if, like Lee-Anne Walters, that's your kid whose lead exposure shot up after the water switch?

And, as Edwards further pointed out, lead in water can have a more immediate and dramatic effect than many other avenues of lead exposure. That's because lead can leach off pipes in big chips and, if the tap water isn't filtered, you can drink down an unnoticed chunk in a glass of water and your blood-lead measurement might shoot up 10 times. He compared it to Russian roulette with a drinking glass, instead of a gun.

Just a few IQ points, a little retarded growth, a greater tendency toward aggressive behavior.

Here's why regulators were dead wrong if their bad decisions were informed by much worse lead poisoning in the past or in other communities today: The U.S. Centers for Disease Control has concluded that there is no – *zero* – level of safe exposure to lead for young children when their bodies and brains are growing at warp speed. That should have been the standard in Flint.

Del Toro knew it. Edwards knew it. Dr. Mona Hanna-Attisha knew it and proved that the water switch was directly linked to a doubling, and, in some zip codes, a tripling of blood-lead levels.

The Flint tragedy is not over, but Edwards – perhaps surprisingly – regards the outcome at this point as a success.

"What happened was tragic, but there's no reason why Flint kids can't have a very good future. Health interventions will ameliorate harm, but I shudder to

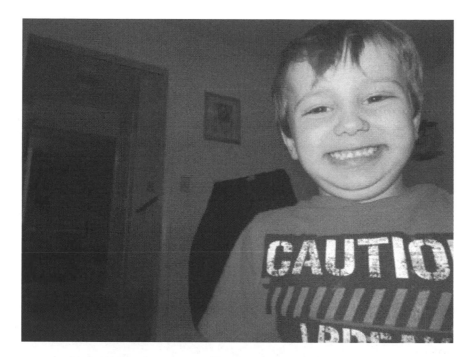

Gavin Walters is a victim of lead-poisoning linked to Flint's water crisis. From April 2014 until early December 2015 when his mom switched to bottled water and sponge baths, Gavin drank and bathed in Flint's city water. Tests showed his blood lead level were above the U.S. Center for Disease Conrol and Prevention level of concern for health-related issues. His mother, Lee-Anne Walters became a champion of the cause of Flint residents. The family now lives in Virginia, but Lee-Anne Walters continues her fight for clean water.

Photo courtesy of Lindsey Smith/Michigan Radio

think what would have happened," he said. "I view Flint as a success. As bad as it was, we got kids protected before the worst harm occurred."

As of this writing, criminal charges are pending against two MDEQ regulators in the thick of the bad decision-making. More charges are expected from a state investigation, and a federal investigation continues. Better answers to why Flint was allowed to happen may emerge at eventual criminal and civil trials.

Until then and beyond then, Flint must serve as the canary – a sad and frightening lesson for regulators, policy-makers, politicians and citizens. As developments warrant, we will update future editions of "Poison on Tap."

Flint lives do matter.

APPENDIX:

- *Executive Summary, Flint Water Advisory Task Force Final Report: Find on-line at http://1.usa.gov/1T8cJLT*
- *Del Toral memorandum warning of high lead levels in Flint (below)*

UNITED STATES ENVIRONMENTAL PROTECTION AGENCY
REGION 5
77 WEST JACKSON BOULEVARD
CHICAGO, IL 60604-3590

REPLY TO THE ATTENTION OF:

WG-15J

June 24, 2015

MEMORANDUM

SUBJECT: High Lead Levels in Flint, Michigan – Interim Report

FROM: Miguel A. Del Toral
Regulations Manager, Ground Water and Drinking Water Branch

TO: Thomas Poy
Chief, Ground Water and Drinking Water Branch

The purpose of this interim report is to summarize the available information regarding activities conducted to date in response to high lead levels in drinking water reported by a resident in the City of Flint, Michigan. The final report will be submitted once additional analyses have been completed on pipe and water samples.

Following a change in the water source, the City of Flint has experienced a number of water quality issues resulting in violations of National Primary Drinking Water Regulations (NPDWR) including acute and non-acute Coliform Maximum Contaminant Level (MCL) violations and Total Trihalomethanes (TTHM) MCL violations as follows:

Acute Coliform MCL violation in August 2014
Monthly Coliform MCL violation in August 2014
Monthly Coliform MCL violation in September 2014
Average TTHM MCL violation in December 2014
Average TTHM MCL violation in June 2015

In addition, as of April 30, 2014, when the City of Flint switched from purchasing finished water from the City of Detroit to using the Flint River as their new water source, the City of Flint is no longer providing corrosion control treatment for lead and copper.

A major concern from a public health standpoint is the absence of corrosion control treatment in the City of Flint for mitigating lead and copper levels in the drinking water. Recent drinking water sample results indicate the presence of high lead results in the drinking water, which is to be expected in a public water system that is not providing corrosion control treatment. The lack of any mitigating treatment for lead is of serious concern for residents that live in homes with lead service lines or partial lead service lines, which are common throughout the City of Flint.

In addition, following the switch to using the Flint River, the City of Flint began adding ferric chloride, a coagulant used to improve the removal of organic matter, as part of the strategy to reduce the TTHM levels. Studies have shown that an increase in the chloride-to-sulfate mass ratio in the water can adversely affect lead levels by increasing the galvanic corrosion of lead in the plumbing network.

Prior to April 30, 2014, the City of Flint purchased finished water from the City of Detroit which contained orthophosphate, a treatment chemical used to control lead and copper levels in the drinking water. When the City of Flint switched to the Flint River as their water source on April 30, 2014, the orthophosphate treatment for lead and copper control was not continued. In effect, the City of Flint stopped providing treatment used to mitigate lead and copper levels in the water. In accordance with the Lead and Copper Rule (LCR), all large systems (serving greater than 50,000 persons) are required to install and maintain corrosion control treatment for lead and copper. In the absence of any corrosion control treatment, lead levels in drinking water can be expected to increase.

The lack of mitigating treatment is especially concerning as the high lead levels will likely not be reflected in the City of Flint's compliance samples due to the sampling procedures used by the City of Flint for collecting compliance samples. The instructions from the City of Flint to residents direct the residents to 'pre-flush' the taps prior to collecting the compliance samples. A copy of the instructions provided by the City of Flint to residents will be included in the final report.

The practice of pre-flushing before collecting compliance samples has been shown to result in the minimization of lead capture and significant underestimation of lead levels in the drinking water. Although this practice is not specifically prohibited by the LCR, it negates the intent of the rule to collect compliance samples under 'worst-case' conditions, which is necessary for statistical validity given the small number of samples collected for lead and copper under the LCR. This is a serious concern as the compliance sampling results which are reported by the City of Flint to residents could provide a false sense of security to the residents of Flint regarding lead levels in the water and may result in residents not taking necessary precautions to protect their families from lead in the drinking water. Our concern regarding the inclusion of 'pre-flushing' in sampling instructions used by public water systems in Michigan has been raised with the Michigan Department of Environmental Quality (MDEQ). The MDEQ has indicated that this practice is not prohibited by the LCR and continues to retain the 'pre-flushing' recommendation in their lead compliance sampling guidance to public water systems in Michigan. A copy of the MDEQ guidance will be included in the final report.

In the case of the Flint resident that contacted U.S. EPA (Ms. Lee-Anne Walters), the initial results from drinking water samples collected by the City of Flint in her home

Page 2 of 5

for lead were 104 ug/L and 397 ug/L. The level of iron in the water also exceeded the capability of the measurement (>3.3 mg/L). The lead results were especially alarming given that the samples were collected using the sampling procedures described above, which minimize the capture of lead. When contacted by U.S. EPA Region 5, the MDEQ indicated that the lead was coming from the Walters' plumbing. Ms. Walters had previously indicated that all of the plumbing in the home was plastic.

Following the confirmation of the initial high lead results, U.S. EPA Region 5 conducted two visits to the Walters' home on April 27, 2015 and May 6, 2015. Based on an inspection of the plumbing and subsequent sampling conducted at the Walters' residence, it was determined that except for a few minor metallic connectors, all interior plumbing, including the pipes, valves and connectors are made of plastic certified by the National Sanitation Foundation (NSF) for use in drinking water applications. Subsequent sampling showed that the faucets in the home appear to be compliant with the new lead-free requirements and are also not the source for the high lead levels. Our inspection of the interior plumbing and analysis of follow-up sampling results demonstrate that the home plumbing network is not the source of the high lead levels found at the Walters' residence. The photographs and all sampling results will be included in the final report.

Based on the U.S. EPA inspection and documentation of the plastic plumbing at the Walters' residence, it was suspected that the high lead was being introduced into the Walters' home plumbing from outside the home, likely from a lead service line. Three portions of the service line were extracted during a subsequent trip on May 6, 2015 and sent for analysis, when the Walters' service line was replaced. Analyses performed to date indicate that a portion of the service line is made of galvanized iron pipe. Inspection of the remaining portion from the water main to the external shut-off valve confirmed that the portion from the water main to the external shut-off valve is a lead service line.

Ms. Walters has also provided U.S. EPA with medical reports on her child's blood lead testing indicating that the child had a low blood lead level (2 ug/dL) prior to the source water switch and an elevated blood lead level following the switch (6.5 ug/dL). Redacted copies of these reports will also be included in the final report.

Subsequent to the discovery of high lead levels in the Walters' drinking water, the water to the Walters' home was shut off on April 3, 2015. The water was briefly turned back on to collect additional samples on April 28, 2015. Since the water had stagnated for an extended period of time, the kitchen tap was flushed for 25 minutes the night before collecting the samples. Three sets of samples were collected at different flow rates (10 at low flow, 10 at medium flow and 10 at high flow).

The drinking water samples collected from the Walters' residence on April 28, 2015 contained extremely high lead levels, ranging in value from 200 ug/L to 13,200 ug/L (see below).

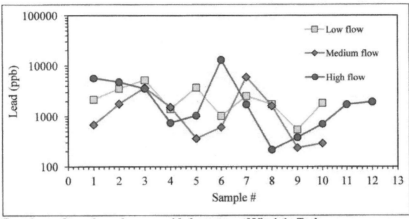

Sample results and graph are provided courtesy of Virginia Tech

Additional sample results from resident-requested samples have also shown lead levels in excess of the lead action level. As with the samples collected by the City of Flint for compliance, the resident-requested samples are also being collected using the 'pre-flushing', so the lead levels captured in these samples likely do not represent the worst-case lead levels in the water and the actual lead levels at these homes may be much higher.

Pending completion of the final report, my interim recommendations are as follows:

1. The U.S. EPA should follow up with the MDEQ and the City of Flint on the recommendation made by U.S. EPA to MDEQ on June 10, 2015 to offer the City of Flint technical assistance on managing the different water quality issues in Flint, including lead in the drinking water. Although there have been two written assessments regarding water quality and operational issues in Flint at the time of this report, they do not address lead in drinking water. The first is an Operational Evaluation Report (OER) produced in November 2014 by Lockwood, Andrews and Newnam, Inc. to assess the factors contributing to high Total Trihalomethane (TTHM) levels in Flint following the source change. The focus of this report is to identify potential causes and remedial actions for lowering TTHM levels. The second report (Water Quality Report) produced by Veolia for the City of Flint on March 12, 2015, is an assessment of Flint's water quality and operations which provides advice to the City of Flint primarily focused on TTHM control and other operational issues. Both reports were written prior to the recent discovery of high lead results in Flint drinking water. As such, the reports do not take into account the potential effects on lead levels in drinking water.

Page 4 of 5

As previously mentioned, the City of Flint currently has no mitigating treatment for lead and is also planning another source water change in the near future. U.S. EPA's Office of Research and Development in Cincinnati has extensive experience in corrosion and corrosion control treatment and distribution system issues and would be a valuable addition to the drinking water advisory group for the City of Flint. Copies of the qualifications and experience for Michael Schock and Darren Lytle have been forwarded to MDEQ.

2. U.S. EPA should review the compliance status of the City of Flint with respect to whether the system is in violation of the LCR requirement to install and maintain optimal corrosion control and whether the MDEQ is properly implementing the LCR provisions regarding optimal corrosion control treatment requirements for large systems. Pursuant to 40 CFR Section 141.82(i), the EPA Regional Administrator may review treatment determinations made by a State and issue federal treatment determinations consistent with the requirements of the LCR where the Regional Administrator finds: (1) A state has failed to issue a treatment determination by the applicable deadlines; (2) A State has abused its discretion in a substantial number of cases or in cases affecting a substantial population; or (3) The technical aspects of a State's determination would be indefensible in an expected Federal enforcement action taken against a system.

3. The U.S. EPA should review whether relevant resident-requested samples are being included by the City of Flint in calculating the 90th percentile compliance value for lead. Recent drinking water tests conducted at homes in Flint for lead that are not part of the compliance sampling pool have revealed high lead levels in the drinking water. The U.S. EPA memorandum signed on December 23, 2004 provides clarification on compliance determinations and states that customer-requested samples are to be included in the 90th percentile lead compliance calculation where the sampling is conducted during the monitoring period from sites and sampling procedures meeting the LCR criteria. Given the prevalence of lead service lines in the City of Flint, should these sample results be from homes with lead service lines, the sample results would be considered compliance samples under the LCR.

Also attached is a timeline of events for Flint, Michigan. Should you have any questions regarding the information or recommendations provided, please let me know.

cc: Liane Shekter-Smith (MDEQ)
Pat Cook (MDEQ)
Stephen Busch (MDEQ)
Michael Prysby (MDEQ)
Marc Edwards (Virginia Tech)
Michael Schock, EPA-ORD
Darren Lytle, EPA-ORD

Page 5 of 5

Interim Report on High Lead Levels in Flint Michigan
Timeline of Events

1. June 2011
   a. The Walters' home was renovated in 2011 and had no plumbing when purchased. Plastic water pipes and plumbing components were installed by the Walters throughout the home. The Walters family moved into the home at 212 Browning Avenue in June 2011.
   b. A whole-home iron filter installed for aesthetic reasons. The iron filter cartridge was changed every 6 months during the time when Flint purchased finished water from Detroit. Subsequent to the switch to the Flint River source on April 30, 2014, the filter was required to be changed every 2-3 weeks and eventually required replacement every 6-14 days due to much higher iron levels.
   c. Tap water treated by the refrigerator filter was consumed in the household from April 2014 through late November/early December 2014. The filters used were not NSF certified to remove lead.
2. October 2012
   a. The Walters had their twin boys' blood lead levels (BLLs) tested and the result for each child was 2 ug/dL.
3. April 30, 2014
   a. The City of Flint switches from purchased Detroit water to treating raw water from the Flint River.
   b. Michigan Department of Environment Quality requires City of Flint to conduct two six-month rounds of monitoring for lead and copper (July-December 2014 and January-June 2015).
4. August 2014
   a. The City of Flint Violates the National Primary Drinking Water Regulations Maximum Contaminant Level (MCL) for E. Coli bacteria (Acute Coliform MCL violation)
5. August 2014
   a. The City of Flint Violates the National Primary Drinking Water Regulations MCL for Coliform bacteria (Monthly Coliform MCL violation)
6. September 2014
   a. The City of Flint Violates the National Primary Drinking Water Regulations MCL for Coliform bacteria (Monthly Coliform MCL violation)
7. Later November/Early December 2014
   a. The Walters family stops drinking water from the tap due to water quality.
8. November 2014
   a. Lockwood, Andrews and Newnam, Inc. produces an "Operational Evaluation Report" to assess the factors contributing to high TTHM levels in Flint following the source change. This report is required by the National Primary Drinking Water Regulations when water tests show TTHM or HAA5 levels in excess of 80 percent of the MCL. The focus of this report is to identify potential causes and remedial actions for lowering TTHM levels.
9. December 2014
   a. The City of Flint Violates the National Primary Drinking Water Regulations MCL for Total Trihalomethanes (Average TTHM MCL violation)
10. February 4, 2015
    a. Walters' child develops skin rashes over entire body after bathing. The video is shown to City of Flint by Ms. Walters.
11. February 11, 2015
    a. The City of Flint tests drinking water iron level at Walters' residence and the level exceeds the capability of the measurement (>3.3 mg/L).
12. February 18, 2015
    a. The City of Flint tests the drinking water at the Walters residence for lead and iron.
    b. Tests reveal high lead in the drinking water (104 ug/L) and iron level once again exceeds the limit of the test (>3.3 mg/L).
    c. The Walters' water is tested after pre-flushing for "3-4 minutes" the night before (see sampling instructions). The sample was collected from the kitchen tap with the iron filter in place.
13. February 25, 2015
    a. EPA Region 5 receives a call from Ms. Walters regarding high lead levels discovered in her home.

b. The City of Flint once again tests the drinking water iron level at the Walters' residence and the result is once again beyond the measurement capability (>3.3 mg/L).
14. February 26, 2015
    a. The Walters have their children's blood lead levels tested and their child's blood lead level is 3 ug/dL.
15. March 2015
    a. The City of Flint increases the Ferric Chloride dosage used in the filtration process to improve the removal of disinfection byproduct precursor material, in an effort to lower the TTHM levels.
16. March 03, 2015
    a. The City of Flint re-tests lead levels in drinking water at Walters' residence. The lead level measured is 397 ug/L. The water is once again tested after pre-flushing for 3-4 minutes the night before but this time with the iron filter removed (see sampling instructions).
17. March 11, 2015
    a. The City of Flint re-tests the iron levels in drinking water at Walters' residence The iron level once again exceeds the limit of the test (>3.3 mg/L).
18. March 12, 2015
    a. Veolia (hired as a consultant by City of Flint) to assess water quality issues, submits "Water Quality Report" to City of Flint which provides recommendations and a roadmap for water quality and operational improvements, primarily focused on lowering TTHMs.
19. March 19, 2015
    a. EPA Region 5 calls MDEQ expressing concern regarding the high lead levels found.
    b. The MDEQ response received via voicemail states that the high lead levels at the Walters' home are due to lead sources in the homeowner's plumbing. In previous and subsequent conversations with Ms. Walters, she stated that the plumbing has always been all plastic. An inspection conducted by EPA Region on April 27, 2015, confirmed that all pipes, fittings and valves in the Walters' home are NSF-approved CPVC pipe (certified for drinking water use) and sequential sampling results following the replacement of the service line found that there are no sources of lead in the home plumbing.
20. March 26, 2015
    a. EPA R5 learns that the local Health Department is looking at whether there is a potential uptick in cases of Legionella in the County, which includes the City of Flint.
    b. Due to recent bacteriological and other distribution system water quality issues, EPA Region 5 contacts EPA ORD (Cincinnati) to discuss possible support for assessing whether the potential uptick in Legionella being assessed by Genesee County, which includes the City of Flint, could be caused by or related to the distribution system upsets from the water quality changes and subsequent flushing events by the City of Flint which can mobilize sediment from within the water mains and dislodge microbial contaminants, including Legionella bacteria from biofilm within the water mains.
    c. EPA ORD indicates that they are available and willing to provide support to the local health department and City of Flint should they conclude there has been an increase in Legionella cases in the county.
21. March 27, 2015
    a. Based on a suspected conflict of interest at the local health department that conducted the February 2015 BLL testing, the Walters' take their child to a healthcare facility in a different location to have his blood lead re-tested. The result from this BLL test (6.5 ug/dL) is significantly higher than the February BLL test (3 ug/dL) and he is found to also be iron deficient as well (anemic).
22. April 3, 2015
    a. The water is shut off at Walters' residence due to the high lead levels.
    b. The Walters' home is provided water via garden hose from neighboring home (hose spigot to hose spigot). The Walters use this water only for bathing, washing dishes and washing clothes.
23. April 27, 2015
    a. EPA Region 5 visits the Walters' home and reviews the internal plumbing, bringing back water samples, iron filter cartridges and relevant photographs.
    b. The internal plumbing at the Walters' residence is confirmed as all plastic as had been stated by Ms. Walters.
24. April 28, 2015
    a. The water at the Walters' residence was turned back on temporarily to collect additional water samples. The water in the service line had been shut off since April 3, 2015.

b. The kitchen tap was flushed at low flow for 25 minutes the night before (on April 27, 2015) the sequential sampling conducted on April 28, 2015.

c. On April 28, 2015, 30 Sequential samples were collected at Walters residence

d. The drinking water samples are sent to Virginia Tech for analysis. All samples are analyzed for Ag, Al, As, Ba, Ca, Cd, Cl, Co, Cr, Cu, Fe, K, Mg, Mn, Mo, Na, Ni, P, Pb, S, Se, Si, Sn, Sr, Ti, U V, and Zn.

e. Extremely high lead levels were found in all samples. The minimum lead value was 200 ug/L; the average lead value was 2,429 ug/L; and the maximum lead value was 13,200 ug/L.

f. A review of the analytical results by Virginia Tech shows lead levels in all water samples correlated with phosphate levels, cadmium levels and uranium levels found in the samples and most of the lead was found to be in particulate form.

g. The correlation between lead and phosphate would be consistent with the dislodging of the pipe scale from the service line outside the home containing lead and phosphate which would have formed during the period of time when Flint was purchasing water from the City of Detroit that was treated with orthophosphate. Additional analyses are being conducted to confirm the chemical compositions.

25. May 6, 2015

a. EPA Region 5 visits Walters' home to collect pipe samples from service line. Three sections of the service line were extracted and sent to Virginia Tech for analysis.

b. EPA inspection reveals that the portion of the Walters' service line from the water main to the external shut-off valve on the corner of Bryant Street and Browning Avenue is made of lead. EPA's inspection also confirms that the portion of the Walters' service line from the home to the external shut-off valve appears to be galvanized iron pipe. Additional analyses are underway at Virginia Tech on the third piece of service line extracted.

c. The service line to the Walters' residence is replaced with a new copper service to the water main in front of the Walters' residence on Browning Avenue.

d. Sample bottles are left with Ms. Walters for collecting sequential samples following the replacement of the service line to the Walters' home.

e. EPA Region 5 collects a set of sequential samples from each of two residences on Bryant Street which are connected to the same main as the Walters' old service line. These samples were analyzed by Chicago Regional Laboratory. The results indicate that home #1 (4526 Bryant Street) does not appear to have a lead service line and lead results in all samples are low. The results from home #2 (4614 Bryant Street) indicate that the portion of the service line from the external shut-off valve to the water main is likely made of lead, which is consistent with the historical practice in Flint. The sampling had a high lead result (peak value) of 22 ug/L.

26. May 6, 2015

a. The City of Flint tests the water at 216 Browning Avenue at resident's request, again using a first-draw, pre-flushed sampling protocol, which yielded a high lead result (22 ug/L).

b. The City of Flint tests the water at 631 Alvord Avenue, yielding a high lead result (42 ug/L).

27. May 13, 2015

a. Water samples are collected at Walters' residence following the replacement of the service line.

b. 15 sequential samples were collected from kitchen tap, 1 sample was collected from the bathroom tap and 2 samples were collected from the water heater.

c. The samples were shipped to the EPA CRL and received on May 14, 2015.

d. All kitchen tap and bathroom tap results for lead and copper were low, confirming that the sources of lead were external to the home. Residual lead was found in the water heater samples (31.7 ug/L), very likely from deposition of lead-containing particulate coming into the home via the old service line which was disconnected and replaced on May 6, 2015.

28. June 2015

a. The City of Flint Violates the National Primary Drinking Water Regulations MCL for Total Trihalomethanes (Average TTHM MCL violation)

ACKNOWLEDGMENTS

In addition to the staff of and contributors to Bridge Magazine, many individuals and organizations helped us with the content for "Poison on Tap."

For the powerful photo used on this book's cover, credit goes to the Flint Journal's chief photographer, Jake May, and his editors at MLive.com. Several of Jake's water-crisis photos appear in the chapters of this book. We also often cited Flint Journal/MLive.com reporter Ron Fonger's many scoops through the book's timeline.

Michigan Radio, the state's public radio network, permitted us to select from any of the water-crisis photos that have appeared on its website. We're especially indebted to Steve Carmody, who rarely let a scene slip by without recording an image. Lindsey Smith's interviews with key players and the documentary "Not Safe to Drink," also helped inform our narrative.

Flintwaterstudy.org (Virginia Tech) gave us full access to the photos it has published on its websites. University staff photographer Logan Wallace, who spent time in Flint in early March 2016 with professor Marc Edwards and his team of researchers, students and volunteers, provided powerful images. One of the most notable was a joyful photo of four Flint crisis heroes – Edwards, Lee-Anne Walters, Miguel Del Toral and Dr. Mona Hanna-Attisha – moments after they met in person for the first time. Edwards' effective use of Freedom of Information Act requests to get critical documents proved vital for us.

Photographer Brittany Greeson, who took a break from college to document the Flint saga, agreed to permit use of her tender photo of Hanna-Attisha with a baby under her care at Hurley Medical Center, and the soulful image of Lee-Anne Walters bathing her lead-poisoned son, Gavin.

Thanks also to: the Karegnondi Water Authority for authorizing use of several photos depicting the construction of the new water line from Lake Huron to Flint; Michigan State University for photos it provided of Hanna-Attisha and the Flintstones; and Dan Crannie, owner of Signs by Crannie, for allowing us to use his signature photo of a night shot of the Flint Vehicle City mounted on the arches marking downtown Flint.

CSPAN, the cable channel that provides public affairs coverage of Congress, politics and Washington, generously licensed our use of screen-capture images from its videos of Flint water hearings held by the U.S. House Oversight and Government Reform Committee in February and March 2016.

MSNBC's Rachel Maddow Show permitted us to use a screen-capture from the host's town hall show with Flint residents in January 2016.

We also thank the citizens of Flint, as well as local, state and federal government officials and others who gave their time for interviews, second-guessing our conclusions and providing records, data and photos.

Finally, we congratulate the work of journalists across Michigan and at various national newspapers, magazines and networks whose coverage helped inform our effort.

ABOUT OUR TEAM

JOHN BEBOW: John's Timeline and Michigan Truth Squad is the heart of "Poison on Tap." His instincts told him that the Flint water crisis was one of the most profound stories of government failure in Michigan history. He knew that Bridge Magazine needed to examine what happened and what the lessons are for the state's citizens and leaders. John is the president and CEO of the Center for Michigan. Before that, he was an investigative reporter at the Detroit News, Chicago Tribune and Detroit Free Press.

DAVID ZEMAN: David is the senior editor of Bridge. He edited the stories that appeared on bridgemi.com and that became the basis for "Poison on Tap." David worked for two decades at the Detroit Free Press as an investigative reporter and editor. His team won a Pulitzer Prize and other awards for uncovering the Kwame Kilpatrick scandal.

CHASTITY PRATT DAWSEY: Chastity's work humanized the narrative of "Poison on Tap." She was among the first reporters outside Flint to document the frustration of citizens in her report "Cringe over troubled water." Before joining Bridge, Chastity covered the Detroit Public Schools for more than a decade. Her reports in the Detroit Free Press led to the creation of the Detroit Blight Authority and cost two superintendents their jobs.

MIKE WILKINSON: Mike is Bridge's computer-assisted reporting specialist and wrote a critical piece that gave Flint's crisis broader perspective. He found that thousands of Michigan children have been exposed to more lead than those in Flint. Before he joined Bridge, Mike had a similar position at the Detroit News.

RON FRENCH: Ron, a senior Bridge writer, reported that the Flint water crisis had quickly became a hot topic in college business school and public affairs classes. Before Bridge, Ron was an award-winning reporter at the Detroit News.

PHIL POWER: The Center for Michigan's founder and chairman, Phil left his career as a community newspaper publisher to form the Center in 2006. His columns about the crisis in Flint provide insight into executive decision-making and public policy.

NANCY NALL DERRINGER: In "Poison on Tap," Nancy wrote about the first criminal charges in the Flint crisis and the huge commitment of cash for Flint from 10 foundations. She has been a journalist in the Detroit area and at The News-Sentinel in Fort Wayne, Ind.

TED ROELOFS: Ted is a regular contributor to Bridge. He wrote a handful stories about the implications of the Flint crisis beyond Flint. He worked at the Grand Rapids Press for about 30 years.

COLLEEN ZANOTTI: Colleen assembled the graphics for "Poison on Tap." Her work has appeared in dozens of publications, including Bridge Magazine.

HEATHER LEE SHAW: Heather designed the covers and pages of "Poison on Tap." She is a partner at Mission Point Press, the book's publisher.

DOUG WEAVER: Doug was the primary copy editor for "Poison on Tap." He is business manager and a partner at Mission Point Press.

BOB CAMPBELL: Bob was the editor of "Poison on Tap." His first book, "Storm Struck," was a bestseller for Mission Point Press. Bob was a reporter and editor at the Detroit Free Press for 30 years.

ANNE STANTON: Anne also helped copy edit "Poison on Tap." Anne is the editorial director and a partner at Mission Point Press.

Made in the USA
San Bernardino, CA
05 June 2016